OCCUPATIONAL LUNG DISEASES

LUNG BIOLOGY IN HEALTH AND DISEASE

Executive Editor: **Claude Lenfant**

Director, Division of Lung Diseases
National Institutes of Health
Bethesda, Maryland

Volume 1 IMMUNOLOGIC AND INFECTIOUS REACTIONS IN THE LUNG, *edited by Charles H. Kirkpatrick and Herbert Y. Reynolds*

Volume 2 THE BIOCHEMICAL BASIS OF PULMONARY FUNCTION, *edited by Ronald G. Crystal*

Volume 3 BIOENGINEERING ASPECTS OF THE LUNG, *edited by John B. West*

Volume 4 METABOLIC FUNCTIONS OF THE LUNG, *edited by Y. S. Bakhle and John R. Vane*

Volume 5 RESPIRATORY DEFENSE MECHANISMS (in two parts), *edited by Joseph D. Brain, Donald F. Proctor, and Lynne M. Reid*

Volume 6 DEVELOPMENT OF THE LUNG, *edited by W. Alan Hodson*

Volume 7 LUNG WATER AND SOLUTE EXCHANGE, *edited by Norman C. Staub*

Volume 8 EXTRAPULMONARY MANIFESTATIONS OF RESPIRATORY DISEASE, *edited by Eugene Debs Robin*

Volume 9 CHRONIC OBSTRUCTIVE PULMONARY DISEASE, *edited by Thomas L. Petty*

Volume 10 PATHOGENESIS AND THERAPY OF LUNG CANCER, *edited by Curtis C. Harris*

Volume 11 GENETIC DETERMINANTS OF PULMONARY DISEASE, *edited by Stephen D. Litwin*

Volume 12 THE LUNG IN THE TRANSITION BETWEEN HEALTH AND DISEASE, *edited by Peter T. Macklem and Solbert Permutt*

Volume 13 EVOLUTION OF RESPIRATORY PROCESSES: A COMPARATIVE APPROACH, *edited by Stephen C. Wood and Claude Lenfant*

Volume 14 PULMONARY VASCULAR DISEASES,
edited by Kenneth M. Moser

Volume 15 PHYSIOLOGY AND PHARMACOLOGY OF THE AIRWAYS,
edited by Jay A. Nadel

Volume 16 DIAGNOSTIC TECHNIQUES IN PULMONARY DISEASE (in two parts),
edited by Marvin A. Sackner

Volume 17 REGULATION OF BREATHING (in two parts),
edited by Thomas F. Hornbein

Volume 18 OCCUPATIONAL LUNG DISEASES:
RESEARCH APPROACHES AND METHODS,
edited by Hans Weill and Margaret Turner-Warwick

Other volumes in preparation

IMMUNOPHARMACOLOGY OF THE LUNG,
edited by Harold H. Newball

SARCOIDOSIS AND OTHER GRANULATOMATOUS
DISEASES OF THE LUNG,
edited by Barry L. Fanburg

OCCUPATIONAL LUNG DISEASES

RESEARCH APPROACHES AND METHODS

Edited by

Hans Weill

Tulane University School of Medicine
New Orleans, Louisiana

Margaret Turner-Warwick

Cardiothoracic Institute
Brompton Hospital
London, England

MARCEL DEKKER, INC. New York • Basel

Library of Congress Cataloging in Publication Data

Main entry under title:

Occupational lung diseases: research approaches and methods.

(Lung biology in health and disease ; v. 18)
Includes bibliographical references and indexes.
1. Lungs–Diseases. 2. Occupational diseases.
I. Weill, Hans, II. Turner-Warwick, Margaret, III. Series.
RC756.L83 vol. 18 616.2'4s 81-15249
ISBN: 0-8247-1362-1 [616.2'4075] AACR2

MARCEL DEKKER, INC.
270 Madison Avenue, New York, New York 10016

Current printing (last digit):
10 9 8 7 6 5 4 3 2

PRINTED IN THE UNITED STATES OF AMERICA

CONTRIBUTORS

Eric D. Bateman, MBChB, MRCP* Clinical Lecturer, Department of Medicine, Cardiothoracic Institute, Brompton Hospital, London, England

Geoffrey Berry, M.A. (Cantab) FIS Scientific Staff, MRC Pneumoconiosis Unit, Penarth, South Glamorgan, Wales, United Kingdom

Cooley Butler, M.D. Associate Professor, Department of Pathology, University of New Mexico School of Medicine, Albuquerque, New Mexico

Peter Cole, B.Sc, M.B., FRCP Senior Lecturer and Honorary Consultant Physician, Department of Medicine, Cardiothoracic Institute, Brompton Hospital, London, England

Morton Corn, Ph.D., M.S., B.Ch.E. Professor and Director, Department of Environmental Health Engineering, The Johns Hopkins University School of Hygiene and Public Health, Baltimore, Maryland

J. E. Cotes, M.A., D.M. (Oxon), FRCP Reader, Respiration and Exercise Laboratory, Department of Occupational Health and Hygiene, The University of Newcastle upon Tyne, Newcastle upon Tyne, England

Robert J. Davies, M.A., M.D., MRCP Consultant Physician and Senior Lecturer, Academic Unit of Respiratory Medicine, St. Bartholomew's Hospital, London, England

Venkatram Dharmarajan, Ph.D., C.I.H.† Assistant Professor, Department of Medicine, Pulmonary Disease Section, Tulane University School of Medicine, New Orleans, Louisiana

Robert J. Emerson, B.A., Ph.D.‡ Research Assistant, Department of Medicine, Cardiothoracic Institute, Brompton Hospital, London, England

---

Present Affiliations

* University of Cape Town and Groote Schuur Hospital, Cape Town, South Africa

† Corporate Industrial Hygiene Department, Mobay Chemical Corporation, Pittsburgh, Pennsylvania

‡ Pulmonary Unit, Department of Medicine, The University of Vermont College of Medicine, Burlington, Vermont

Geoffrey B. Field, M.B., B.S.(Sydney), M.D.(NSW), FRACP, V.Sc.(Med) Senior Staff Physician, Department of Thoracic Medicine, The Prince Henry Hospital, Little Bay, Sydney, New South Wales, Australia

Bryan H. Gandevia, M.D. FRACP Associate Professor, Department of Thoracic Medicine, University of New South Wales; Chairman, Department of Thoracic Medicine, The Prince Henry Hospital, Little Bay, Sydney, New South Wales, Australia

Reed M. Gardner, Ph.D. Professor, Department of Medical Biophysics and Computing, University of Utah and LDS Hospital, Salt Lake City, Utah

John C. Gilson, CBE, FRCP* Director, MRC Pneumoconiosis Unit, Penarth, South Glamorgan, Wales, United Kingdom

Henry W. Glindmeyer III, D.Eng. Assistant Professor, Department of Medicine, Tulane University School of Medicine, New Orleans, Louisiana

Yehia Hammad, B.Sc., D.P.H., M.Sc., D.Sc. Associate Professor, Pulmonary Diseases Section, Department of Medicine, Tulane University School of Medicine, New Orleans, Louisiana

John L. Hankinson, Ph.D., B.E.E., M.S.E.E. Chief, Clinical Investigation Branch, Department of Health and Human Services, National Institute for Occupational Safety and Health, Morgantown, West Virginia

Roland H. Ingram, Jr., M.D. Director, Respiratory Division, Department of Medicine, Peter Bent Brigham Hospital, Harvard Medical School, Boston, Massachusetts

Robert N. Jones, M.D. Associate Professor, Department of Medicine, Tulane University School of Medicine, New Orleans, Louisiana

Reynold M. Karr, M.D.† Assistant Professor, Department of Medicine, Tulane University School of Medicine, New Orleans, Louisiana

Jerome Kleinerman, M.D. Professor and Chairman, Department of Pathology, Mount Sinai School of Medicine, New York, New York

J. Corbett McDonald, M.D., FRCP, FFOM‡ Professor and Head, TUC Centenary Institute of Occupational Health, London School of Hygiene and Tropical Medicine, London, England

E. R. McFadden, Jr., M.D. Associate Director, Pulmonary Division, Peter Bent Brigham Hospital, Harvard Medical School, Boston, Massachusetts

---

Present Affiliation

* Now retired.

† 3202 Colby Avenue, Everett, Washington, 98201

‡ Professor and Head, Institute of Occupational Health and Safety, McGill University, Montreal, Canada

A. J. Newman Taylor, M.Sc. (Oxon Med), M.B., B.S., MRCP Consultant Physician, Department of Medicine, Brompton and London Chest Hospitals, and Honorary Senior Lecturer in Clinical Immunology, Cardiothoracic Institute, Brompton Hospital, London England

Frederick D. Pooley, B.Sc., M.Sc., Ph.D., MAIME, MIMM, FGS., C. Eng Reader, Department of Mineral Exploitation, University College of Cardiff, Cardiff, Wales, United Kingdom

John E. Salvaggio, M.D. Henderson Professor of Medicine, Department of Medicine, Tulane University School of Medicine, New Orleans, Louisiana

Margaret Turner-Warwick, M.A., D.M., FRCP, Ph.D. Professor, Department of Thoracic Medicine, Cardiothoracic Institute, Brompton Hospital, London, England

Hans Weill, M.D. Professor, Department of Medicine; Chief, Pulmonary Diseases Section, Tulane University School of Medicine, New Orleans, Louisiana

Merlin R. Wilson, M.D.* Clinical Associate Professor, Department of Medicine, Tulane University School of Medicine, New Orleans, Lousianna

---

Present Affiliation
* Director, Clinical Reference Laboratory, Tulane University School of Medicine, New Orleans, Louisiana.

FOREWORD

Most of us who are asked to name how the great advances in modern medicine and surgery have come about, would probably respond by listing some Nobel laureates and the discoveries closely linked with their names: for example, Roentgen and X-rays; Koch and the tubercle bacillus; Fleming and penicillin; Enders and culture of polio virus; Banting and insulin. Yet, once in awhile, an event that is ineligible for a Nobel Prize has had just as important an impact on medical advance as one that was eligible and won an award. One such event was Abraham Flexner's 1910 report "Medical Education in the United States and Canada" that resulted in a considerable decrease in the number of American medical schools and a considerable increase in their quality and in the scientific content of their curricula. Another was the opening of the Johns Hopkins Medical School in 1893, staffed by four professors, each outstanding as a scientist in his specialty and each believing in joining scientific research, medical education, and patient care.

Sometimes a book or a series of books has had a strong influence on the advance of medical science. One such book was the first edition of Osler's *Medicine* (1892) because Osler's emphasis on how little physicians knew for sure led John Rockefeller's adviser on philanthropy to recommend the building of the great Institute for Medical Research, which opened in 1904 and for decades was the foremost institution for research in basic medical sciences in the United States. Another was the first (1941) edition of Goodman and Gilman's *Pharmacological Basis for Medical Practice* that revolutionized teaching and research on the action and use of drugs; as one professor of pharmacology stated in 1941, no professional pharmacologist could from then on teach at a lower level than that of the superb text used by his students!

In the field of respiration and the lungs, there are some classic monographs and a comprehensive *Handbook of Physiology* that have heightened the interest of scientists, students, and physicians in this subject and stimulated them to enter pulmonary research. One can safely predict that this new series of monographs, "Lung Biology in Health and Disease," will have an even greater impact on young (and older) researchers because it is the first truly comprehensive, monumental work in this field. It does not deal just with cellular processes or just with clinical problems but with the entire spectrum of basic sciences and of lung function, metabolic functions, and respiratory defense mechanisms. The series will also include volumes that apply modern biological knowledge to elucidate mechanisms of pulmonary and respiratory disorders (immunologic, infectious, and genetic disorders, physiology and pharmacology of airways, genesis and resolution of pulmonary edema, and abnormalities of respiratory regulation). Other volumes will deal with the biology of specific pulmonary diseases (e.g., cancer, chronic obstructive pulmonary disease, disorders of the pulmonary circulation, and abnormalities associated with occupational and environmental factors) and with early detection and specific diagnosis.

This series shows the lung as a challenging organ, with many problems calling for innovative research. If it attracts some imaginative, creative, and perceptive young scientists to attack these difficult problems, the tremendous effort in writing, editing, and publishing these volumes will be well worthwhile. The volumes cannot win the Nobel Prize, but someone may who was challenged by them.

Julius H. Comroe, Jr.
San Francisco, California

PREFACE

The requirements for an interdisciplinary approach to the investigation of occupational lung diseases is well-illustrated by the biomedical, physical, chemical and biometric fields from which the contributors of this monograph are drawn. It is particularly gratifying that this group of internationally recognized experts have thought it worthwhile to produce the first book which deals specifically with the ways in which new knowledge is acquired in this important field. The table of contents provides convincing evidence of the wide range of approaches that have added to our data base in the understanding of lung disorders of occupational origin. Overall objectives in this research and of problems encountered along the way are discussed in the first chapter.

The contributors were asked to review the important methods and approaches in the field, and it was suggested that this monograph will not be a "cookbook" with detailed techniques, nor that it necessarily have textbook completeness in terms of covering every possible method now being applied to this type of research. Rather, that they be discriminating and emphasize those approaches which are now or are likely to be productive in the future in terms of our understanding of causation and mechanisms of occupational lung disease. The contributors were encouraged to illustrate how certain approaches have addressed and answered specific scientific questions in their own research. The reader of this monograph will undoubtedly agree that they have met this charge superbly.

Those likely to benefit from this monograph will include academicians who are looking for research opportunities in this important area of lung diseases with particularly unique possibilities for prevention. Government and public health authorities who have the responsibility of evaluating scientific data which relate to occupational lung diseases should find much in this book to help them discharge their responsibilities in arriving at informed decisions. Finally, the investigator in this field who may have limited experience in a number of the disciplines covered in the monograph, and who will have need to either interpret results from these other fields or apply such methods to scientific questions which may have been raised in the course of his own research, will certainly find this volume useful for frequent reference.

The editors wish to express their appreciation first to all of the contributors on both sides of the Atlantic. We also wish to thank Claude Lenfant who proposed this topic to us and whose friendly encouragement led to the completion of this project. Finally, a most thorough job of subject and author indexing was cheerfully accomplished by Kathleen Rhodes and Gil Sharon. We are indeed grateful to them.

Hans Weill
Margaret Turner-Warwick

INTRODUCTION

> We live in an age remarkable for its vast discoveries, for its wonderful developments in knowledge; developments which are giving us great control over the material world, annihilating time and space. At one moment, discoveries obtrude upon our notice in a gentle light; at another, they burst forth with the most brilliant meteoric glare, dazzling us with their splendor and awakening profound and wondrous anticipation of the future.
>
> *S. S. Fitch, 1853*

Such an interesting statement, although written years ago, seems to appropriately describe the state (and the role) of research vis-à-vis occupational lung diseases today.

Occupational lung diseases, especially those resulting from mineral dust inhalation, were known by Greek and Egyptian physicians of the B.C. era. During the romantic period consumption was believed to be caused mostly by effeminacy among the intellectuals and wealthy and by work abuse and exposure in laborers and in the less privileged classes of the society. Today, we have greater awareness concerning occupational lung diseases and we now know that this group of diseases require medical knowledge and cannot be attributed to syndical and societal factors. Thus, it is not surprising that by and large, the initial search and studies in this field are now based on pathogenetic processes, as reflected in nearly all authoritative treatises dealing with these disorders and are organized on the basis of etiology.

This monograph, the eighteenth of the series "Lung Biology in Health and Disease," gives a new dimension to the study of occupational lung diseases: it is concerned with research approaches and methods. The series is indeed very priviledged to have gained the editorship of Drs. Hans Weill and Margaret Turner-Warwick, who are both leaders in the field and bring to this volume years of experience marked by innovative and pioneering work. Further, they have enrolled an international authorship of great reputation and achievement. To the editors and to the authors, I express appreciation and gratitude for their contribution. No doubt, this volume will "awaken profound and wondrous anticipation of the future."

Claude Lenfant, M.D.
Bethesda, Maryland

CONTENTS

OCCUPATIONAL LUNG DISEASES

1

Occupational Lung Diseases

The Scope of the Problem

MARGARET TURNER-WARWICK

Cardiothoracic Institute
Brompton Hospital
London, England

I. Introduction

Any aerosolized material which remains in suspension in the air we breathe will be inhaled by those exposed, and its penetration into the airways or to the gas-exchanging parts of the lung will depend largely upon its size. Inhaled aerosols are of many forms and include fogs, fumes, gases, suspensions, and droplets. A very wide variety of agents are included under each of these major headings. Occasionally, ingested material and agents absorbed through the skin may also reach and damage the lung.

While the potential hazard of the immediate working environment may have been reduced in recent years with regard to certain traditionally culpable agents such as some of the inorganic dusts, there is an endless multitude of potential inhalation hazards which are the consequence of the continued exploration of new materials and processes in our Utopic search for a better living environment. Unfortunately, improved amenities of living do not always equate with a better working environment for those employed in the implementation of this better life. While the hazard of the immediate working environment of the operator is probably the largest and most important consideration, other more indirect exposures are also of concern to the community as a whole. These include exposure of workers employed incidentally in a contaminated area—for example, riveters employed in the shipbuilding industry, working in asbestos-laden atmospheres, or neighborhood exposures including those living close to industry or in contact with contaminants derived from the factory environment, for instance those cleaning contaminated workers' clothing.

A number of recently published textbooks have summarized the currently available facts about those industrial related pulmonary disorders which have to date been investigated in any depth. In the present volume we shall try to extend the horizons of the subject and consider particularly the research tools and methodology available to examine environmental hazards, the particular problems which have to be solved, and the critical limitations which have to be recognized and accepted.

II. Some Inherent Problems of Occupational Medicine

Some of the problems which will be tackled in this volume may be summarized.

1. The range and types of damage to the lung are great, and this means that appropriate methods have to be designed to detect different varieties of disordered structure and function. No single method can be expected to be applicable as a universal detector of all types of abnormalities.

2. There are many reasons why a new environmental hazard is overlooked for remarkably long periods of time. Awareness of these factors can lead to earlier detection.

3. There are many problems associated with the positive identification of an offending casual agent, even when a particular environment is suspected.

4. When a specific agent has been identified, there are major problems in defining the ways in which it causes lung damage, in other words, in clarifying the nature of pathogenesis.

5. The problems of identifying dose responses and threshold limits below which no hazard exists are great.

6. Before epidemiological studies of any type are undertaken, major problems have to be resolved concerning suitable definitions of disease and appropriate defining criteria to be used in case detection.

7. Establishing defining criteria presents especially difficult problems when attempting to identify early cases or indeed subclinical disordered function of the lung.

8. All current epidemiological methods have major inherent problems, and these will be identified and discussed in detail. In particular, accurate monitoring of the dose of an inhaled agent is of central importance and the value of much epidemiological information depends critically upon this. Obtaining accurate information about the amount of any contaminant in the environment involves complex technology and indeed constitutes an entire scientific discipline of its own.

9. Perhaps the single most difficult problem of all is that of defining appropriate controls.

10. Not least of the practical problems in occupational medicine is that dependent upon observations which to a large extent have to be made in the field. In this respect the challenge is far greater than for those working in a tightly controlled hospital environment. Both types of study are, however, essential; neither is less good than the other; rather they form complementary approaches. The problems they are able to solve are, however, different.

11. Many different types of investigation are appropriate in the investigation of problems in occupational medicine. Some are short term, perhaps involving a single before-and-after exposure study. Others may be long-term, extending over many years; these may be necessary to identify the total burden of disease in a work force and to define the long-term consequences of a particular form of exposure. Clinical and epidemiological methods of investigation of occupational disease are complementary and answer different questions. Neither is inferior to the other, but they have to be used appropriately.

12. Once the problems of the scientist have been resolved, others emerge. For instance, if difficulties arise through the use of words between experts, this is a minor problem compared to the misunderstandings which arise when scientists attempt to communicate with management, unions, lawyers, or the public.

13. When all is said and done, the community through its politicians has to consider whether the advantages to the community of a particular product as a whole outweigh the hazard which may be inevitable during the course of its production. In the final analysis this may prove to be the greatest problem of all.

III. The Range and Types of Lung Damage

The airways are often the major target organ, but even within this part of the lung many types of damage occur. Airway *hyperreactivity* may develop (i.e., occupational asthma), but many varied patterns of such hyperreactivity are now identified and their pathogeneses are thought to be different. *Hypersecretory chronic bronchitis* with sputum production may be the main symptom, or obliterative changes (*obstructive chronic bronchitis*) may develop affecting larger or smaller airways. Under certain circumstances destructive emphysema may develop and cause physiological obstruction due to airway collapse on expiration. Acinar involvement, in other words damage to the gas-exchanging parts of the lung, may also be of many different types. Diffuse and acute involvement occurs with agents inducing pulmonary edema and this may progress to widespread fibrosis when alveolar wall damage has been severe. Chronic and insidious widespread fibrosis is well documented with certain inorganic dusts and as an end-stage result of injury from many organic materials. Nodular lesions in the acini may also be acute and reversible or may be chronic. Widespread granulomas occurring with exposure to organic dusts and to special material such as beryllium as well as focal fibrotic nodules in pure nonanthracotic silicosis are well recognized. In certain individuals much more extensive lesions develop, notably the conglomerate lesions of silicosis or the progressive massive fibrosis of coal workers.

The pleura may be particularly affected, especially in asbestos workers, and lesions of this type complicate interpretation of physiological measurements and, by masking the intrapulmonary shadows, confound the interpretation of the chest radiograph.

Certain agents, especially radioactive materials and asbestos, induce lung or pleural tumors, the early detection and prevention of which require entirely different methods of investigation to those required to study obstructive or restrictive disorders of the lung.

IV. Problems of Initial Awareness of a Potential Hazard

There are many excusable reasons why a respiratory hazard may be overlooked for long periods of time by even astute observers. Minor respiratory symptoms are extremely common and tend not to be reported. Affected workers are apt to leave work which causes chest symptoms without necessarily giving a medical explanation and indeed they may be barely aware of it themselves. Suspicion of damaging environmental agents is often blunted by the overwhelming symptoms directly and properly attributable to the habit of smoking cigarettes.

The lag period between exposure and symptoms adds further difficulties. The lag may be hours, weeks, months, or years. Many workers developing occupational asthma develop their symptoms at night ("nonimmediate" asthma) and its association with a particular occupation is overlooked. Asthma may also persist for weeks after cessation of exposure (for instance toluene diisocyanate or grain dust) so that the conventional history of freedom from symptoms at weekends or holidays is no longer obtained. Under certain circumstances, as in byssinosis, asthmatic symptoms actually improve on continued exposure and provide an especially misleading history to the unwary.

Pulmonary fibrosis usually develops after very prolonged exposures and of course can develop years after removal of exposure. The lag between minimal exposure and the development of disease is perhaps most marked with asbestos-related mesotheliomas. The problem of obtaining accurate environmental information retrospectively, sometimes over several decades, obviously poses immense difficulties.

V. Identifying Causal Agents

A central problem in occupational lung disease is that directed at ascertaining that a particular structural or functional derangement of the lung is *caused* by a certain inhaled agent. The problem is real because many changes in the lung are not pathognomonic and an identical or nearly identical condition may be found in unexposed individuals. A few examples will make this clear. Bronchial asthma in atopic individuals occurs in about 5% of the adult population, but asthma is also frequently associated with work-related inhaled agents. In some instances an inhaled agent especially affects atopic individuals, either because of their predilection to immunologic sensitization or because atopic individuals have hyperreactive bronchi which respond more readily to irritants of any type. These facts may explain to a large extent the very long delay which has occurred in medicine before occupational asthmas have been studied and defined in any detail. Indeed, such studies are only now beginning to be undertaken on a substantial scale.

A second example is that of granulomas in the lung. The clinical and pathological features of chronic beryllium disease mimic sarcoidosis closely and in spite of certain differences, for example the reactivity to Kveim antigens, the results of these tests are not considered specific enough to be of absolute value in individual cases. Thus there may be no way of being absolutely certain whether a patient has beryllium-related chronic granulomatous disease or is suffering from nonoccupational sarcoidosis. In an analogous way there is no way of proving with certainty whether a worker has asbestos-related alveolar wall fibrosis, i.e., asbestosis, or nonoccupational cryptogenic fibrosing alveolitis. The fact that the lungs contain asbestos fibers and asbestos bodies proves no more than that the worker is telling the truth and has in fact worked with the material. Rule-of-thumb reasonable assumptions regarding cause and effect in an individual are necessary to implement the law in most countries, but it is wise to remember that they remain assumptions. Much time would be saved if lawyers and doctors agreed alike that proof (in the individual case) is often not possible and that the law of reason and precedent has to be accepted.

Methods are of course being developed to strengthen the case with regard to causal agents in asthma and hypersensitivity pneumonitis. Where bronchial challenge tests in the laboratory reproduce the clinical symptoms and a physiological disorder similar to those observed in the working environment, then there is a strong likelihood that cause and effect have been established. Such tests do not of course elucidate the mechanism of lung damage.

VI. Problems of Pathogenesis

It is well recognized that a simple agent may cause many different types of injury to the lung and it is therefore probable that many factors determine the type of damage seen in an individual case. Asbestos dust, for instance, causes in different individuals intrapulmonary alveolar wall fibrosis (asbestosis), benign diffuse pleural thickening with or without calcification, localized pleural plaques with or without calcification, and mesothelioma of the pleura and peritoneum and is also a strong contributory factor in the development of lung cancer. Not uncommonly more than one type of pathology is seen in the same individual. Thus, understanding pathogenesis includes an understanding of the conditions necessary to determine the different types of lesions induced by the same inhaled agents.

Detailed investigation of immunologic responses to certain agents, especially various organic dusts, have shown several distinct potential methods of induction of lung damage. For instance there is evidence that certain organic dusts (e.g., *Micropolyspora faeni,* or avian proteins) stimulate antibody formation and may induce an immune complex Arthus reaction, but they may also sensitize T lymphocytes with the potential of consequent lumphokine-mediated tissue damage. Additionally, recent evidence suggests that some materials (e.g., *M. faeni*) activate complement by the alternative pathway and can therefore induce tissue damage in unsensitized individuals on their first exposure to the agent. The importance of immunologic information lies in the fact that not only may mechanisms of tissue damage be defined, but also the special reactivity of the host may be identified. This, under some conditions, may be as important as the dose of the inhaled agent.

A large body of literature has now accumulated on the use of animal models to dissect the multiple components involved in the pathogenesis of occupational agents. Great difficulties have been encountered in using such models. For example, it is difficult to ensure that the conditions of exposure are similar to the human working environment not least because nasal clearance mechanisms in animals are very different from those in humans and the anatomy of their airways and hence particle penetration is also different. Other host factors relating to species may also be important. The very long exposure times necessary to induce several of the occupational fibroses and tumors present special problems in animal models. In spite of these, carefully designed animal models can provide information complementary to human studies. For example, study of the critical dimensions of particles inducing certain types of lesions, such as mesotheliomas, has been largely worked out in animal studies.

VII. Identification of Dose Responses

The many aspects of this subject will be discussed in great depth in several chapters in this book. Dose responses are of fundamental importance partly because they are relevant to the problem as to whether there is a threshold limit below which all individuals are free from hazard. They also have a bearing on whether a disease is mainly dependent upon the dose of inhaled agent and is thus potentially controllable, or whether it is apparently dose independent, suggesting that either host factors and individual susceptibility are of greater importance (or that measurements of dose have for some reason been technically inadequate). The fact must not of course be forgotten that even in those instances where a clear dose response is demonstrated, on the ascending slope of the dose-response curve, every point represents a proportion of the population who have been affected but equally represents another who have not. Again the explanation of these two populations may lie in accuracies of dose measurements in the exposed individuals or in a variation of host susceptibility. This fact, universal in medicine, indicates that dose and host are always involved—such is the heterogeneity of the human.

The problems of establishing threshold doses in practical terms are fraught with difficulties besides that of subject variation in susceptibility because they are inevitably linked with problems of defining and identifying subclinical minimal disease in individuals or populations. In practice it is obviously extremely difficult to establish clear criteria for disease in its earliest stages, and this compounds the problem of identifying subclinical disordered structure or function of the lung.

Dose-response relationships are also difficult to establish when there is a large latent period between exposure and evidence of disease. Under these circumstances, details of exact exposure may be difficult or impossible to obtain retrospectively and approximations are always the subject of controversy. Prospective epidemiological studies would seem to be the only real way of solving the problem, but longitudinal prospective studies over long periods of time are the most difficult to maintain and complete. In addition, monitoring methods are apt to change during the course of such studies, as are the industrial processes themselves. Interpretation of the data obtained is further complicated by the compounding effects of cigarette smoking which in many instances is quantitatively far greater than the subtle changes induced by minimal levels of other agents in the working environment.

VIII. Epidemiological Methods

The advantages and disadvantages of different types of epidemiological studies to detect morbidity and specific mortality will form a major part of this volume. Special problems relate to these types of study of lung disease. The criteria for the earlier disturbance of function have to be defined and the correct yardsticks used for measuring them. When new hazards with unknown damaging consequences are being studied the wrong tools can easily be used. Inevitably, surveys have to be conducted largely in the field and methods of approprirate simplicity have to be developed. These must be noninvasive, acceptable to the workforce, rapid, and often suitable for application on a very large scale.

One of the major difficulties in the scientific field is how to obtain the correct controls; clearly, these may be of many different types. Comparison between groups exposed to different doses may sometimes provide more useful information than attempts to identify an appropriate nonexposed group. The whole subject of controls is one of the most difficult and controversial topics in the whole of medicine.

IX. Nonmedical Problems

In the field of occupational medicine (as in all others), there is great difficulty in obtaining a consensus of definitions of disease and agreement on defining criteria for case collection. Problems arise because there is often failure of understanding that a conceptual definition, for instance that based on pathology, is not applicable directly where living populations are being studied and that indirect defining criteria have to be applied. Much time is also spent trying to establish universal agreement about the definition or the defining criteria for a disorder. Definitions should be the servant and not the master; their usefulness depending upon the questions being asked and the problems to be solved. For example, an agreed definition in terms of pathology may be excellent where a question in such terms is being asked and where the tools to be used are appropriate to this field. Such a definition, however, is useless to the epidemiologist. Uniformity *within context* is required, but universal definitions are unlikely to be practical in the majority of instances.

If the logic behind definitions is misunderstood within the medical and scientific professions, it is even more easily misunderstood by other professional lay bodies, including lawyers, management, unions, politicians, and the public at large. All these have been led to believe over many centuries that the authority of the medical profession enables it to identify disease with precision, that each has a clear-cut cause and pathognomonic characteristics by which it is readily distinguished from another. Moreover, they often assume that the distinction between health and disease is also as clear-cut. Further, and one must admire the touching confidence placed in the profession by nonmedical people, there is often a general belief that the doctor "knows." He knows when disease is present and when it is absent and how it is caused. Unfortunately, this is not so.

If there is misunderstanding with regard to the limitation of medical knowledge and the use of words, there is even greater difficulty in indicating to nonprofessional people that disease in an individual may not be detectable at all, although the disadvantageous implication to a community can be detected in populations using epidemiological tools. Education at a sophisticated level is required so that all those responsible for the development of new techniques and those who handle them can work alongside those who are responsible for monitoring potential hazards. This attitude of partnership should be a universal principle in the development of advanced technology in a civilized world and should never result in polarization of antagonism and mistrust where investigations are conducted in secret and results withheld through fear of misunderstanding or, worse, disguised by professional jargon (nonmedical as well as medical).

In the end the community has to decide whether the advantages of new technological advances outweigh the disadvantages or whether techniques can reduce the hazard to acceptable levels. What is acceptable has to be balanced against the advantages gained; the community as a whole, again, has to be the final arbiter.

X. Conclusion

The importance of occupational medicine lies in the implication it has for society, far beyond the conventional limits of medicine. Much of the subject must appropriately deal with healthy subjects and not sick ones, so that the techniques and methods used are very different from those included within the conventional training of doctors. This volume attempts to discuss and evaluate the strengths and the limitations of these. No attempt is made to achieve a systematic or comprehensive account of occupational lung diseases. It is more an attempt at an orientation, including some pointers for the future in this relatively new and growing field of uncontroversial importance.

2

Clinical Techniques

BRYAN H. GANDEVIA

The Prince Henry Hospital
Sydney, New South Wales, Australia

I. Introduction

From the time of Ramazzini (1633-1714) until the twentieth century symptoms and signs were the only clinical and epidemiological criteria available for the diagnosis of occupational respiratory diseases during life. Radiography eventually allowed objective assessment, with acceptable specificity [1], of the prevalence of silica and coal pneumoconioses, the two commonest industrial pulmonary complaints of the period. The inevitable emphasis on radiographic evaluation led to refinements in methodology which increased the accuracy and sensitivity of the technique for epidemiological purposes; major advances related

The research activities of the Department of Thoracic Medicine, Prince Henry Hospital, have been supported consistently by the Dust Diseases Board (New South Wales) and for special purposes by the National Health and Medical Research Council, the Asthma Foundation of New South Wales, the Australian Tobacco Research Foundation, as well as by industry and trade unions.

to the control of observer variation and the development of quantitative (grading) procedures. As a result, some understanding was obtained of the relationships among radiographic response, exposure, and functional status. These advances, together with improved measures for environmental appraisal and control, provided a rational approach to the design of appropriate surveillance programs and permitted the setting of reasonable confidence limits for the incidence of new cases in the future.

No such systematic approach to the nonpneumoconiotic respiratory diseases is yet apparent, although in an age of increasing technological complexity these are becoming of greater importance than the "classic" pneumoconioses. Not only concern for occupational health but also more liberal trends in workers' compensation demand more attention to these disorders. Where aggravation of preexisting (nonoccupational) disease is compensable (as in Australia) the question arises as to the possibility of occupationally induced excess of chronic nonspecific respiratory disease in industrial populations. Some modern disorders are hypersensitivity reactions, which introduce a new dimension both to epidemiological surveys and to environmental dose-response relationships. These conditions may be episodic, with or without a chronic and less reversible component (often a point at issue), posing special problems for epidemiological surveys, whether cross-sectional or longitudinal [2].

Occupational diseases without distinctive radiographic manifestations have two further features in common. There is no single objective means of assessment, such as the chest radiograph offers for silicosis, and all are characterized, or even defined, in terms of symptoms on exposure, or an excess of nonspecific symptoms and signs beyond the levels obtaining in the general (unexposed) population. Schilling's work on byssinosis was perhaps the first to encounter these problems: with McKerrow, he attempted to introduce objectivity by measuring ventilatory capacity before and after exposure [3]. In this condition, as in other "asthmatic" syndromes, differentiation from nonoccupational disorders rests heavily on symptoms, which are subjective, and their time relationships to exposure.

The simplest objective evidence in support of a symptom is a physical sign. There is therefore a need to refine techniques by eliciting and quantitating both symptoms and signs so that they may be used effectively in epidemiological studies. Technical refinement is all the more necessary because, unlike the radiographic signs of silicosis, the prevalence of symptoms and signs, inevitably nonspecific, will not be zero in a "nonexposed" population.

The group of disorders characterized by diffuse interstitial inflammation and/or fibrosis also emphasizes the need for reconsideration of symptoms and signs in epidemiological studies. In pulmonary asbestosis, as well as in conditions such as farmer's or bird fancier's lung, inspiratory crepitations (fine rales) have some discriminatory value in that they are not usually present in the common nonoccupational respiratory disorders. They are also likely to prove more sensitive than radiological or functional change; theoretically, one persistent crepitation reflects involvement of one tiny "respiratory unit," a degree of sensitivity to which other means of investigation cannot aspire. They are therefore of special significance where "early" radiological changes are difficult to detect or are nonspecific, and in situations where lung function tests lack specificity, sensitivity, or discrimination. All these difficulties may be encountered in epidemiological studies directed at identifying interstitial lung disease. The problems are complicated by the fact that no "best" test, functional or radiographic, is likely to emerge: there are grounds for anticipating that either the chest radiograph, gas transfer, the mechanical properties of the lung parenchyma, or the behavior of "small airways" may be chiefly affected in the early stages. The "best" test, in statistical terms, is probably the vital capacity, a test which is totally nonspecific. However, if associated with auscultation for crepitations greater discrimination is acquired; the combination of fine, inspiratory, basal crepitations and a reduced vital capacity in the presence of asbestos exposure suggests asbestosis, whether in the individual or the group, especially if the FEV_1/VC ratio is normal or raised [4].

Over the past decade or so, in the course of investigating a variety of occupational syndromes, we have examined more objective and quantitative means of eliciting symptoms, and we have been concerned to validate symptoms and signs chiefly by reference to functional tests since histologic correlation is not practicable. This chapter summarizes our experience (after discarding some unsuccessful approaches) but it aims to illustrate that symptoms and signs do have some "meaning," at least in functional terms, although this varies from one population to another and from one environmental hazard to another. To some extent, a pragmatic approach to symptoms and signs is inevitable; in any particular survey the design should be such as to allow evaluation of their significance. Put another way, symptoms may be simply considered as a means of subdividing the workforce under investigation; analysis in terms of these symptoms may then reveal their significance in the particular occupational context. Their relevance to any respiratory syndrome depends on a variety of factors, including their prevalence and whatever specificity can be given them (e.g., chest tightness on Mondays, association with a particular task, or absence in weekends). It cannot be expected that, for example, "dyspnea" will have the same significance, in functional or pathological terms, in populations exposed to asbestos, cadmium fume, and toluene-2,4-diisocyanate.

It is also unrealistic to hope that "normal" standards can be developed, or that comparisons can be made with values derived from the so-called "general population." Age, sex, smoking habit, previous respiratory disease, previous exposure to environmental inhalants, not to mention race, family size, socio-economic status, and city or rural habitat, would all have to be taken into account to produce these ideal standards. The impracticality of absolute standards emphasizes the need for appropriate epidemiological design within any given work population. Comparisons need to be made *within* these populations, using as a control group those who are unexposed or minimally exposed but who are otherwise identical (in terms of age, sex, race, socioeconomic status) with the heavily exposed group. A common difficulty is that selection factors are already operative in determining which of these groups the new employee enters; for example, if one finds differences between the exposed and "control" groups in smoking habit, there is probably some hidden reason, quite possibly of relevance to the problem under investigation.

Symptoms are subjective sensations, and they do not have the same connotation when elicited in a questionnaire administered to an actively working population as when they are volunteered by a patient in a clinical consultation. For the most part, symptoms vouchsafed in the former situation will be subclinical. Motivation differs in these circumstances, and is more readily influenced by such factors as financial loss or gain, by the prospects of an altered work environment, or by sociopolitical considerations. Symptoms are influenced by social, economic, cultural, and educational background, as well as by previous experience, and it is inherently unlikely that their prevalence will be directly comparable between studies in different occupational groups. Still less are they likely to afford valid comparisons between occupational groups in different countries. Classification by symptoms is primarily a technique appropriate to a local, defined population; comparisons between populations are complicated by influences other than the occupational inhalant. Thus, for certain purposes, classification by objective indices (such as a loose cough on request; see below) is preferred, although the prevalence of symptoms (e.g., of a productive cough) in groups so defined may well throw light on the attitude of populations to symptoms. In the investigation of a suspected hazard in which symptoms are the defining characteristic, classification by symptoms is inevitable, but their validity must be examined in terms of some objective indices, such as lung function tests, or perhaps by radiographic changes [5]. Physical signs are limited in number, and their prevalence is not usually high, so that, with some exceptions, as when interstitial disease is suspected, they are of little discriminatory value.

These considerations have some bearing on questionnaire design, to which much attention has been directed. Questions relating to symptom perception carry a greater error (assessed by variability in response) than more factual or objective questions such as those related to smoking habit [6], a finding which suggests that questions regarding symptoms should be as specific, and as "objective," as possible (see below). The approach to symptoms indicated above implies that there are limitations to comparisons between surveys of different population groups which cannot be overcome no matter how the questions are worded (sharpened). However, it also implies that within one survey population comparisons between subgroups in terms of symptom prevalence may have reasonable sensitivity, reflected, hopefully, in objective data. This places the emphasis not so much on a question which is "standardized" internationally but one which is appropriate to the syndrome, the population, and the hazard under investigation. A measure of flexibility in the symptom questions to be asked seems unavoidable, and indeed the rigidity of the standard questionnaire is a feature which, while perhaps appropriate to insidious-onset dust diseases with diagnostic radiographic appearances, limits their usefulness in the varied non-pneumoconiotic disorders. This is not an argument for a nonstandard format to all questions or for ad hoc changes with every survey. Flexibility does not include scope for bad design or bad wording nor does it exclude attention to the other factors which may influence answers, such as variability between observers (where self-completion forms are not used), the order of questions, and the use of qualifying phrases or subsidiary queries. Appropriate observer training [7] and measures to control or assess observer variation are essential, whatever the details of methodology.

Against this background, the major respiratory symptoms and signs may now be reviewed. For reasons inherent in the foregoing discussion, we do so from the viewpoint of methodology rather than by attempting to demonstrate their meaning in absolute terms, although illustrative examples of their significance in industrial studies are briefly mentioned. Many of the problems relating to the evaluation of symptoms and signs and their relationship to objective data are examined in a nonoccupational context by Fletcher et al. [8] and by Van der Lende [9].

II. Description of Tables 1 and 2

Tables 1 and 2 are referred to at many points in the text, and it is appropriate at the outset to describe their construction; the abbreviations used are set out in Table 3. They are based on 590 "healthy" males in active employment, and comprise two complete industrial populations which, at the time of the studies, we deemed to have suffered no environmental respiratory hazard in their employment. The definition of each of the symptoms and signs is described in the relevant section of the text. The lung function tests represent a selection of indices from a comprehensive range applied on site in a mobile laboratory [10]. The values shown in the tables are the means of values adjusted for age, or for

Table 1 Symptoms in Relation to Lung Function[a]

	Whole series (± SD)	Current smokers	Dyspnea	Cough > 3/12	Chest tightness < 1/wk	Chest tightness > 1/wk	Asthma history
N	591	401	32	143	71	43	42
Current smokers %	67.9	100	79.4	89.6	76.0	72.7	53.3
Age	34.2 (10.6)	34.7	38.7*	37.6*	36.1	37.2*	29.4*
FEV_1	3.71 (0.57)	3.70	3.28*	3.56*	3.65	3.25*	3.21*
VC	5.02 (0.56)	5.02	4.82*	4.98	5.04	4.98	4.84*
$FEV_{1\,(\%VC)}$	74.0 (9.2)	73.5	66.9*	71.3*	72.9	64.4*	67.1*
FRC	3.53 (0.64)	3.56	3.83*	3.60	3.70*	3.74	3.79*
TLC	6.96 (0.74)	6.99	7.00	7.01	7.04	7.23*	7.16
$RV_{(\%TLC)}$	27.6 (6.3)	27.8	30.9*	28.7*	27.8	30.4*	31.4*
$CC_{(\%TLC)}$	40.3 (7.8)	41.2*	45.0*	41.1	42.0	42.4	43.0

$\dot{V}_{max(50\%\ TLC)}$	2.76 (1.26)	2.60*	2.10*	2.33*	2.56	1.92*	2.42
PEF	7.97 (1.62)	7.92	6.93*	7.53*	7.84	6.91*	6.76
T_L	31.6 (5.1)	30.3*	29.0*	30.7*	29.9*	29.5*	31.4
R_L	2.36 (1.27)	2.36	3.01	2.65*	2.54	3.15*	2.97*
C_L	0.347 (0.116)	0.352*	0.343	0.351	0.363	0.376	0.391*
PL_{max_i}	34.1 (9.9)	34.2	31.8	33.6	33.2	31.5	31.1*
$PL_{(90\%TLC)}$	16.2 (3.4)	16.2	15.6	15.9	16.0	15.3	15.0

[a]Values for individual lung function tests have been adjusted for age or age and height as appropriate. The asterisk (*) indicates significant ($P < 0.05$) difference from mean value for whole series (column 1).

Table 2 Physical Signs in Relation to Lung Function[a]

	Whole series (± SD)	Productive cough	Rales	Rhonchi	Rales, rhonchi
N	591	142	98	40	12
Current % smokers	67.9	88.7	80.4	80.0	53.8
Age	34.2 (10.6)	38.1*	39.0*	38.7*	42.2*
FEV_1	3.71 (0.57)	3.49*	3.64	3.31*	3.14*
VC	5.02 (0.56)	4.95	4.98	4.92	4.68*
$FEV_{1\,(\%VC)}$	74.0 (9.2)	70.0*	73.2	66.8*	65.6*
FRC	3.53 (0.64)	3.68*	3.56	3.71	4.13
TLC	6.96 (0.74)	7.10*	6.96	7.14	7.52
$RV_{(\%TLC)}$	27.6 (6.3)	29.9*	28.0	30.9*	35.7*
$CC_{(\%TLC)}$	40.3 (7.8)	43.4*	40.6	43.7*	45.5*
$\dot{V}_{max(50\%TLC)}$	2.76 (1.26)	2.03*	2.54	1.79*	2.18
PEF	7.98 (1.62)	7.27*	8.04	7.41*	7.12
T_L	31.6 (5.1)	30.5*	31.2	31.0	31.0
R_L	2.36 (1.27)	2.78*	2.37	3.29*	4.34*
C_L	0.347 (0.116)	0.360	0.350	0.332	0.325
PL_{max_i}	34.1 (9.9)	32.2*	33.1	34.5	30.5
$PL_{(90\%TLC)}$	16.2 (3.4)	15.3*	15.7	16.6	14.6

[a]Values for individual lung function tests have been adjusted for age or age and height as appropriate. The asterisk (*) indicates significant ($P < 0.05$) difference from mean value for whole series (column 1).

Table 3 Abbreviations Used in Tables 1 and 2*

FEV_1	Forced expiratory volume in one second (litres)
VC	Vital capacity (liters)
$FEV_{1\,(\%VC)}$	Forced expiratory volume in one second as percentage of vital capacity.
FRC	Functional residual capacity (liters)
TLC	Total lung capacity (liters)
$RV_{(\%TLC)}$	Residual volume as percentage of total lung capacity
$CC_{(\%TLC)}$	Closing capacity as percentage of total lung capacity
$V_{max(50\%\ TLC)}$	Maximum expiratory flow at 50% of total lung capacity
PEF	Peak expiratory flow (liters/sec)
T_L	Single breath gas transfer factor (ml CO min^{-1} $mmHg^{-1}$)
R_L	Pulmonary resistance during tidal breathing : Mead-Whittenberger method (cmH_2O $liters^{-1}$ sec^{-1})
C_L	Static deflation pulmonary compliance (liters/cm H_2O)†
PL_{max_i}	Transpulmonary pressure at maximum inspiration (cm H_2O)
$PL_{(90\%\ TLC)}$	Static transpulmonary pressure at 90 per cent of total lung capacity.

*Gas volumes and flows are expressed at BTPS conditions.

† Measured as the slope of the static deflation pressure-volume curve over the litre above FRC.

Note: Other measured parameters of lung function have been omitted as not contributing to the present descriptive review.

age and height where the effect of the latter is significant. As this procedure obscures an age effect in relation to symptoms and signs, mean age for each symptom or sign grouping is also shown. Smoking exerts an important effect, more on the development of symptoms and signs than on lung function, and more with advancing years. Although it is possible to allow for the effects of smoking by statistical means, I have chosen not to do so for present purposes, because the aim of this essay is to evaluate the symptoms and signs themselves rather than to examine their cause. Although we are not concerned to describe the effects of smoking, its influence may be gauged by noting the prevalence of smokers in each symptom or sign group. However, smoking significantly affected a limited number of functional tests in this series (closing capacity, flow at 50% of total lung capacity, transfer factor and pulmonary compliance). For simplicity, standard deviations are shown only for the series as a whole; although not relevant in the present context, significant differences in variance, implying perhaps a nonhomogeneous group, may be as important as differences between the mean value shown for those with the stated characteristic compared to the mean value for those without that characteristic. This has been done merely to simplify tabulation; as the number with each characteristic and the total number are shown, the mean value for the remainder can readily by calculated. The approach adopted here is not necessarily that used in analyzing the data from a particular study, when it may well be appropriate to use more complex or sophisticated statistical methods.

III. Dyspnea

Intuitively it may be accepted that a question relating to exercise tolerance is slightly more objective than a question relating to breathlessness. There are three questions of which several variants are in common use:

1. Are you able to keep up with others of your own age walking up hills and stairs?
2. Are you more breathless than others of your own walking up hills and stairs?
3. Are you more breathless on exertion than others of your own age?

The first seeks factual experience rather than a comparative impression of a sensation. We have not evaluated questions of these types, partly because in an initial attempt the order of the questions was found to exert a significant influence, and partly because persistent dyspnea or lowered exercise tolerance is an uncommon, and hence an insensitive, symptom in a working population. In one survey, those claiming to be "more breathless on exertion" weighed significantly more (nearly 8 kg) than those without this symptom, indicating a further complicating factor. In the present (tabulated) series, as assessed by the question "Do you get short of breath on exertion more easily than others of your own age?", dyspnea was present in only 5.4% of subjects. On the other hand, it was a highly significant symptom in terms of respiratory function (Table 1). The pattern of the findings is consistent with airways obstruction, small airway dysfunction, and possibly mild impairment of gas exchange, but over 80% of the subjects admitting to dyspnea were smokers, and the subjects were also older than the average.

The number of subjects whose exercise tolerance is limited on the flat is negligible in the occupational populations we have studied. The value of the symptom would increase with increasing age and disability in the population, perhaps one subjected to a major hazard in high concentration over a long period. Such a situation is now found only where socioeconomic conditions determine or permit an exposure beyond conventionally acceptable limits.

A more sensitive and quantitative method of assessing dyspnea in predominantly healthy workers is desirable. We have recently investigated a "line" method, where the left end of a 10 cm line represents "I cannot breathe at all" (zero), and the other end indicates "My breathing is perfectly normal" (100 mm) [11]. The subject is asked to mark his position on the line, and breathlessness, or lack thereof, is expressed by the distance along the line from zero. In a series of 126 subjects (25% drawn consecutively from a current survey and the remainder from patients attending hospital mostly with chronic respiratory disease), the correlation coefficients for this figure with forced expiratory volume at one second (FEV_1) and forced expiratory ratio (FER: FEV_1/VC) were 0.74 and 0.59 respectively ($P < 0.001$). The slope of the regression lines for patients and for survey subjects was identical. The line scores were then arbitrarily ranked from I (81-100 mm; i.e., breathing close to normal) to V (1-20 mm; close to inability to breathe at all) and related to five grades of dyspnea based on exercise tolerance as identified by the British Medical Research Council (MRC) questionnaire. The results are related to FEV_1 measurements (expressed as a percentage of predicted normal values) in Figure 1. The findings reflect the discriminatory value of grading dyspnea by the line method, but they also indicate the insensitivity (in terms of FEV_1) of the standard questionnaire in relation to the severity of dyspnea likely to be encountered in occupational epidemiology. When FER was plotted against dyspnea grade, the differences between grades according to the questionnaire were again less well defined than between grades according to the line method. We have not yet employed the line method in an extensive population survey but it seems to offer some advantages over the questionnaire method. Sensitivity toward the healthy end of the scale, a difficulty in any epidemiological survey, may be improved by modifying the statements at either end of the line.

We have also tested a method of assessing dyspnea based on paired statements relating to severity (as employed for cough; see below). The approach was promising, but modifications are needed to make it less time consuming and also as effective as the line method.

If limitation of exercise tolerance is a specific issue in any group under study (it is commonly relevant only to individuals) the inclusion of an exercise test in the survey procedures becomes obligatory, as it would be unwise to draw inferences from the history, however obtained, and from the results of lung

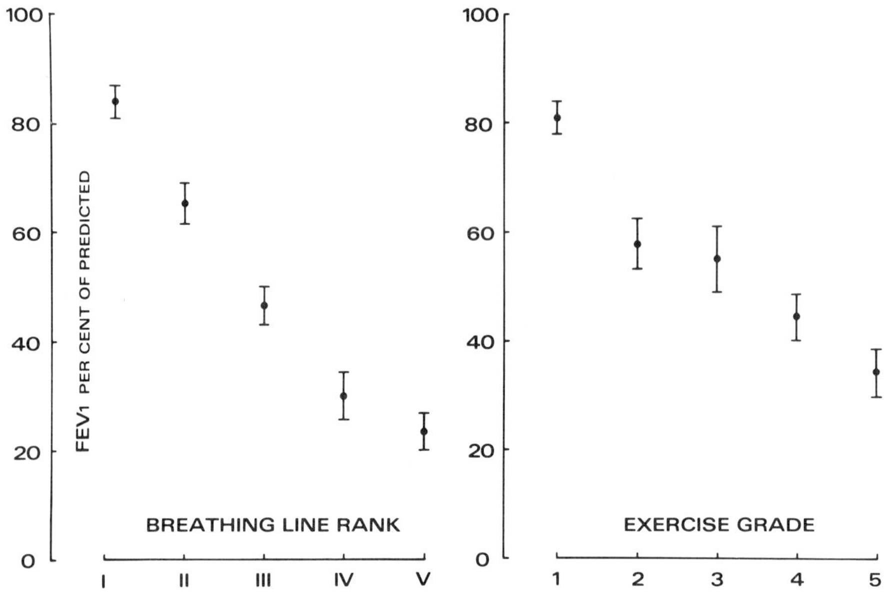

Figure 1 The relationship of FEV_1 (expressed as a percentage of predicted normal values) to breathing line ranks (I to V) and to exercise grades (1 to 5). Values shown are mean ± SE. See text for discussion.

function tests at rest. Such a situation might call for a statistical sampling procedure. Exercise procedures range from the simple to the complex, but where the latter incorporate measurements of arterial blood gas tensions the test probably falls outside the limits of the epidemiological approach.

IV. Cough and Sputum

In principle, subsidiary questions are better than qualifying phrases in a primary symptom question. This is well illustrated by the qualifying phrase "in winter" or "in bad weather" in the MRC questions relating to the presence or absence of cough and sputum. Such qualifying phrases lack meaning in many parts of the world. Lebowitz and Burrows [6] propose a series of questions to avoid this difficulty, commencing with "Do you ever have a cough when you don't have a cold?", although even then the word *ever* may be introducing a qualification. In the past, we have simply asked a part of the MRC question: "Do you usually have a cough?" (*usually* being defined as 3 or 4 days a week or 3 or 4 months of the year) [12]. However, in Table 1, a history of cough/sputum implies an answer of "yes" to the questions "Do you have a cough/phlegm for as much as 3 months in the year?"; the "3 months" qualification is intended as an overall estimate and not to mean that the cough is present continuously over 3 months. Nearly a quarter of the series admitted to cough. The chief significance of a positive answer (Table 1) appears to be that 90% of the sufferers were smokers, drawn more from the older subjects. However, there were some significant functional differences between those with and without cough (± sputum), reflected in a relative increase in airway resistance (and correlated indices). In an occupational group of nearly 150 subjects studied by us on two occasions 4 years apart there was an overall increase in cough prevalence from 26 to 28%, but with about 12% of the series losing the symptom and 14% acquiring it; the absolute value of a symptom with such variability is open to question.

More information, of a semiquantitative kind, is obtained from a cough questionnaire based on a series of six statements each reflecting a "degree of severity" of cough [13]. The statements are presented in random order to the subject in selected pairs on a card, and he is asked to select which statement in each pair is more appropriate to his cough status. At the conclusion, he has automatically placed himself in one of 10 uniquely ranked categories; inconsistencies are uncommon and readily detected. The questionnaire takes about 5 min to apply and does not require medically qualified personnel. Figure 2 represents the findings in a series of aluminum smelters. Group I claimed to be asymptomatic on exposure to smelting fume, while group III give a history of recurring chest tightness, often with wheezing, of breathing difficulty, during or after certain operations; the symptoms were consistent with a syndrome known from clinical experience. Group II had similar symptoms but less often than once a week. In group I a cough grade greater than 3 is a function of smoking. Group III is clearly different in terms of this index of respiratory malfunction; it includes nonsmokers with a grade of cough severity not encountered in group I. Group II is nonhomogeneous, as it also was in respect to other parameters of respiratory function. In this situation, the cough questionnaire not only distinguishes normal from abnormal but it also permits an assessment of the relative contributions of smoking and the occupational environment.

In the nonpneumoconiotic occupational disorders, cough, often periodic or episodic, is of more diagnostic value than phlegm production, which may deserve more attention, perhaps along the lines of a phlegm score, as suggested by Fletcher et al. [14].

Clinical experience of certain types of occupation respiratory disorder, such as byssinosis and occupational "asthma" or "bronchitis," suggests that this symptom is distinct from wheezing or asthma although all may be related

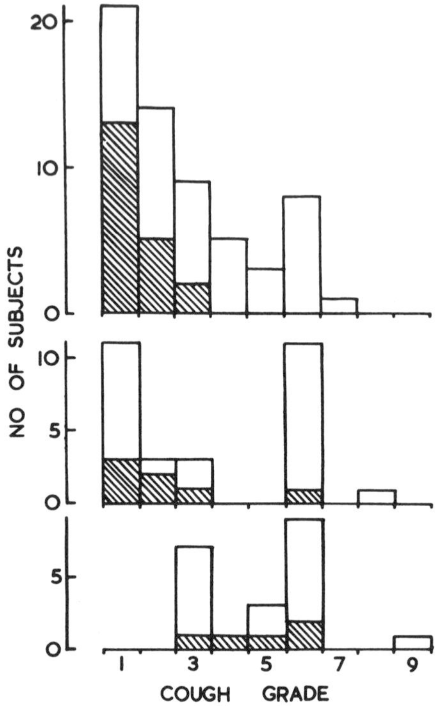

Figure 2 The numbers of asymptomatic subjects (top), subjects with infrequent wheezing or chest tightness (center), and subjects with frequent wheeze or tightness (bottom) on occupational exposure in relation to cough grade (1 to 9). Shaded areas represent nonsmokers. (Reproduced with permission from Gandevia [24]. Copyright 1974 by the New York Academy of Sciences.)

physiologically and pathogenetically. Rather than ask leading questions (such as whether this occurs on Monday mornings or in relation to specific processes) we have asked whether, if this symptom is present, it occurs more or less often than once a week.

Table 1 indicates that when chest tightness occurred less often than once a week it had little functional or occupational significance, and 76% of this group were smokers. Occurring more frequently, the symptom was associated with smoking in 74% of cases, and with above-average age, but also with functional changes in the direction of airways obstruction. In the 4 year follow-up survey previously mentioned [p. 23] of a population with no relevant respiratory hazard, the overall prevalence of chest tightness (more than once a week) increased from 4 to 6%, but 1% had "lost" the symptom.

In occupations with a respiratory hazard, as illustrated in Figure 2, the pattern may change. Approximately 19% of this population of aluminum smelters had chest tightness more often than once a week (bottom row), and 26% less often (center); the comparable figures from the series shown in Table 1 (with no hazard) are 7 and 12%, respectively. The associated functional changes in the population exposed to a hazard were similar but more impressive than the changes recorded in Table 1. In this study, bronchial reactivity to histamine, 1.0 mg/ml (using FEV_1 change and a standardized inhalation procedure), was, on average, greater in group III than in the asymptomatic group I. Although the mean values did not differ significantly, the standard deviation was significantly higher in the group claiming chest tightness. These findings are consistent with those described above for cough grade from the same survey, and also illustrated in Figure 2.

Our evidence suggests that this symptom deserves enquiry but requires careful evaluation especially in relation to its frequency and to smoking habit. Its significance will vary according to the environmental inhalant and the syndrome of which it forms a part.

V. Productive Cough upon Request

An objective index of sputum production is especially desirable in an occupational context. The collection of a morning sputum specimen [15] had too high a lapse rate in our hands, and as it is unsupervised the validity of the result is open to doubt whether the containers are returned empty or full. We have used the "loose cough sign" as an index of sputum production [16]. The subject is instructed to take a big breath and cough hard: the cough is adjudged "loose" (productive) or "dry" (unproductive) simply by its sound. The test is quick and the lapse rate zero, even where there are language difficulties. The test has been validated by reference to sputum volume and it has also been related to the distribution of grades of cough severity [13]. Observer variation (which occurs in about 10% of positive coughs and a lower proportion of negative ones) has not been decreased by tape recording of the cough. In practice, it has distinguished better than the history those subjects showing a decrease in FEV_1 over the working day in response to several inhalants, and its prevalence has varied significantly in different occupational groups. In Australia, the association with smoking increases with age [17]; smoking is the major determinant but there is a background prevalence in nonsmokers of approximately 10% at all ages, including young children [18]. These relationships will not necessarily be found in other countries and circumstances [19-21]. Epidemics of acute respiratory illness might conceivably influence apparent prevalence in comparisons between populations, but comparisons within a single occupational population surveyed within a short period are not invalidated, especially as any acute infective influence of bronchial secretion is more likely to occur in those with some chronic respiratory abnormality, or in smokers.

In the present series (Table 2), 24% had a loose cough (89% of whom smoked), a finding associated with significant changes in a wide range of lung function tests, including those related to lung elastic recoil. It seems that the test selects from the smokers a group showing more widespread and significant functional changes. This group thus exerts an important influence on the lung function data obtained in an occupational survey, so that it warrants careful consideration, especially where comparisons are contemplated between different populations.

The significance of sputum production, its assessment by subjective and objective means, and its relationship to ventilatory capacity are described and evaluated by Fletcher and his colleagues [8] in their prospective study of chronic bronchitis in postal workers. Similar information should be sought in other occupational groups.

VI. Rales and Rhonchi

We have recorded fine, bubbling, inspiratory, or expiratory "moist" sounds heard toward the bases on more than a single breath as "fine rales." Trained observers have shown good agreement but observer variation can be high, especially, in our experience, if transient rales (audible on only one or two breaths) are accepted as a positive finding. The sign was positive in 17% of the present series, chiefly in older smokers. Interestingly, it is not associated with significant functional abnormality. One hypothesis to account for this is that it is a very sensitive sign of peripheral airway disorder, insufficiently diffuse to produce abnormality in functional tests. In support of this view is the finding that about half of one series of proteolytic enzyme workers were found to have fine rales, and, contrary to experience in other occupational studies (including the present series), there was no positive association between the presence of rales and a productive cough on request [22]. As aerosol challenge with proteolytic enzymes produced fine rales in some cases [23], the epidemiological finding was presumably significant.

Expiratory wheezes, or high-pitched rhonchi, are relatively infrequent (6.8%; Table 2) and are associated with the expected functional evidence of airways obstruction. The combination of rales and rhonchi, by no means confined to smokers, is uncommon but is associated with relatively severe airway narrowing (Table 2). Identification of this combination in individual cases may therefore be worthwhile in an epidemiological survey.

The fine rales, as described above, may be distinguished from fine, dry, "crackles" best heard at the bases laterally; the latter are typically confined to inspiration and may show a crescendo effect, increasing in number as inspiration proceeds. These are heard in interstitial lung diseases, including asbestosis. The work of Leathart [24] and Harries [25] suggests they are an "early" diagnostic feature of asbestosis, and the sign warrants inclusion in any survey of asbestos workers. This is especially true if lung function tests are restricted to the simpler tests, since these are nonspecific. In a study of 114 asbestos workers in Singapore [4], the presence of rales of this type was associated with a significant mean decrease in FEV_1 and FVC of about 0.4 liters, the combination affording a basis for at least a provisional diagnosis of asbestosis. Similar findings, but including a semiquantitative approach to the "scoring" of these adventitiae, have been reported from the United States [26].

Electronic recording of breath sounds and waveform analysis are receiving exploratory attention as an epidemiological tool in the study of working populations. It is hoped that observer variability can be reduced by the improved standardization presumably available when such records are made. Necessary equipment includes an electronic stethoscope, such as is used in phonocardiography, a preamplifier, and a tape recorder. Additional electronic capability will depend on the analyses required. Preliminary attempts at recording breath sounds in our field studies have not been satisfactory.

VII. Past or Present History of Asthma

Table 1 reflects the answers to the question "Have you ever had asthma?" A past or present history of asthma is clearly associated with detectable changes in a wide range of pulmonary function tests (Table 1) in this series, where there was no occupational risk of asthma. The findings may be taken to reflect the "background" effects of asthma in any working population, with the reservation that potentially asthmatic subjects may tend to select an occupation without a respiratory hazard. Nonetheless, the association of this symptom with functional changes is such that a history of asthma should be sought. When there is a significant influence of occupational asthma, its prevalence, as well as its influence, will presumably be greater than in this series.

VIII. Atopic Status

Between 10 and 30% of the population are atopic on symptomatic grounds, depending on what entities are accepted as reflecting atopic status. "Hay fever" is the best predictor of atopic status in terms of positive skin tests, and as this diagnosis when made by the subject is probably reasonably accurate (despite overlap with perennial rhinitis) it may suffice as a simple questionnaire index of atopy. We find a higher proportion of positive answers to the question "Do you often sneeze or get an itchy running nose?" than if "hay fever" is merely listed among past illnesses. This question also allows qualifying questions regarding the influence of season, tasks, or specific inhalants, occupational or otherwise; these symptoms often precede the onset of occupational asthma. Hay fever was significantly associated with the respiratory syndrome of aluminium smelters, but no relationship has been demonstrated in workers with a variety of other substances [22]. More information is clearly required: the relevance of atopy may vary with the nature of the inhalant, its capacity to induce immediate-type sensitivity, and the severity of exposure. Atopy may confuse the epidemiological situation further by influencing selection for, or survival in, a given occupation.

Atopic status is probably best assessed for epidemiological purposes by objective indices such as prick test reactions to two or three common inhalants, or serum IgE levels [27].

IX. Specific Symptomatology

In some occupational respiratory syndromes there are aspects of the history which are strongly suggestive of an occupational cause. The classic example is the Monday tightness of byssinosis; others include improvement over days off or holiday periods, immediate onset of symptoms on exposure, or, in some cases, nocturnal or continuous symptoms on regular daily exposure [28]. It is difficult to devise an appropriate questionnaire without asking such leading questions as "Is your breathing worse on Monday?", or "better on days off." Furthermore, such questions can sometimes be misleading in their implications or interpretation, as when a subject develops occupational asthma which becomes persistent, even through days off, or when he has no immediate reaction but develops symptoms only after work or in the early hours of the morning. Our present approach is to ask, in relation to chest tightness, whether it occurs more or less often than once a week; the significance of the distinction has been discussed. This at least appears to produce a group with reasonably definite symptoms and a group which includes some with "real" and some with "doubtfully relevant" symptoms. Subjects may admit to chest tightness but deny asthma, which they have not had previously, and which their doctors are commonly reluctant to diagnose. Indeed, the dominance of cough, often an associated symptom, frequently leads to a clinical label of bronchitis; the cough questions previously outlined can sometimes be correlated with chest tightness.

The alternative epidemiological approach is that which the clinician normally uses, and which we have successfully used in relatively small populations when personal interview with all exposed subjects is feasible. Conventional standard questions are asked regarding asthma, wheezing, chest tightness, and hay fever, requiring an answer of yes or no. Finally the question is asked "Does the dust/fume/vapor upset you in any way?" It is surprising what remarkable symptoms emerge, with headache and constipation likely to be prominent, but if respiratory symptoms are not mentioned, or follow after a list of others, the clinician is unlikely to accord them the same significance as if they were immediately volunteered. If respiratory symptoms are not mentioned, the questions are asked "Does the material affect your chest/breathing/nose in any way?" The clinical approach does not commend itself to the statistician but if a hazard is suspected but unproven it should at least supplement any standard questionnaire in a selected sample of the population. A view of the natural history of a disorder within the limitations of a cross-sectional survey also requires a similar style of interview, based on clinical philosophy but employing standard questions as far as possible. This applies especially in the investigation of acute or subacute recurrent syndromes, particularly when the hazard is not obvious or well-recognized; the occupational basis may be no more than suspected. These syndromes may affect upper or lower respiratory tract, together or singly, and they include "influenza-like" syndromes with fever and malaise. Leading symptoms questions are unavoidable, but such a questionnaire needs to be supplemented by critical clinical queries, especially as to time relationships (of symptoms to one another, of symptoms to task or work area).

The usefulness of the clinical approach to the epidemiological situation is illustrated by an outbreak of asthma, affecting about 25% of employees, in an industry processing poppies to produce morphine in a finely divided state. An allergist, after seeing several of the more severe cases, directed attention to the incoming poppies as a likely cause, although he did not have the opportunity to inspect the site and note that the early stages of the processing were remarkably free of dust. After the standard questionnaire had been administered, those with symptoms of any kind were interviewed in a clinical setting. It emerged that in all cases the first attack had occurred while handling the pure morphine in a finely divided dry state, and subsequently environmental control measures in this area resolved the problem. It is of interest that the employees themselves blamed an intermediate process where organic solvents were acting as a nonspecific respiratory irritant. It is difficult to see how this problem could have been resolved by questionnaire without asking a question (which did not occur to us at the time) such as "Where were you at the time of your *first* attack?" It is doubtful whether this question would be understandable or answered consistently as part of a standard questionnaire, certainly if self-administered, especially as the responders, in the context of other work-oriented questions, may infer that the answer should involve a work area.

X. Interrelationships between Symptoms and Signs

Symptoms and signs show a variety of associations between themselves, and these associations vary in different circumstances. For example, in the series shown in Tables 1 and 2, 82% of subjects with an unproductive cough on request had no abnormality on auscultation of the chest, by comparison with only 52% among those whose cough was productive. Rales occurred twice and rhonchi four times as often in those with a loose cough. There were also highly significant interrelationships between the symptoms of cough, chest tightness, and a complaint of dyspnea. These interrelationships will necessarily vary from one respiratory hazard to another [29], just as the prevalence of individual symptoms and signs will vary. The varying prevalence of rales and the presence or absence of a relationship to smoking has already been mentioned. In the present context, the precise interpretation of these interrelationships is not the issue so much as the way in which permutations and combinations of symptoms, signs, and often other objective data may be meaningfully employed in an occupational survey. It is likely that a more sophisticated approach could be developed by the use of appropriate statistical methods, including cluster analysis, to aid in the recognition and characterization of newly identified occupational respiratory syndromes.

XI. Summary and Conclusions

In this chapter I have presented a case for the importance of symptoms and signs in the investigation particularly of the nonpneumoconiotic disorders. I have also attempted to show that the elicitation of symptoms such as dyspnea and cough may be made more objective and sometimes given a semiquantitative basis. If possible an objective index, such as the cough sign, should be associated with a subjective symptom (such as a history of cough and sputum); both provide somewhat different but perhaps complementary information, perhaps especially with respect to time [9]. Comparisons within an occupational population may well employ symptoms, or a symptom complex, as a defining characteristic of a group, and indeed this approach must be used when an occupational respiratory syndrome is itself defined in symptomatic terms. Similarly, within a homogeneous working population which can be classified according to level of exposure to a known hazard (either cumulative, peak, or long-term levels may be relevant, depending on the hazard and the syndrome), the prevalence of symptoms and signs are of considerable significance.

Comparisons between populations pose problems of greater complexity as the significance of symptoms and signs, which are often nonspecific, will vary from one hazard to another, and attitudes to symptoms are not constant from one population to another. Comparisons, especially international ones, should begin with classification on objective criteria (clinical, functional, or radiologic) rather than symptoms; symptom frequency may then be examined in groups so defined.

The small size of some occupational populations exposed to a respiratory hazard stresses the need not only for collective experience but also for refinement of techniques for eliciting symptoms and signs. The validity and discrimination of the methods used require evaluation in the whole range of environmental circumstances; survey design and analysis in any particular situation should incorporate approaches to this evaluation.

Although there is a core of information, similar to that obtained in available standard questionnaires, which is required in all surveys, it is doubtful if symptom questions can be standardized to a form appropriate to all environmental hazards and their associated syndromes. Nonetheless, once the principle of flexibility is accepted, considerable scope exists for standardization of approach in terms of methodology and statistical evaluation; there is little doubt that the contribution to be made by symptoms and signs to many occupational respiratory problems has been underestimated and underinvestigated.

Acknowledgments

In the preparation of this review I am particularly indebted to Mr. Peter Owen, scientific officer to the Department of Thoracic Medicine, Prince Henry Hospital, for his assistance with the statistical analysis and to Professor H. J. H. Colebatch for many discussions of the issues involved.

References

1. Terms such as specificity, validity, discrimination, and sensitivity as applies to tests used in epidemiology are defined and discussed by the International Labour Organisation: Respiratory function tests in pneumoconiosis: Report and related papers, Geneva, ILO, 1966. (See also Ref. 2.)
2. Gandevia, B., Assessment of lung function in occupational surveys, *Bull. Physiopathol. Respir. (Dancy)*, **6**:537–560 (1970).
3. McKerrow, C. B., M. McDonald, J. C. Gilson, and R. S. F. Schilling, Respiratory function during the day in cotton workers: A study of byssinosis, *Br. J. Ind. Med.*, **15**:75–83 (1958).

4. Chew, P. K., M. Chia, S. F. Chew, J. M. J. Supramaniam, W. Chan, C. H. Chew, Y. K. Ng, and B. Gandevia, Asbestos workers in Singapore: A clinical, functional and radiological survey, *Arch. Environ. Health,* **26**: 290–293 (1973).
5. Musk, A. W., and B. Gandevia, Respiratory function and the chest radiograph: An epidemiological study of the significance of minor radiographic abnormalities, *Aust. N.Z. J. Med.,* **8**:7–13 (1978).
6. Lebowitz, M. D., and B. Burrows, Comparison of questionnaires: The B.M.R.C. and N.H.L.I. respiratory questionnaires and a new self-completion questionnaire, *Am. Rev. Respir. Dis.,* **113**:627–635 (1976).
7. Fairbairn, A. S., C. H. Wood, and C. M. Fletcher, Variability in answers to a questionnaire on respiratory symptoms, *Br. J. Soc. Prev. Med.,* **13**:175–193 (1959).
8. Fletcher, C., R. Peto, C. Tinker, and F. E. Speizer, *The Natural History of Chronic Bronchitis and Emphysema.* Oxford, Oxford Univ. Press, 1976.
9. Van der Lende, R., *Epidemiology of Chronic Non-specific Lung Disease (Chronic Bronchitis).* Assen, van Gorcum & Co., N.V., 1969.
10. Field, G., P. Owen, and B. Gandevia, Mobile laboratory for respiratory surveys in industry, *Med. J. Aust.,* **1**:867–869 (1976).
11. Thind, G., G. Field, and B. Gandevia, in preparation.
12. Ferris, B., Epidemiology standardisation project, *Am. Rev. Respir. Dis. (Suppl.),* **118**:1–120 (1978).
13. Field, G. B., The application of a quantitative estimate of cough frequency to epidemiological surveys, *Int. J. Epidemiol.,* **3**:135–143 (1974).
14. Fletcher, C. M., R. Peto, and C. M. Tinker, A comparison of the assessment of simple bronchitis by measurements of sputum volume and by standardized questions on phlegm production, *Int. J. Epidemiol.,* **3**:315–319 (1974).
15. Elmes, P. C., A. C. Dutton, and C. M. Fletcher, Sputum examination and the investigation of "chronic bronchitis," *Lancet,* **1**:1241 (1959).
16. Hall, G. J. L., and B. Gandevia, Relationship of the loose cough sign to daily sputum volume, *Br. J. Soc. Prev. Med.,* **25**:109–113 (1971).
17. Gandevia, B., A productive cough upon request as an index of chronic bronchitis: The effects of age, sex, smoking habit and environment upon prevalence in Australian general practice, *Med. J. Aust.,* **1**:16–20 (1969).
18. Hall, G. J. L., B. Gandevia, H. Silverstone, J. Searle, and H. Gibson, The interrelationships of upper and lower respiratory tract symptoms and signs in seven-year-old children, *Int. J. Epidemiol.,* **1**:389–403 (1973).
19. Anderson, H. R., Respiratory anomalies in Papua-New Guinea children: The effects of locality and domestic wood smoke pollution, *Int. J. Epidemiol.,* **7**:63–72 (1978).
20. Chia, M., N. K. Virabhak, Y. K. Ng, S. K. Lee, J. M. J. Supramaniam, W. Chan, P. Martin, and B. Gandevia, Upper and lower respiratory tract disorders in eight-year-old Singapore children: An investigation of survey techniques, *Singapore Med. J.,* **13**:307–312 (1972).

21. Cullen, K. J., T. A. Welborn, M. S. Stenhouse, M. G. McCall, and D. H. Curnow, Ventilatory capacity and productive cough in a rural community, *Br. J. Prev. Soc. Med.,* **23**:85–90 (1969).
22. Gandevia, B., Pulmonary reactions to organic materials: Clinical history, physical examination and x-ray changes, *Ann. N.Y. Acad. Sci.,* **221**:10–26 (1974).
23. Mitchell, C. A., and B. Gandevia, Acute bronchiolitis following provocative inhalation of "Alcalase"—a proteolytic enzyme used in the detergent industry, *Med. J. Aust.,* **1**:1363–1367 (1971).
24. Leathart, G. L., Pulmonary function tests in asbestos workers, *Trans. Soc. Occup. Med.,* **18**:49–55 (1968).
25. Harries, P. G., *The Effects and Control of Diseases Associated with Exposure to Asbestos in Devonport Dockyard.* Gosport, U.K. Royal Navy Clinical Research Working Party, Institute of Naval Medicine, 1971.
26. Mitchell, C. A., M. Charney, and J. B. Schoenberg, Early lung disease in asbestos-product workers, *Lung,* **154**:261–272 (1978).
27. Pepys, J., *Hypersensitivity Diseases of the Lungs due to Fungi and Organic Dusts.* Basel, S. Karger, 1969.
28. Gandevia, B., Occupational asthma, *Med. J. Aust.,* **2**:332–335 (1970).
29. Mitchell, C. A., and B. Gandevia, Respiratory symptoms and skin reactivity in workers exposed to proteolytic enzymes in the detergent industry, *Am. Rev. Respir. Dis.,* **104**:1–12 (1971).

3

Radiography

JOHN C. GILSON

MRC Pneumoconiosis Unit
Penarth, South Glamorgan
Wales, United Kingdom

ROBERT N. JONES

Tulane University School of Medicine
New Orleans, Louisiana

I. Introduction

The subject of this chapter is the use of chest radiographic data as response variables in the study of occupational lung diseases. Restrictions on the subject and length of this volume preclude consideration of the range of radiographic appearances seen in various disorders. For the qualitative distinctions between various disorders, the reader can refer to textbooks of radiology [1,2] or chest diseases [3-7], or to review articles [8-15]. For details of quantitative relationships of a radiographic feature to dosage of a noxious inhalant, or to other response variables such as pulmonary function testing, disability, or death, the reader must search the current medical literature. The perspective on these relationships changes with almost every addition of data from population studies. We are concerned here with quantifying the changes in the pattern of shadows in the chest radiograph produced by inhaled dust. Most of the work has been on disorders caused by mineral dusts, although similar approaches have been tried for study of other conditions.

II. Obtaining Radiographs for Population Studies

A. Personnel

High-quality radiographs can be obtained with a wide variety of equipment. Its correct and integrated use is of greater influence on the final product than is the excellence of any one component in the system [16–19]. The technologist (radiographer) must therefore be well trained, so that he or she knows which parts of the whole system (exposure factors, film-screen combination, development) are likely to be responsible for imperfections in the finished product. The physician will only obtain films of consistently high quality by explaining his or her requirements to the technologist and maintaining a constant exchange of comments with the technologist about film quality. A major factor in poor film quality is the failure to maintain this dialogue.

B. Mobile or Static Equipment

Mobile radiographic systems are no longer limited to the production of miniature photofluorograms, but can produce standard chest radiographs of high quality. Automatic developing equipment is essential and is incorporated into the mobile unit. The major difficulty in setting up such a unit is the large cost for a system that will have only intermittent use. In operation, the equipment requires particularly careful maintenance and calibration because of variations in temperature. The remaining difficulty is the adequacy of the available power supply. This may be satisfactory in large industrial plants, but not so at other sites. The problem can be solved with the use of a mobile generator; batteries or capacitors may be substituted, but usually impose some limitation on the range of possible exposure factors.

C. X-ray Tube Potentials and Use of Grids

Whether static or mobile, the generator should have a minimum capacity of 300 mA at 125 kV, and preferably a capacity of 150 kV. The generator must be full wave rectified and preferably three phased. A rotating anode tube is essential with as small a focal spot as possible, consistent with the anticipated load, but in any case not exceeding 2 mm in diameter [20].

When the potential exceeds 100 kV, or the subject is more than 22 cm in thickness (anteroposterior chest measurement), a grid is required to reduce scatter or secondary radiation from soft tissues. This secondary radiation reduces the sharpness of shadows cast upon the film. A moving or fixed grid may be used. When a fixed type is used, it should be one such that the lines on the film cannot or can only just be detected. A 10:1, 100 lines per inch grid is satisfactory. The older types of grids produce lines which can cause confusion in detecting small opacities.

D. Recommended Ranges of Kilovoltage

There is still some controversy over the relative merits and disadvantages of using high (120-150 kV) or conventional (65-75 kV) kilovolt techniques. The principal advantages claimed for the higher kilovolt technique are an increased proportion of acceptable films and a better definition of parenchymal and pleural detail because of reduction in the density of rib shadows. At higher kilovolt levels, the adsorption of calcium is reduced and the ribs are correspondingly less dense. Areas of abnormal calcification in lungs or lymph nodes may also be less easily seen. The contrast range is usually reduced in higher kilovolt films and this might influence the ease of detection of small opacities. Most of the advocates of the higher kilovolt technique will concede that with meticulous attention to detail, excellent films may be obtained using the lower kilovolt range. It is now common to use kilovoltages in the range 90-110, and grids are required with this range. Even this modest increase in kilovoltage entails a substantial reduction in the dose of radiation given to the subject [17].

There remains a need for definitive study of the effects of conventional and higher kilovolt techniques on reading levels for rounded and irregular small opacities.

E. Exposure Control

The radiographic exposure may be controlled by manual manipulation of current and exposure time for a given kilovoltage, or by automatic exposure devices (commonly called phototimers). Phototimers terminate exposure after receiving a specified amount of radiation. These operate on the photoelectric or ionization chamber principle, they may be placed in front of or behind the film, and may vary in speed of response (see Reference 16, pp. 125-134). Phototimers are to be regarded as aids in obtaining consistently better radiographs, not as substitutes for careful thought and technique. The ease in obtaining correct film exposure is balanced by the need for repeated calibration.

The exposure time should be 1/60 sec or less, and should not exceed 1/25 sec. Longer exposures produce detectable movement which increases the apparent size of small pulmonary opacities, while also reducing their sharpness of outline.

In many epidemiological studies where chest radiographs are taken, it may be anticipated that future films will be required. To make these as comparable as possible, it is helpful to keep a record of the exposure factors used in the initial examination. Some modern sets automatically provide such a record. A record of the weight and chest thickness of the subject is also helpful.

F. Timing of Exposure

The film should be exposed at the point of maximum inspiration and before the Valsalva effect of holding the breath against a closed glottis occurs. This is usually achieved by close observation of the subject by the technologist. Equipment is not available for triggering the start of the exposure from the cessation of inspiratory flow. This can be combined with a device to ensure that exposure occurs at a chosen point in the cardiac cycle. No one has yet provided quantitative assessments of the importance of these devices in improving consistency of technique.

In serial films of groups of the same individuals, it is not uncommon to observe systematic change in the height of the diaphragm between two cross-sectional surveys. This can be important because one of the effects of a poor inspiration is crowding of the vascular shadows at the bases. These may be wrongly recorded as a low category of small irregular or rounded opacities.

G. Films and Intensifying Screens

Medium-speed films and matched screens are best to ensure adequate image detail [20]. High-speed film may cause a grainy appearance which is difficult to detect the smallest of the opacities due to inhalation of dust. Intensifying screens and cassettes should be matched carefully for survey work. One of the causes of lack of sharpness in the radiograph is poor screen-film contact due to worn or damaged cassettes; periodic testing is therefore a requirement for high-quality work. Dusty and damaged screens will cause recurrent artefacts which can seriously interfere with film assessment.

H. Film Size and Positioning

It would seem a platitude to state that the whole of the chest should be visible on the radiograph, but the very commonly used 14 × 17 in. film does not ensure this. Trials under survey conditions have shown that films of 40 × 40 cm (15¾ × 15¾ in.) are of adequate dimensions for 95% of individuals [21]. Turning a 14 × 17 in. film to the horizontal position is not convenient when large numbers of films are being classified. Under survey conditions, it will often not be possible to take a second film if the first one is unsatisfactory. The 40 × 40 cm films are now generally available, and are increasingly used for research and surveillance of occupational lung disease. The need to include both costophrenic angles in all films of asbestos-exposed groups has hastened the use of this size film.

Projection of the shadows of the scapulae over the lung fields is the commonest positioning fault. These shadows can cause difficulty in detecting the extent and width of pleural thickening.

Radiographs are best taken with the subject stripped to the waist; some clothing casts a granular pattern which interferes with the classification of small opacities. Garments provided by the department of radiology should be checked for radiolucency.

A collimator to confine the x-ray beam to the area being examined is essential. It should have adjustable diaphragm and a light beam for centering. Evidence of the adequacy of the collimation is the presence of "cone cuts" just outside the area of the lungs. Collimation reduces unnecessary radiation and greatly improves film quality by reducing scatter from the shoulders and axillae.

I. Film Processing

Automatic processing equipment is a requirement for high consistency of film quality in survey radiography, in which there is a special need to avoid bias due to technical differences. The processing equipment needs daily calibration. Higher developing temperatures produce smaller tolerances in development time, and increased likelihood of grainy film. It may therefore be preferable to work at lower temperatures, even though this involves some slowing of output. When the best possible comparability of films is required, the new film (dry) should be compared with the previous one before the individual leaves. Incorrect exposure cannot be fully compensated by alterations in film processing.

J. Assessment of Film Quality

As a general rule, exposure is about right if the intervetebral spaces of the thoracic spine are just visible through the mediastinal structures. If the spine details are easily seen, the film is overexposed. If no structures are seen through the heart, the film is underexposed. It is desirable to be able to see the pulmonary vessels behind the left heart shadow.

In practice, the shape and size of the individual is a major factor in the quality of the film obtained. In about 5% of subjects, it is impossible to obtain a really high-quality radiograph. This is easily demonstrated in longitudinal studies of the same population in which unacceptable films are found year after year in the same individuals.

Unfortunately, although most radiologists could assent to the general description of an ideal film given above, there is often very poor agreement on assessing the quality of particular films. Perhaps the biggest factor in this is human adaptability. Readers adapt to reading grossly overexposed or underexposed films, or films having almost any other imaginable defect of quality. Most readers have never received formal training in film quality. There is lack of agreed terminology for describing film defects. The development of objective standards for film quality is in its infancy, but is likely to proceed rapidly now that portable microdensitometers are becoming available. With such instruments, the following criteria are recommended by Dr. Russell Morgan, and have recently received general approval from participants in an international workshop*:

1. The hilar regions should exhibit a minimum of 0.2 units of optical density above the fog level of the film.
2. Parenchymal regions should exhibit a maximum of 1.8 units of optical density above fog.
3. The gross image contrast, defined as the difference in optical density between the darkest parts of the parenchyma and the lighter parts of the hilar regions, should be within the range of 1.0 to 1.4 units of density.

In practice, in the classification of films for mineral pneumoconiosis, it has been common to record the overall quality as good, acceptable, poor, and unreadable. It may prove helpful to record the principal defect such as too white (underexposed), too black (overexposed), movement, or other defects (usually poor film-screen contact). An assessment can also be made of whether the defects do or do not impair ability to see details of the parenchyma and pleura separately. This may be relevant because an overexposed film may still permit a fairly confident assessment of the pleura when little can be seen of the details of the lung parenchyma. A moderately underexposed film may still permit assessment of the parenchyma while leaving the pleural shadows indistinct.

The effect of poor radiographic technique in survey work is an increase in random or systematic error. The relationship between technique and the assessment of abnormality has interested several investigators [22–25], and is relevant to the problems of inter- and intraobserver variation (see below).

III. Reading the Film

A. Objectives

When a film is obtained in an occupational study, it should be immediately examined to detect and record abnormalities relevant to the subject's health.

---

*Sponsored by the U.S. National Institute of Occupational Safety and Health, and the American College of Radiology, Washington, D. C., September 1978.

This is the discharge of an obligation to the subject, although the report may go (with his or her consent) to a physician. This is a clinical procedure, the reading is interpretative, and it should take into account all relevant nonradiographic information available to the reader. Such things as age, smoking, dust exposure, and past history of illness should be used to interpret the film. If available, previous radiographs should be used for comparison. The second, or epidemiological, reading of the film is of quite a different type, and the two forms of assessment cannot be combined. The purpose of the second reading is to extract as much information as possible from the pattern of shadows, and to relate this strictly radiographic data to other variables such as age, past dust exposure, smoking habits, lung function, immunologic variables, etc. This is achieved by a quantitative and semiquantitative comparison of the film against a set of standard radiographs and a series of written definitions in a classification. The procedure is therefore one of pattern recording, with a minimum of interpretation of the significance of shadows in terms of pathology or disease entities. The procedure is therefore ideally carried out with the reader having no knowledge of the individual's age, dust exposure, etc. Indeed, it is desirable to mix films of the study population with films of nonexposed individuals to reduce bias due to preconceived ideas of the radiographic effects of exposure.

B. Single Film

When classifying groups of films in cross-sectional studies, either for research or routine surveillance, there are a number of practical points which require attention.

Randomization of Films

In most surveys, it will be found that the serial order in which the films are taken is related in some recognizable way to past exposure. The elderly or disabled may come early because they are more easily available without disturbance to the running of the factory or the mine. All persons in a discrete dust exposure category may be examined in the same session. Bias of reading level may be introduced by classifying many abnormal or normal films at one time. To reduce this effect, the whole group of films should be randomly mixed by dealing into piles before they are presented to the readers.

Film Identification

As little identifying information as possible should appear on the films. Name, age, occupation, and name of the factory, mine, or other industrial unit are undesirable because they are potential sources of bias to the reader. A number to identify the subject and the date of the radiographic examination should be sufficient. The technologist, clinician, and epidemiological reader should all avoid making any marks on the film to draw attention to particular features.

Batch Size

It is desirable to read all the films in a particular survey over a short period (a few days) and in as large a batch per day as may be done without fatigue. This procedure helps to reduce bias; for example, some readers tend to overread at the start of a session. There are also diurnal and longer fluctuating cycles of reading levels for individual readers. The number of films which can be assessed per day will vary with the experience of the reader and the amount of abnormality in the films. It may range from less than 100 to over 400 films [26].

C. Serial Films

Special problems arise when assessing serial films of the same individuals. There may be a pair or one or more intermediate films. There is an extensive literature on this topic, recently reviewed by Liddell and Morgan [27], which may be consulted for details. Several methods have been suggested and tested.

Random Readings

All of the films are mixed and classified without knowledge of dates or identity. Theoretically, this gives an unbiased estimate for each film. The extent of progression (or regression) can be obtained for the group. Random variations in reading will show progressions and regressions which may not be real. In practice, the reader is not likely to remain completely blind as to the date of all the films; there are almost always differences in technique over the interval and there is usually a change in the color of the film base. Despite its limitations, this is a method which should be included in most studies because it is the least biased. It can serve as a check on the results of side-by-side comparisons.

Side-by-Side Readings

There are many varieties of this, for example, side-by-side with and without knowledge of the dates of the films; the first film may be on the left or the right viewing box, or put up randomly. Various other methods of attempting to confuse and mislead have been tried. No clear evidence for adopting one particular method has emerged. This is in part due to there being no good series where there was no technical difference over the interval and where there was good evidence about an external variable such as measured dust exposure to relate to the radiographic progression. At present the choice usually made is to put up the films in serial order, that is, left to right, with knowledge of dates. This method has the advantage of letting the reader make allowances for differences in technique or changes in the subject, including the level of the diaphragm. This comparison is seen as being within the individual, instead of against an external standard as in the random reading method. More sophisticated methods of reading in pairs are usually invalidated by the reader acquiring additional information about the sequences during the reading. Changes other than that related to pneumoconiosis will affect the appearance of the film (weight changes being the most important). Smoking and age itself have to be included in the analysis, although these should not be known at the time of classifying the pairs.

In reading serial films in pairs, it is often considered sufficient to record change on a 5 point scale: definite regression, possible regression, no change, possible progression, and definite progression. The alternative method of recording the full classification of each film separately seems to have little advantage; in practice, possible or even definite progression may be recorded without a certain change of category in the classification.

When several films of the same individual are available, there are many ways in which the diads (pairs), triads, tetrads, etc., could be assessed for progression. In general, the use of the earliest and latest film of good quality provides most of the information. Intermediate films may be of use for estimates when the first or last film is not comparable to the other member of the pair. The use of multiple intermediate films to analyze the shape of the radiographic progression curves usually fails because of random errors in the assessment process, the numbers available, and the long intervals required to assess progression in the mineral dust diseases.

In summary, when pairs of films are available, they are at present best read both randomly and in pairs with knowledge of the film order. The results of both types of assessment can then be related to the independent variables such as dust exposure. In time, it will become apparent which method is the more sensitive means of detecting change or the first appearance of abnormality.

D. Optimal Conditions for Viewing the Film

Epidemiological reading requires attention to small differences in patterns. For this work, the viewing conditions are extremely important. Exclusion of excessive levels of ambient light is highly desirable. The viewbox should be sufficiently bright and all panels should have equal illumination. The least requirement is two separate well-matched viewing boxes. A simple and better viewing box has two color-matching 80 W fluorescent tubes, 150 cm in length, mounted 10 cm behind an opal screen, 3 mm thick. This will give a uniformly illuminated screen along the whole length of 160 × 40 cm. It will take four of the 40 × 40 cm films. The reader should be able to view the film at a distance of 25 or 30 cm and at least twice this distance. In some radiology departments, the viewboxes are mounted on the wall at the back of a desk or table, effectively preventing close viewing. The experienced reader leans forward and backward several times in viewing each film; a comfortable chair and proper height of the viewbox are important in limiting fatigue. It is helpful to have the viewbox tilted slightly away from the reader.

The use of another person to record the reader's judgments is essential in large surveys to avoid the distraction of repeatedly looking away from the film to record its features. Conditions of relative quiet are needed to prevent lapses of attention during classification.

E. Recording

Whatever classification scheme is used, the result will be a recording of classified shadows. The recording sheet may be noncoded, "precoded," or designed for optical scanning devices. The spatial organization of these sheets is very important and should be designed with simplicity and accuracy of recording in mind. Where there are mandatory negative entries, these should all be organized in one column or row so that they may be easily checked for omissions. If the recorder is to write, for example, the letter A, B, or C in a box or space, then those letters should appear in parentheses under the box so that a numeral or incorrect letter will not be accidentally entered. Proper identification of the film should also be easy to check from its prominent position on the recording sheet.

At the end of reading each batch of films, the recording sheets must be checked for completeness and accuracy. Whatever the classification, there will be opportunities to check for obvious inconsistencies: for instance, an abnormality cannot be simultaneously present and absent. In large surveys, the reading session is essentially the only stage at which inconsistencies can be corrected by another look at the film. It has been shown [26] that with a good recording sheet and alert recorders, the errors (including omissions) can be reduced to less than 0.5%, but published works show that the errors have often been much greater.

IV. Classifying Radiographic Appearances

A. Past Schemes

Historically, there have been two contrasting approaches to this problem. The earlier approaches attempted a synthesis of all the abnormal features—parenchymal, pleural, and others—to produce a grading of severity of pneumoconiosis. These earlier schemes were primarily for clinical use for assessing the severity of disease for compensation purposes. The first widely used international scheme of this type was that recommended after the first International Labour Office (ILO) Conference on Pneumoconiosis in Johannesburg, in 1930 [28]. The scheme was partially radiographic and partially clinical.

After World War II, there was a rapid expansion of epidemiological research applied to chronic diseases in general, starting with respiratory and occupational disease in particular. By that time, coal workers' pneumoconiosis (CWP) had been shown to differ in many ways, including radiographically, from silicosis [29]. The research on coal workers' pneumoconiosis led to a new approach to classification of the chest radiograph. The radiograph was now used as one of several indices of response to inhaled dust, the others being tests of lung function, standardized questionnaires about respiratory symptoms, and serologic and other blood studies. It was thus necessary to apply to the radiograph similar criteria of usefulness to those applied to the other tests, i.e., reproducibility, validity, sensitivity, and simplicity.

The classification developed for the studies of coal workers' pneumoconiosis in the late 1940s, known as the Cardiff-Donai scheme, provided the basis for the ILO 1950 recommendations following the Sydney conference. The principles formulated at that time have been used in the subsequent revisions. These principles included:

1. The scheme should be largely descriptive of appearances, with as little interpretation as possible in terms of pathology, disease entities, or disability.
2. The scheme should provide a quantitative measure of the continuum of change of appearances from normality to the most advanced stages.
3. The scheme should take into account the natural history of the pneumoconioses as far as these are known.
4. Tests of reproducibility by the same and other users on both a short- and long-term basis should be made available.
5. The scheme should be tested for validity by showing that it has good power of discriminating between those with and without past dust exposure.

It may be of interest to recall that in the early 1950s "linear patterns" in the radiographs were not included in the scheme because tests in coal miners showed that they had poor validity. The distinction in the 1950 scheme between small and large pneumoconiotic opacities was made because of differences in their natural histories in CWP [30].

The 1950 ILO scheme applied primarily to CWP. The 1958 revision by experts for ILO widened its scope to most types of pneumoconiosis, excluding asbestosis [31]. The 1968 revision [32] added precision to a number of the definitions in the text but still did not include asbestosis. By 1971 when the ILO held its next pneumoconiosis conference in Bucharest, the UICC/Cincinnati (1970) scheme had been published [33]. This was specifically aimed at classifying films of asbestos workers, and was conceived as an extension of the ILO schemes. The ILO U/C classification (1971) recommended in Bucharest integrated the 1968 and 1970 schemes into one comprehensive classification covering all types of pneumoconiosis [34].

B. Current Schemes

The 1971 ILO U/C classification is the current scheme but is now in the process of review and change. The ILO reviews the classification at about 10 year intervals. A revision was presented at the ILO conference on pneumoconiosis in Caracas, November 1978. If ratified by the council of the ILO, this revision will be the "ILO 1980" classification.

The present system (and the proposed revision) have general instructions calling for one initial interpretation—whether the radiograph demonstrates any features of dust diseases. If it contains one or more features that are possibly due to dust, the radiograph is classified. The current classification provides descriptions of two kinds of small opacities (rounded and irregular) and requires the recording of size, profusion, and extent of these opacities. There is a separate grading scheme for opacities larger than 1 cm. Pleural thickening is recorded as to presence in the costophrenic angle, and as to site, width, and extent on the chest wall. Pleural calcification is separately recorded as to site and extent. Ill-defined diaphragm is recorded as present or absent, and ill-defined cardiac outline according to extent. Symbols are used for other abnormalities resulting from dust, or for recording the features of other diseases. A set of standard radiographs (obtainable from the International Labour Office, Safety and Health Branch, CH1211, Geneva 22, Switzerland) accompanies the instructions for use of the classification. These films provide examples of the kinds of radiographic abnormalities classified, and show differing levels of profusion of small opacities according to the categories described. Lower limit standards are included for such features as pleural thickening and ill-defined diaphragm.

The general and specific instructions for its use, and some explanatory notes, are contained in the official publication. A widely circulated issue of *Medical Radiography and Photography* [35] includes the instructions and photographs of the 1971 standard films; the photographs are not suitable for use as standards in film reading.

All classifications are compromises between the desirable goals of describing exhaustively the range of possible radiographic appearances, and remaining simple enough to be reliable and useful in application to large numbers of films. A classification cannot simultaneously meet extreme requirements in either direction, and so cannot be "perfect." The ILO U/C system is no exception, and certain difficulties in its use have become widely appreciated. One difficulty lies in getting agreement on the kind of small opacity, rounded or irregular, that is present [36]. A preponderance of either kind of opacity has meaning with respect to both etiology and prognosis. There is also difficulty in arriving at the category of profusion of small opacities in films showing marked inhomogeneity of profusion in various zones of the lungs. The ILO 1980 revision recommends changes from the present system which are aimed at meeting some of these difficulties. One recommendation is that a single profusion grade, using the appropriate standard film, should be given for small opacities, regardless of kind. The kind of small opacity (i.e., shape) is described by using any two of the six letters defining shape (p, q, r) for rounded, and (s, t, u) for irregular. Thus (qq) indicates that all the small opacities are rounded and (qt) that they are predominently rounded but with some irregular, and vice versa for (tq). Thus a wide range of shapes of small opacities can be easily recorded using the standard films as references for the appearance of the different shapes. These modifications do not relate to the problem of averaging profusion over lung zones. Research is just beginning on the grading of profusion separately in each of four quadrants. Other recommendations in the 1980 scheme include the grading of pleural thickening and calcifications separately for each side of the chest. The system has been simplified by downgrading ill-defined diaphragm or ill-defined cardiac outline to the status of symbols (to be recorded only when present). Several items recorded as symbols have been slightly changed. Pleural thickening in the interlobar fissure has been added, in light of evidence that it is a feature of populations exposed to asbestos [37]. Although the 1980 revision treats pleural thickening in greater detail, there is still no confirmed method of separating visceral and parietal thickening. This would be highly desirable because they may have quite different prognostic significances.

In the current (1971) system, classification of large opacities is associated with a problem of large interobserver variation. The 1980 system will not include changes in definition of these opacities, but will drop the distinction between those with well-defined and ill-defined outlines. The major source of variability, however, seems to arise from failure of the reader to separate pneumoconiotic from nonpneumoconiotic large opacities. It is difficult to accept the proposition that the interobserver variability arises because shadows 1 cm and over in diameter are missed by experienced readers. Since differences are likely to be due to different understandings of what is a pneumoconiotic opacity, this observation raises the question of whether the initial instruction to classify only appearances thought to be pneumoconiotic is the best compromise. The alternative of classifying all appearances was rejected in earlier revisions of the scheme, and again in 1979, on the basis that there are many similar appearances due to other conditions which are not properly classified under schemes for pneumoconiosis. This view has been supported by work done by the American Thoracic Society (with support of the Division of Lung Diseases of the U.S. National Heart, Lung and Blood Institute). This work explored the possibility of using the ILO 1971 scheme as the basis of a general classification for the chest radiograph. It was clear that extensions to the ILO scheme were necessary to cover many patterns not seen in pneumoconiosis. A scheme incorporating these extensions, called "ATS-DLD-78" [38], includes measurement of lung size, and more complete description of large opacities, including nonpneumoconiotic large opacities. Despite the inclusion of very desirable features and the careful construction of this alternative classification, it may in the end not be widely used. The ILO system has the great advantage of being applicable to the health surveillance of large working populations, an enterprise mandated under the laws of many countries. This combination of social, political, and economic reasons to overcome the financial barriers of population radiography simply does not exist for many diseases, no matter how suited they are to such study. Another important advantage of the ILO schemes has been continuity. As time passes, more information on the validity of earlier schemes is acquired. For example, it may take 20 years or more to establish the mortality experience of persons with different types and severities of radiographic patterns. It is therefore likely that some parts of earlier ILO schemes will continue to be used in longitudinal studies and in ongoing surveillance projects.

V. Interobserver and Intraobserver Variation

As long as classification involves subjective assessment, it will necessarily involve inter- and intraobserver variations [39]. This is comparable to the situation in many other clinical assessments, for example, variations in interpretation of signs from the physical examination, or in interpretation of electrocardiograms. At the inception of the UICC/Cincinnati classification, it was shown [26] that the observer variability was comparable to other clinical assessments. Interobserver variation is easy enough to detect, but may be rather difficult to characterize [26,36,40–42]. Figures 1 and 2 are contrived to show different patterns of interobserver variability in two readers categorizing the profusion of small opacities according to the 12 point scale in the ILO U/C system. The main diagonals show films on which there was complete agreement, and the distances from this diagonal along row or column show the degree of disagreement. Figure 1 shows the operation of a bias along scales of similar length and Figure 2 shows truncation of the entire scale by one reader. Simplifications as to which reader is more or less sensitive than the other may obscure rather complex relationships such as these. The inter- and intraobserver variations are related to the distribution of abnormality in a particular set of films. At one extreme, if all the films are reported 0/0 (few or no small opacities), the observer variation is 0. Also, by recording very little abnormality, the observer may achieve good reproducibility but low sensitivity when tested against an independent variable such as dust exposure. The tabulations shown in Figures 1 and 2 are widely used to express inter- and intraobserver variation. The percentage of perfect agreements (the diagonal boxes) and that of those with ±1 subcategory on the 12

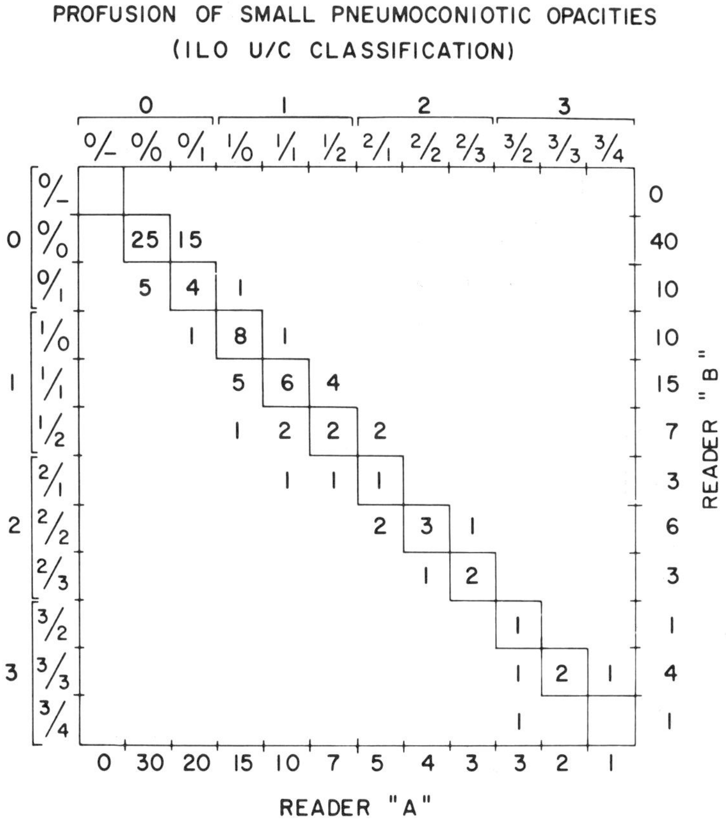

Figure 1 Contrived distributions for two (hypothetical) readers classifying 100 films by the ILO scheme. Small pneumoconiotic opacities are tabulated by profusion grade, ignoring size and shape. Reader B shows a middling tendency (see text), but both readers operate along scales of equal length, shown by identical numbers of films placed in categories 0, 1, 2, and 3.

point scale are often used. These may be standardized to a 30% abnormality rate [26].

Intraobserver variation is usually less than interobserver variation. A few individuals seem to have much more difficulty in using the classification than other trained observers. Experienced and well-trained observers often show a marked bias in relation to each other, but fairly comparable intraobserver variation.

Recognition of the problems of variability and bias has led to general agreement on the need for multiple readers [43]. There is no agreement, how-

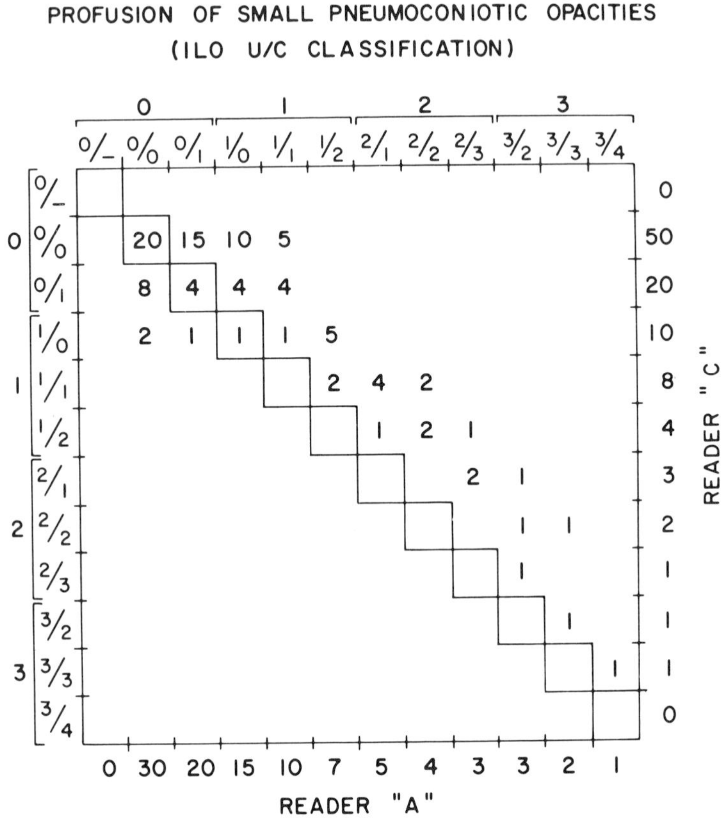

Figure 2 Distributions for two (hypothetical) readers, contrived as in Figure 1. Reader C evidently operates along a shorter scale than Reader A.

ever, as to how best to reconcile differences between readers. Minimizing intra-observer variability ought to begin with the training of readers. Descriptions and standard films are not entirely adequate for training, and the experienced reader can be extremely helpful to the novice. Even among experienced readers, discussions after independently reading a group of films are good in bringing small groups closer together. This aids in the consistent use of conventions in interpretation, whether these conventions are prescribed by the system or are necessary because of peculiarities of the films under study. It is also helpful to provide each reader with the tabulation of his or her individual readings, compared to the readings of the remainder of the group. Individuals can quickly appreciate any systematic deviation from the judgments of the other readers. Sets of previously read films, introduced into each batch of films under study,

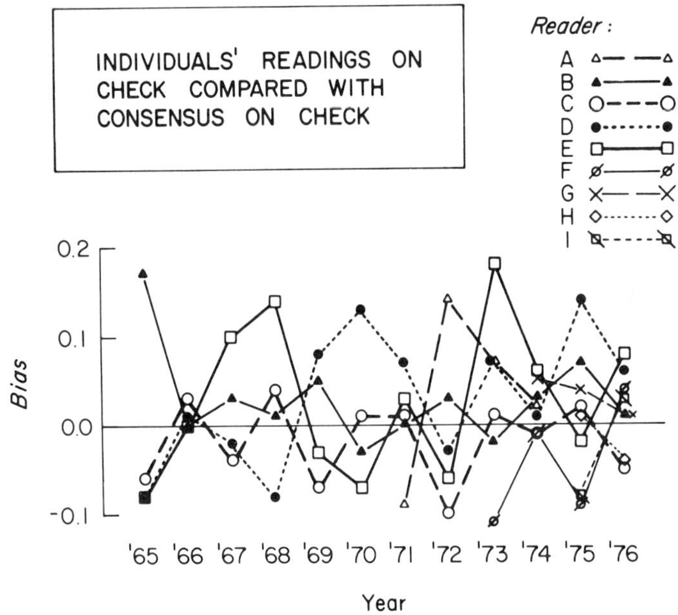

Figure 3 Fluctuations in bias, a measure of the average difference between the readings of the individual reader and the consensus.

can serve to provide the reader feedback during the actual reading trial [44]. When used as "trigger films," the reader classifies the film without knowledge of his or her previous reading, but is immediately afterward shown the previous reading. This enables the reader to detect any drift in reading level during the course of the reading session. Two types of trigger films are useful: an external set chosen to show the range of severity of abnormalities; and an internal set chosen from films being studied, consisting mainly of normal films and those showing low levels of abnormalities. These will be indistinguishable from the remainder of the study films. A consensus reading session for both the internal and external trigger films, prior to the main reading trial, can be used to reduce interobserver variability—particularly with respect to unusual features of the films in that study. This is the only recommended use of consensus readings. When consensus readings are used to arrive at a single judgment for each individual study film, too many data are lost in comparison to preserving the judgments of several readers [45]. Consensus readings also involve difficulty in avoiding biases of nonradiographic sorts. Finally, the process is inordinately time consuming and may be stressful to those doing it. The loss of information by consensus reading is shown by comparing two films. One was read as 0/1, 0/1, and 0/0 by three readers independently; on consensus the reading was re-

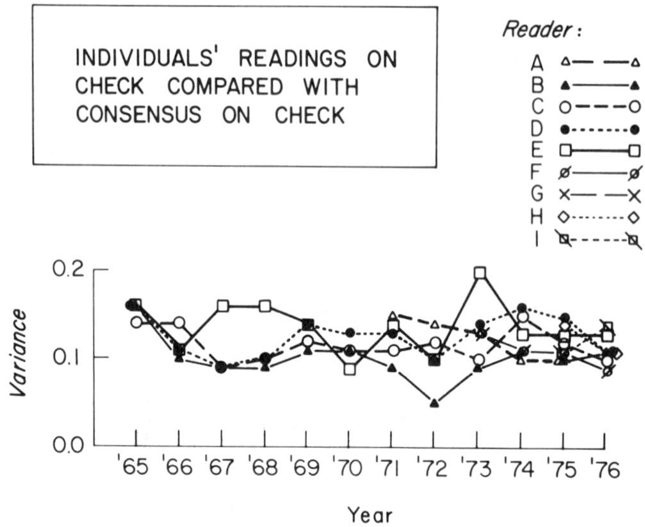

Figure 4 Fluctuations in variance, a measure of the spread of differences between the readings of the individual reader and the consensus.

corded as 0/0 and therefore the same as a film read 0/0 by all three readers. The first film is clearly likely to be in fact further along the continuum of small opacities than is the second film.

Intra- and interobserver variation is kept at its lowest level in groups constantly using the classification and undertaking informal and formal tests of variability [26]. The most comprehensive and protracted study is that by the U.K. National Coal Board Radiological Centre. Figures 3, 4, and 5 display data from the Periodic X-ray Service of the National Coal Board. Figure 3 and Figure 4 show, for nine readers over 11 years, changes in the individual's bias and variance relative to the group. The tests are made yearly with 360 films, made up of 260 from the current year and 100 from the previous year. The figures show the remarkable consistency and the way individuals' biases cycle above and below the mean. The application of this periodic surveillance of coal workers' pneumoconiosis to individual mines is shown in Figure 5. A progression index (a measure of the average level of progression for a defined subpopulation) is derived from the serial films of coal-face workers at each mine. If the readings are consistent on a long-term basis, the index should be the same for each mine when the films are reread after an interval. Figure 5 shows that the repeat progression index ranks the mines in a similar but not quite identical order.

The most appropriate way of using multiple readings is not universally

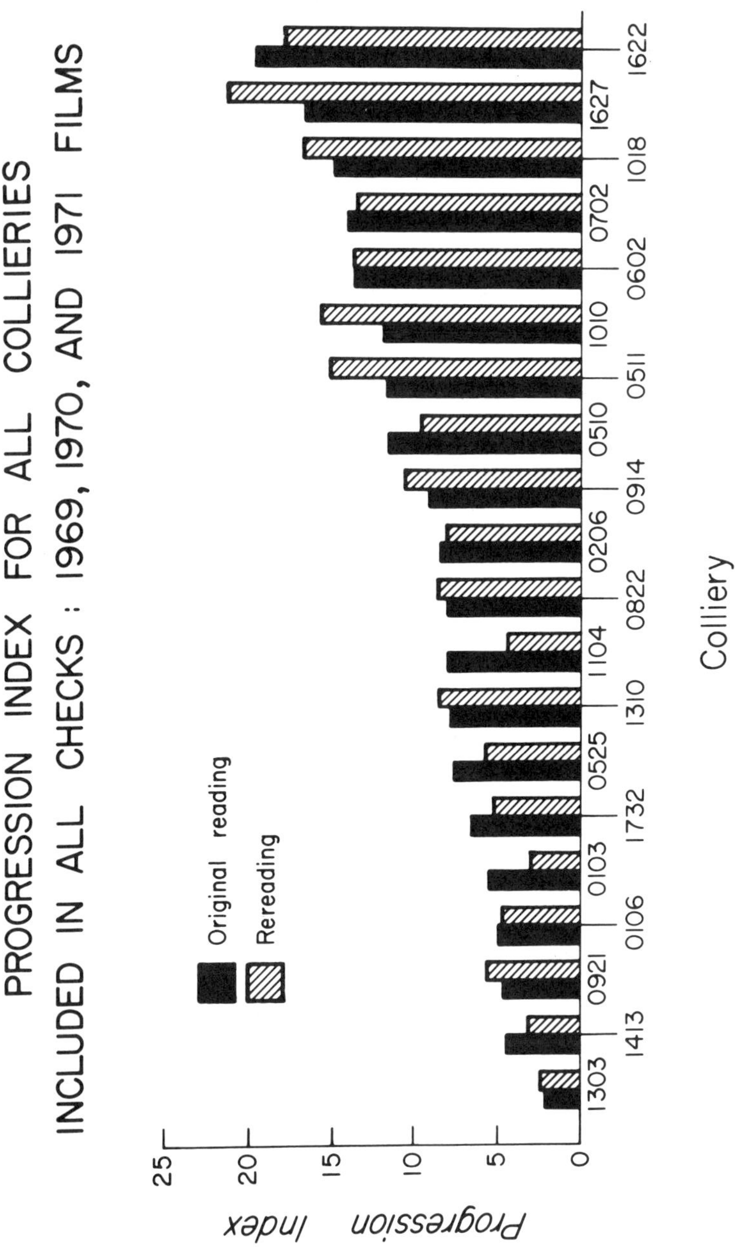

Figure 5 Effect on rank order of mines produced by reclassifying serial films for progression of pneumoconiosis.

agreed upon. Some authors use a simple integer scale such as −1, 0, 1, 2, etc., for 0/−, 0/0, 0/1, 1/0, etc. This assumes that the width of the subcategories is the same. In fact, this may not be so; indeed, the definition of the subcategories would lead one to expect a "middling" effect such as that reported by Morgan et al. [46]. Middling effect is the term applied to the phenomenon whereby more films are categorized as 1/1, 2/2, or 3/3, than in the subcategories on either side of these (for example, the data of Reader "B" in Fig. 1). If the films were not purposely selected for resemblance to "midcategory" standard films, then the reader is behaving as if the central subcategories are, in fact, wider than the adjacent subcategories. It is clear that experienced readers disagree over the proportion put in the various subcategories. It may be that some apply the criteria strictly while others put into 1/0 or 1/2 those films which have fewer or more small opacities than the standard category, 1/1 film. This may be one cause of observer variation needing further study. Oldham [47] has produced evidence about the width of the subcategories, showing that they are not uniform, but he was able to fit a transformed scale which seemed to have wide applicability in different types of pneumoconiosis. Oldham's paper and later contributions by Fox and colleagues [48,49] and Jacobsen [50], should be consulted for fuller discussions on the methods of using data obtained from applying the ILO classification.

There is a need for more research into the best way of combining multiple readings in the same body of data, particularly where there is external information, such as dust exposure, with which to test the sensitivity and validity of the different methods [51].

The later ILO classification schemes include the means of recording most of the pattern changes for all types of mineral pneumoconiosis. However, most of the published papers using these schemes report only a limited amount of the information recorded. There is now an opportunity to test the various components in more depth for reproducibility, sensitivity, and validity.

VI. Comparability of Data

The ILO classifications are intended for use with the posteroanterior (PA) film alone. The investigator must be cautious in using extra films for a cross-sectional study. If a survey of asbestos workers includes oblique films for assessment of pleural abnormalities, the PA film should first be read separately. The results of this separate reading will allow comparability with prior and current studies employing only the PA view. The added information from the oblique films may then be used for comparison to exposure and other response variables in the study population, and the two sets of radiographic prevalence data can be compared for sensitivity and specificity in the study population. The use of prior films to refine judgments about the abnormalities seen on the current films also leads to higher estimates of disease prevalence. This arises because of the bias against regression; abnormalities clearly seen on the penultimate film will be considered to be present on the last film, even if they cannot be clearly seen because of deficiencies in technique. The use of films of sizes significantly different from the standard radiograph is not recommended. Photofluorograms using 100 × 100 mm film may be applicable where disease prevalence rates are low and considerations of cost are paramount [44]. Even when extra films obviously allow refinement of prevalence data, the potential gain of information, e.g., from oblique views, must be balanced against increased study cost (in time and materials), production time loss in a working population, and extra radiation dosage.

Some principles involved in use of radiographic data in relation to other variables are discussed in Chapter 17. The existence of elegant techniques for such comparisons does not mean that the analytic techniques for reduction of radiographic data are settled and universally accepted. There is no consensus on how best to use information from multiple readings, whether by different readers or by the same reader at different times. There is still disagreement, as mentioned above, regarding analysis of readings of serial films.

VII. The Future

At present, there is no obvious substitute for the radiograph as a practical, sensitive, and relatively specific indicator of the pulmonary reaction to inhaled mineral dusts. The radiographic examination is brief, convenient, and not uncomfortable. The incremental dose of radiation is extremely small so that the risk-benefit comparison for a single PA radiograph is favorable. The resulting film is permanent and transportable, and can be viewed by many persons at many different times.

Today's films may be better analyzed by future techniques for extracting information from the pattern of density gradients. There have been great improvements in the ability of machines to quantify these gradients over a large range of densities and over very short distances of spatial separation. This gives hope for the application of powerful computer technology to the problem of pattern discrimination [43]. There seems to be no practical limit to the sensitivity of today's automated systems. A modern computer could easily compare any number of dots of finite area to each of its neighbors on an x-ray film. The need is for development of programs capable of being as selective as the human reader is when he or she views the pattern.

Improvements in chest radiography, however, need not be so dramatic to have an appreciable effect on epidemiological studies. The epidemiologist should be cautious in accepting and endorsing technical refinements. There are large populations classified according to the current or compatible older systems that are now showing substantial mortality rates. The ability to correlate radiographic appearances with mortality is extremely valuable. Even an improvement in precision of the measuring systems may on balance be detrimental if comparability to older studies is lost, and one must begin anew waiting for the appearance of significant morbidity and mortality in the exposed population.

In terms of present systems, too little attention has been given to the relationship of radiographic appearances to other factors. In particular, there has been little research on the effect of smoking per se (as separate from aging) on radiographic appearances. There is only a small amount of information from carefully studied groups regarding the background levels of various abnormalities in unexposed portions of the general population.

Computerized axial tomography (CAT) is an example of a technique that is not currently applicable in large surveys, but may be very useful in assessing the sensitivity of more widely used methods. Recent surveys in rural areas of Turkey suggests that certain relatively specific pleural abnormalities are not confined to persons heavily exposed to asbestos in the workplace or in urban environments [52]. This raises the possibility that there are large groups of persons with pleural disease undetectable on standard radiographs. The ability of CAT to identify pleural plaques can be used to examine the sensitivity of standard radiographs [53] and perhaps to detect new and unsuspected circumstances of exposure to noxious inhalants. The use of the high-kilovolt (200 kV) xeroradiography technique has recently been claimed to demonstrate pneumoconiotic small opacities invisible with current techniques [54]. Such a claim must be validated by relatively large surveys relating the abnormality to indices of exposure. Such surveys should naturally try to assess the losses of information of other types, as well as the gain of information related to the abnormality in question. The recognition that most advances in technology involve costs as well as benefits, and that one of the costs can be a loss of some types of scientific data that must be weighed against a gain of other data, will provide good perspective on efforts to improve the epidemiological use of chest radiography.

References

1. Felson, B., *Chest Roentgenology*. Philadelphia, W. B. Saunders Co., 1973.
2. Shanks, S. C., and P. Kerley, *A Text-Book of X-Ray Diagnosis*. Philadelphia, W. B. Saunders Co., 1973, pp. 253–304.
3. Fraser, R. G., and J. A. P. Paré, *Diagnosis of Diseases of the Chest*. Philadelphia, W. B. Saunders Co., 1970.
4. Fishman, A. P., *Pulmonary Diseases*. New York, McGraw-Hill, 1979.

5. Baum, G. L., *Textbook of Pulmonary Diseases,* 2nd ed. Boston, Little, Brown, 1974.
6. Parkes, W. R., *Occupational Lung Disorders.* London, Butterworths, 1974.
7. Morgan, W. K. C., and A. Seaton, *Occupational Lung Diseases.* Philadelphia, W. B. Saunders Co., 1975.
8. Pancoast, H. K., and E. P. Pendergrass, A review of pneumoconiosis—further roentgenological and pathological studies, *Am. J. Roentgenol.,* **26**: 556–614 (1931).
9. Greening, R. R., and J. H. Heslep, The roentgenology of silicosis, *Semin. Roentgenol.,* **2**:265–275 (1967).
10. Bristol, L. J., Pneumoconioses caused by asbestos and other siliceous dusts, *Semin. Roentgenol.,* **2**:283–305 (1967).
11. Sander, O. A., Berylliosis, *Semin. Roentgenol.,* **2**:306–311 (1967).
12. Morgan, W. K. C., and N. L. Lapp, Respiratory disease in coal miners. State of the art, *Am. Rev. Respir. Dis.,* **113**:531–559 (1976).
13. Ziskind, M., R. N. Jones, and H. Weill, Silicosis. State of the art, *Am. Rev. Respir. Dis.,* **113**:643–665 (1976).
14. Becklake, M. R., Asbestos-related diseases of the lung and other organs: Their epidemiology and implications for clinical practice. State of the art, *Am. Rev. Respir. Dis.,* **114**:187–227 (1976).
15. Vix, V. A., Roentgenographic manifestations of pleural disease, *Semin. Roentgenol.,* **12**:277–286 (1977).
16. Thompson, T. T., *A Practical Approach to Modern X-Ray Equipment.* Boston, Little, Brown, 1978.
17. Christensen, E. E., T. S. Curry, and J. E. Dowdey, *An Introduction to the Physics of Diagnostic Radiology,* 2nd ed. Philadelphia, Lea & Febiger, 1978.
18. Ter-Pogossian, M. M., *The Physical Aspects of Diagnostic Radiology.* New York, Harper & Row, 1967.
19. Ridgway, A., and W. Thumm, *The Physics of Medical Radiography.* Menlo Park, California, Addison-Wesley, 1968.
20. Jacobson, G., H. Bohlig, and R. Kiviluoto, Essentials of chest radiography, *Radiology,* **95**:445–450 (1970).
21. Audsley, W. P., S. M. Latham, and C. E. Rossiter, Film sizes for radiography of the chest, *Radiography,* **36**:70–72 (1970).
22. Fletcher, C. M., and P. D. Oldham, The problem of consistent radiological diagnosis in coalminers' pneumoconiosis; an experimental study, *Br. J. Ind. Med.,* **6**:168–183 (1949).
23. Liddell, F. D. K., The effect of film quality on reading radiographs, *Br. J. Ind. Med.,* **18**:165–174 (1961).
24. Wise, M. E., and P. D. Oldham, Effect of radiographic technique on readings of categories of simple pneumoconioses, *Br. J. Ind. Med.,* **20**:145–153 (1963).
25. Reger, R. B., and W. K. C. Morgan, On the factors influencing consistency in the radiographic diagnosis of pneumoconiosis, *Am. Rev. Respir. Dis.,* **102**:905–915 (1970).

26. Rossiter, C. E., Initial repeatability trials of the UICC/Cincinnati classification of the radiographic appearances of pneumoconiosis, *Br. J. Ind. Med.*, **29**:407–419 (1972).
27. Liddell, F. D. K., and W. K. C. Morgan, Methods of assessing serial films of the pneumoconioses: a review, *J. Soc. Occup. Med.*, **28**:6–15 (1978).
28. International Labour Office, Records of the International Conference held at Johannesburg, South Africa. In *Studies and Reports*. Series F, No. 13 (Silicosis), Geneva, International Labour Office, 1930.
29. Fletcher, C. M., K. J. Mann, I. Davies, A. L. Cochrane, J. C. Gilson, and P. Hugh-Jones, Classification of radiographic appearances in coalworkers' pneumoconiosis, *J. Fac. Radiol. Lond.*, **1**:40–52 (1949).
30. Gilson, J. C., and P. Hugh-Jones, Lung function in coalworkers' pneumoconiosis. In *Medical Research Council Special Report Series*. No. 290, London, HM Stationery Office, 1955, p. 9.
31. International Labour Office, Meeting of experts on the international classification of radiographs of the pneumoconioses, *Occup. Safety Health*, **9**: 1-8 (1959).
32. International Labour Office, *International Classification of Radiographs of Pneumoconioses* (Revised, 1968). Occupational Safety and Health Series, No. 22, Geneva, International Labour Office, 1970.
33. UICC Committee, UICC/Cincinnati classification of the radiographic appearances of pneumoconioses, *Chest*, **58**:57–67 (1970).
34. International Labour Office, *ILO U/C International Classification of Radiographs of Pneumoconioses 1971*. Occupational Safety and Health Series, No. 22 (Revised), Geneva, International Labour Office, 1972.
35. Jacobson, G., and W. S. Lainhart, ILO U/C International Classification of radiographs of the pneumoconioses, *Med. Radiogr. Photogr.*, **48**:67–110 (1972).
36. Liddell, F. D. K., Radiological assessment of small pneumoconiotic opacities, *Br. J. Ind. Med.*, **34**:85–94 (1977).
37. Solomon, A., L. M. Irwig, G. K. Sluis-Cremer, R. Glyn Thomas, and R. S. J. DuToit, Thickening of pulmonary interlobar fissures: Exposure-response relationship in crocidolite and amosite miners, *Br. J. Ind. Med.*, **36**:195–198 (1979).
38. American Thoracic Society, Use of chest radiography in epidemiological studies of nonoccupational lung diseases, *Am. Rev. Respir. Dis.*, **118**: 89–111 (1978).
39. Beers, Y., *Introduction to the Theory of Error*. Cambridge, Massachusetts, Addison-Wesley, 1953.
40. Ashford, J. R., A problem of subjective classification in industrial medicine, *Appl. Statist.*, **8**:168–185 (1959).
41. Liddell, F. D. K., An experiment in film reading, *Br. J. Ind. Med.*, **20**:300–312 (1963).
42. International Labour Office, Radiologic classification of the pneumoconioses: An Anglo-American radiograph reading exercise, *Arch. Environ. Health*, **12**:314–330 (1966).

43. Weill, H., and R. Jones, The chest roentgenogram as an epidemiologic tool, *Arch. Environ. Health,* **30**:435–439 (1975).
44. Sheers, G., C. E. Rossiter, J. C. Gilson, and F. A. F. Mackenzie, UK naval dockyards asbestosis study: Radiological methods in the surveillance of workers exposed to asbestos, *Br. J. Ind. Med.,* **35**:195–203 (1978).
45. Oldham, P. D., Observer error—a potential asset, *Proc. R. Soc. Med.,* **61**: 447–449 (1968).
46. Morgan, W. K. C., M. R. Peterson, and R. B. Reger, The "middling" tendency, *Arch. Environ. Health,* **29**:334-337 (1974).
47. Oldham, P. D., Numerical scoring of radiological simple pneumoconiosis. In *Inhaled Particles III.* Proceedings of an International Symposium organized by the British Occupational Hygiene Society 1970, Vol. II. Edited by W. H. Walton. Unwin Brothers, Ltd., Old Woking, Surrey, 1971, pp. 621–632.
48. Fox, A. J., Classification of radiological appearance and the derivation of a numerical score, *Br. J. Ind. Med.,* **32**:273–282 (1975).
49. Lloyd Davies, T. A., A. T. Doig, A. J. Fox, and M. Greenburg, A radiographic survey of monumental masonry workers in Aberdeen, *Br. J. Ind. Med.,* **30**:227–231 (1973).
50. Jacobsen, M., Quantifying radiological changes in simple pneumoconiosis, *J. R. Statist. Soc.,* **24**:229–249 (1975).
51. Rossiter, C. E., L. J. Bristol, P. H. Cartier, J. C. Gilson, T. R. Grainger, G. K. Sluis-Cremer, and J. C. McDonald, Radiographic changes in chrysotile asbestos mine and mill workers of Quebec, *Arch. Environ. Health,* **24**: 388–400 (1972).
52. Baris, Y. I., A. A. Sahin, M. Ozesmi, I. Kerse, E. Ozen, B. Kolacan, M. Altinors, and A. Goktepeli, An outbreak of pleural mesothelioma and chronic fibrosing pleurisy in the village of Karain/Urgup in Anatolia, *Thorax,* **33**:181–192 (1978).
53. Rigler, L. G., An overview of the pleura, *Semin. Roentgenol.,* **12**:265–268 (1977).
54. Glyn Thomas, R., and G. K. Sluis-Cremer, 200 kv xeroradiography in occupational exposure to silica and asbestos, *Br. J. Ind. Med.,* **34**:281–290 (1977).

4

Standardization of Spirometry with Special Emphasis in Field Testing

REED M. GARDNER

University of Utah and LDS Hospital
Salt Lake City, Utah

HENRY W. GLINDMEYER III

Tulane University School of Medicine
New Orleans, Louisiana

JOHN L. HANKINSON

National Institute of Occupational Safety and Health
Morgantown, West Virginia

I. Introduction

The hazardous effect of some airborne pollutants on the respiratory system have resulted in increased interest in the measurements of lung function. The hazardous effects of dust from coal mines [1], hard rock mines [2], and the cotton industry [3] have been recognized and have resulted in an improved working environment in these industries. In addition, chemical vapors and gases, as well as particulates from other industries [4,5], have also been shown to adversely affect the lung. Determining dose-response relationships of these occupational stimuli requires an accurate medical and employment history as well as environmental characterization and quantitative pulmonary function testing. To be most useful, these pulmonary function tests must be accurate, precise (repeatable), sensitive to the environmental stimuli, and readily applicable at the occupational site. This chapter will focus on the standardization of pulmonary function tests and define variables which affect their accuracy and utility in the study of occupational medicine.

The usefulness of pulmonary function testing to quantify the hazardous effects of occupational pollutants have been limited by several factors.

Table 1 Pulmonary Function Test

	Factors influencing test			
Parameter	Pulmonary	Nonpulmonary	Advantages	Disadvantages
Spirometry				
FVC	Elastic recoil of lung Caliber of larger and smaller airways	Poor initial effort Insufficient recording time Poor sustained effort Leaks Calibration errors Calculation errors	Minimal equipment Repeatability Well-documented	Effort dependent, especially near TLC and RV
FEV_1	Same as FVC	Same as FVC Time zero determinations	Same as FVC	Effort dependent, especially near TLC
FEF25–75	Same as FEV_1 but measures the effect of smaller airways	Same as FVC	Same as FEV_1 but not as repeatable Sensitive to smaller airways than the FEV_1 [9–11]	Same as FVC since FVC determines location of 25% and 75% points
$\dot{V}$%FVC [29]	Same as FEF25–75 and sensitive to smaller airways when flow is measured at smaller volumes	Same as FVC	Same as FEF25–75 but not as repeatable	Same as FEF25–75 Necessary to display flow-volume loop

MVV	Same as FVC Air trapping	Poor sustained effort Frequency of breathing not standardized Leaks Calculation errors Calibration errors	Minimal equipment	Effort dependent Hard on patient
He-O_2 Flow-volume maneuver [32,33]				
$\dot{V}_{iso}$%FVC	Same as FEF25–75 but sensitive to smaller airways Affected by distribution of ventilation	Same as FVC Dependent on number of breaths of He-O_2	Minimal equipment	Effort dependent Not very repeatable
$V_{iso}\dot{V}$ [34]	Same as $\dot{V}$%FVC and sensitive to smaller airways	Same as $\dot{V}_{iso}$%FVC	Same as $\dot{V}_{iso}$%FVC	Same as $\dot{V}_{iso}$%FVC
FRC	Elastic recoil of total respiratory system	Patient anxiety affects level of FRC Leaks Calibration errors Calculation errors	Fairly repeatable	Different methods sometimes yield different results (i.e., washout, dilution) Tidal breathing often affected by subject anxiety

Table 1 (Continued)

	Factors influencing test			
Parameter	Pulmonary	Nonpulmonary	Advantages	Disadvantages
				Test time consuming (test can last 15 min before equilibration or washout occurs
RV	Air trapping	Poor effort Leaks Calibration errors Calculation errors	N_2 washout technique is quick and repeatable (patient can breathe at abnormally high frequency and volume)	Effort dependent in reaching RV when test is initiated
Closing volume [34,35]				
CC, CV, ΔN_2, slope of phase III	Distribution of ventilation	Same as FVC Sensitive to flow rate Sensitive to volume history	Looks at small airways	Hard to measure Effort dependent Often difficult to interpret
Diffusion capacity [36]				
$DL_{CO_{sb}}$	$\dot{V}/\dot{Q}$ ratio of lung Total lung capacity Affected by a change of cross-sectional area or thickness of air-blood interface	Same as FVC	Easier than steady-state method but not comparable	Not specific Expensive and sophisticated equipment that requires sophisticated and frequent calibration

	Can be affected by decrease of available hemoglobin			
Plethysmography [37,38]				
TGV	Not influenced by air trapping Same as FRC	Same as FRC and RV; however, box heightens anxiety, and this sophisticated system needs relatively sophisticated calibration methods	Test takes only a few seconds; however, calibration and setup can be time consuming	Calibration difficult High anxiety of patient yields abnormal patient FRC level Expensive equipment
Raw [39–41]	Caliber of larger airways	Same as TGV Dependent on panting frequency Dependent on lung volume	Same as TGV	Not very repeatable Same as TGV Very difficult maneuver for patient Forced oscillation more repeatable [41]

1. Choice of test: There are a wide variety of tests available (see Table 1). Deciding which test to use and interpreting the results of the test presents a major methodological problem. Most pulmonary function tests are relatively nonspecific and they are dependent on many uncontrolled variables which affect not only population studies but even results on the same subject on repeated tests. The scientific community is still looking for an ideal test which will provide early detection and measurement of degradation of pulmonary function. At the present time, however, the forced expiratory spirogram appears to be the best single test available.

2. Instrument standardization: The literature is replete with information which is of marginal value because of inadequate instrumentation. Contradictory results obtained from similar studies are often caused by systematic differences between instruments.

3. Instrument calibration: Quality control to ensure instrument stability and accuracy is necessary in any research study but it becomes especially important in longitudinal studies which may continue for several years. Because of varying and often unfavorable conditions that prevail during testing outside the usual "laboratory" environment, careful and frequent calibration tests must be performed in the occupational setting.

4. Standardization of test procedure: Few lung function tests have been adequately standardized [6,7]. There is still much to be done in the standardization of testing procedures so that results can be interpreted and verified from similar testing done by different investigators in different locations. Utilization of a different testing procedure in itself may cause differences in results which could incorrectly be attributed to occupational exposure. Because of the transient situation and the demanding conditions usually encountered in field testing, technicians performing the tests must have special training.

5. Uniform measurement and computation methods: Even if tests are performed with adequate instruments and accepted procedures, the tests can be quickly invalidated by inadequate measurement and computational methods. In addition, the computerized options available with many instruments often produce erroneous results.

6. Data interpretation: Interpretation of pulmonary function results requires consideration of many factors such as smoking history, sex, height, and race, as well as occupational factors. Care must be used when integrating results from several pulmonary function tests, because when a greater number of tests is used, the probability that all test results will be normal decreases rapidly. This observation is especially important since some subjects never learn to perform the pulmonary tests adequately, and unfortunately most of the tests of lung function are dependent on subject cooperation and effort.

7. Special problems in field testing: Environmental factors such as temperature, electrical power source, and available space are usually suboptimal and

must be compensated for. Efficient test scheduling in occupational studies requires reliable instrumentation and competent technicians to minimize wasted time for the test subjects. In order to maintain cooperation of the study group and their management, it is important to develop efficient, effective testing procedures and perform them at a predetermined time interval.

Because the factors listed above are limiting research progress, and as a consequence are limiting our understanding of occupational lung disease, recommendations and standards are beginning to be made in each of these problem areas. Since spirometry is the most widely used, and one of the most practical and specific tests of lung function, the majority of this chapter will be devoted to spirometric testing.

II. Available Tests and What They Measure

One of the most difficult aspects of conducting occupational studies is deciding which test to employ. To evaluate the available tests, one must consider (1) what they measure (pulmonary versus nonpulmonary factors); and (2) advantages and disadvantages of the test, which includes factors such as equipment costs, testing time, and repeatability of results. Table 1 lists these factors for spirometry, the helium-oxygen flow-volume maneuver, lung volumes, closing volumes, diffusing capacity, and body plethysmography. Chapter 5 provides a review of the various pulmonary function tests [8]. In general, the more sensitive tests are less repeatable and require more sophisticated instrumentation. Spirometry, the least expensive in terms of equipment, requires minimal testing time, and some of the parameters measured from the forced vital capacity (FVC) maneuver are sensitive to small airway disease [9,10]. These parameters include the volume of air exhaled during the first second of the FVC maneuver (FEV_1), the FEV_1/FVC ratio, the average flow rate measured during the middle half of the FVC (FEF_{25-75}), and the instantaneous flow rates measured at specific lung volumes ($\dot{V}_{\%FVC}$). Of these parameters, the FEV_1 is the least sensitive to small airway abnormalities, but is the most repeatable [11].

The unique spirographic patterns produced by normal subjects and subjects with different types of pulmonary pathology make spirometry useful in discriminating between obstructive and restrictive lung disease. Table 2 describes the parameters measured from a forced vital capacity for subjects with obstructive and restrictive disease. Five of the six parameters discriminate between these defects; only the FEV_1 is substantially reduced in both. If the parameters of flow are based on total lung capacity instead of the forced vital capacity, they too would be substantially reduced in both diseases.

Table 2 Forced Spirographic Patterns

Parameter	Obstructive	Restrictive
FVC	Mild reduction with prolonged expiration	Reduced
FEV_t	Reduced	Reduced
FEV_1/FVC	Reduced	Normal or increased
FEF_{25-75}	Reduced	Near normal
FEF_{75-85}	Reduced	Near normal
$\dot{V}$%FVC	Reduced	Near normal

III. Standardization of Instrumentation

The value of spirometry as a test for following a worker's lung function over time is dependent upon standardization of spirometers, test procedures, and measurement techniques. Since the introduction of the FVC maneuver in 1947, instruments which were originally designed to record slow volume changes were being used to record dynamic events. Over the years these instruments have become more sophisticated and a wide variety of designs have been introduced. Presently, there are more than 100 different types of spirometers on the market. These instruments can be divided into two basic categories depending on whether they measure volume directly or detect flow indirectly. The designs for volume-measuring instruments include water-sealed, dry rolling-sealed; and bellows-type spirometers. The water-sealed spirometer consists of a bell seated in an annulus of water. As the subject blows into the spirometer, the bell rises in order to accommodate the volume blown into it. The bell is counterweighted or made of plastic in order to reduce the effect of gravity. The dry rolling-sealed spirometer consists of a canister within a canister sealed by a Teflon membrane. As the subject blows into the spirometer, the Teflon membrane rolls and the spirometer canister separates in order to accommodate the added volume. This design reduces the effect of gravity since the displacement of the piston is in the horizontal plane. The bellows-type spirometer also moves in a horizontal plane, thereby reducing the effect of gravity. For all three designs of volumetric spirometers, the simple expansion of the system as air is introduced into the spirometer is related to volume, and can be displayed as such on a recorder.

The designs for flow-detecting devices include the pneumotachygraph, hot wire, and turbine. The pneumotachygraph is a pressure sensor. Differences in pressure occur with changes in flow and can be related to changes in volume. With the hot wire, a wire is heated to several hundred degrees Fahrenheit. As air is blown across the wire, it is cooled, and this change in temperature changes the resistance of the wire. The resistance is then monitored electronically and related to flow. The final design for flow-detecting devices is the turbine, which simply spins as air passes across it. The faster the rotation of the turbine, the greater the flow of air.

In addition to sensing devices, a spirometer should have a display of volume versus time or flow versus volume during the entire forced expiration. All six spirometer designs discussed previously can be linked to a recorder so that a graphical output can be obtained. Recorders commonly used with spirometers include kymographs, chart plates, XYT recorders, and oscilloscopes. These recorders can sometimes be connected to computers. Usually, volume or flow thresholds are used to initiate the computer memory. These thresholds vary from 10 to 200 ml for volume, or from 1 to 300 ml/sec for flow. Obviously, some of these may allow too much of the signal to escape, and therefore should be tested to assure that the entire forced vital capacity is captured and recorded by the computer. Finally, the computer can produce a digital display, printout, or some type of permanent storage. It is often assumed that the cost of these computers is related to the accuracy of their output; however, due to poor programming, one often finds little correlation between the two. Obviously, there are many different designs of spirometers attached to different types of recorders and computers. Some of these instruments have been evaluated and reported on in the literature. Though some reports are favorable, others have shown variations in spirometer volume measurements in excess of 20% [12]. Because of the wide variety of instruments and the variability of their accuracy, the American Thoracic Society initiated the Snowbird Workshop on the Standardization of Spirometry in January of 1977 [13]. This workshop produced a document on standardization of spirometry which has been updated and revised several times and is now an American Thoracic Society statement [14].

The following lists primary measurements made with a spirometer and the instrument requirements, recommended by the ATS, necessary for these measurements.

1. The vital capacity (VC) is the maximum volume of air exhaled from the point of maximum inspiration. Instruments which measure vital capacity should be able to accumulate volume for at least 30 sec. To make this measurement, spirometers should have volumes of at least 7 liters measured at body temperature and pressure saturated (BTPS) and should be capable of measuring this volume over a flow range from 0 to 12 liters/sec. The accuracy required for this measurement is at least ±3% of reading or ±50 ml, whichever is greater.

The rationale for this requirement is that vital capacity is a time-independent measurement. Thirty seconds is generally the maximum time in which a subject can extend exhalation. Studies of populations show that for vital capacity and forced vital capacity, a 7 liter volume will allow measurement of more than 95% of the population [14,15]. Accuracy of ±3% or ±50 ml, whichever is greater, was determined by intertest variability and the day-to-day variability for the same subject [15,16]. Instrument errors should ideally be smaller than the subject variability, which is about 3%, and minimum resolution of 50 ml is a reasonable lower resolution limit for adults when very small volume test results are obtained.

2. The forced vital capacity (FVC) is the vital capacity obtained with a maximal forced expiratory effort. As with the vital capacity, the volume recommended for instrumentation is at least 7 liters with capacity for measuring flows between 0 and 12 liters/sec. Also, the instrument must be capable of accumulating volume for at least 10 sec [14]. A 10 sec interval is required so that most obstructed subjects have adequate time to complete their expiration.

3. The timed forced expiratory volume (FEV_t) is defined as the volume of air exhaled in a specified time during the performance of an FVC maneuver. For example, an FEV_1 is the volume of air exhaled during the first second of the FVC. This measurement and its ratio, obtained when it is divided by the forced vital capacity (FEV_1/FVC), are good indicators of obstructive lung disease. Requirements and their rationale for this measurement are similar to those for forced vital capacity measurement. Volume accuracy should be within ±3% of reading or ±50 ml, whichever is greater [14]. An important requirement of this measurement is that the start of the test, time zero, is to be determined by the back-extrapolation method. The start of test, by back extrapolation, is obtained by the extrapolation of peak flow to maximum inspiration.

This test is dependent on resistance to airflow, e.g., blowing through a drinking straw into a spirometer will yield a different FEV_1 than blowing through a 1 in. diameter tube. The resistance to airflow should be less than 1.5 cmH_2O per liter/sec at flow rates of 12 liters/sec [14].

4. The FEF_{25-75} measures the forced expiratory flow during the middle half of the FVC. Requirements for instrument accuracy for this test are ±5% of reading or ±100 ml/sec, whichever is greater. This measurement has a greater subject standard deviation than the FVC or FEV_1 because two, rather than one, volume-time measurements are made [14].

5. Flow or instantaneous forced expiratory flow, $\dot{V}$, can be measured either electronically or mechanically. When flow-volume loops or other measurements of flow are made, the flow measurement should be accurate to within ±5% of reading or ±0.2 liters/sec, whichever is greater [14]. Flow range should be 0 to 12 liters/sec.

6. A permanent graphical record of the forced vital capacity is one of the most important requirements which evolved from increasing recent interest in standardization of the instruments used for spirometry. The Snowbird Workshop recommended that instruments used to record the FVC and FEV_1 should provide at least a tracing of volume and time or volume and flow during the entire forced expiration. For the volume-time tracing, the recorder must be capable of displaying the entire FVC maneuver, at constant speed, from maxi-

mum inspiration for at least 10 sec after the start of the maneuver. If the paper record is made it must have at least the following characteristics: (1) paper speed of 2 cm/sec, with higher speeds preferable; (2) volume sensitivity of at least 10 mm of chart per liter of volume; and (3) flow sensitivity of at least 4 mm of chart per liter/sec of flow (all specifications are measured in BTPS). The participants at the Snowbird Workshop felt that the spirogram represented the best method of ensuring that this "effort-dependent" test was properly performed. Most forced vital capacity spirograms are displayed as a volume-time tracing. In order to determine the quality of the start of the FVC test and achieve reliable results by back extrapolation to determine time zero, the recorder should be "up to speed" before the forced expirogram is begun. The 10 sec record requirement is based on data which show that most obstructed subjects can complete the test in 10 sec [14,15]. The requirements of chart speed and volume sensitivity are based on earlier recommendations and the need to have accurate visual resolution on the record.

Although not specifically recommended, a thermometer installed in the spirometer is extremely important for volume-measuring devices [17] since the air blown into the relatively cool spirometer is condensed. This can yield a 1% volume decrease for every 2°C difference between body and spirometer temperature. Two conditions common in occupational testing have emphasized this point:

1. Uncontrolled temperature conditions in the occupational setting, such as cold temperatures in a mine or hot temperatures in a mill, can greatly affect results.
2. Rapid testing of many subjects can increase the spirometer temperature. Therefore, the spirometer can easily warm up several degrees during a testing session.

Even spirometers which comply with these standards can produce significantly different results. For instance, the accuracy for the FEV_1 requires a maximum measurement error of ±3% or ±50 ml, whichever is greater. Since the annual decline for the FEV_1 is approximately 1% per year, acceptable spirometers can produce results with a mean difference six times this predicted annual decline. Even instruments from the same manufacturer can produce systematically different data. Therefore, it is not only important to obtain an acceptable instrument, but to employ the same type of spirometer, and, if possible, the same instrument when repeated testings are required. This is especially true if the study protocol demands testing the subject before and after a work shift.

IV. Calibration Techniques

To obtain accurate results, spirometry system "calibration checks" should be conducted at least at the beginning of every day and "complete calibration" should be performed at least every week. The most important calibrating device currently available is a calibrating syringe with a volume of at least 3 liters with ±1% accuracy, traceable to the National Bureau of Standards. It may be necessary to deviate slightly from the calibration procedures listed below, depending on the type of spirometer. Since some flow-detecting devices are affected by humidity, the manufacturer should provide the appropriate "multiplying" factor to compensate for the effects of using "cool," "dry" air in the syringe rather than the warm, moist expired gas. It is also important with volume-measuring devices that the air inside the calibrating syringe be at the same temperature and relative humidity as the air inside the spirometer. Otherwise, some heat transfer may occur after the syringe is emptied into the spirometer and the gas inside the spirometer may expand or contract.

Calibration Check Procedure

1. The first step in evaluating a spirometer already owned, or where purchase is being considered, is comparison of manufacturer's specifications with the ATS recommendations. It is important to observe that a 10 liter spirometer which has an accuracy specification of ±3% of full scale, that is, ±300 ml, will not meet the ATS recommendation of ±3% of reading or ±50 ml, whichever is greater.

2. Check for any leaks in the tubing or spirometer; this is particularly important for volume-measuring devices.

3. Simulate a normal and obstructed patient by injecting the air from a 3 liter calibrating syringe into the spirometer in approximately 2 sec (normal) and 6 sec (obstructed). The spirometer "corrected" volume output should read between 2.91 and 3.09 for a 3 liter syringe. Also observe if there are adequate recorder volume and time sensitivities based on the spirometer recommendations.

4. A forced expiration should be performed with relatively low flow rates at the end of the maneuver to determine if the spirometer prematurely terminates its volume measurement or if it continues to show an increase in volume as you approach residual volume. Premature termination at low flows is a particular problem with currently available flow-measuring devices.

5. Check the "start of test" determination for any unusual sensitivity. These artefacts can occur when the subject is shaking the mouthpiece and tubing while straining to completely inhale at the start of the FVC maneuver. When this occurs, the FEV_1 may be zero or unusually low due to the false start.

6. The recorder's timing accuracy should be checked with a stopwatch simply by observing the time displacement over an appropriate time period.

7. The automatically determined FEV_1 should be compared with several hand-determined FEV_1 values using volume-time tracings and the back-extrapolation method. This comparison is necessary to test that the instrument is using a start-of-test determination method equivalent to the back-extrapolation method.

8. Perform any other calibration check procedures which may be recommended by the manufacturer. These procedures should be simple enough for a technician to follow and complete enough to ensure that the spirometer is functioning within the recommendations.

9. Finally, it is good practice to have a technician perform a few FVC maneuvers at the beginning of each session to serve as quality control values. These data can also provide information concerning the variability of the repeat tests performed in your laboratory.

V. Standardization of Test Procedures

The Snowbird Workshop also dealt with the need to standardize spirometric testing procedures. Standardized procedures and measurement techniques were suggested in order to produce spirometric data compatible between instruments and laboratories and from one time period to another.

Standardized methods of spirometric testing are as follows: The subjects are to be instructed in the FVC maneuver and the appropriate technique demonstrated. A minimum of three acceptable FVC maneuvers should be performed. Acceptability is determined by the technician's observation that the subject understood the instruction and performed the test properly. This includes observation of a smooth continuous exhalation with a good start and apparent maximal effort and without (1) coughing; (2) valsalva maneuver (closed glottis); (3) early termination of expiration (in a normal subject this will be before completion of the breath, and in an obstructed subject this should be assumed to take place if the expiratory time is less than 6 sec); (4) a leak; (5) an obstructed mouthpiece (obstruction due to tongue being placed in front of the mouthpiece, dentures falling in front of the mouthpiece); (6) an excessive variability among the three acceptable curves, e.g., the FVC of the two best of three acceptable curves should not vary by more than 5% or 100 ml, whichever is greater; and (7) an unsatisfactory start of expiration characterized by excessive hesitation or false starts. Unsatisfactory starts prevent accurate back extrapolation to determine time zero. To achieve accurate time zero the extrapolated volume on the volume-time tracing spirogram should be less than 10% or 100 ml, whichever is greater.

The FVC maneuver can be performed by either a closed or open circuit method. For the closed circuit method the subject inhales the maximal inspiration from the spirometer. For the open circuit method, the subject inspires maximally, places the mouthpiece in his or her mouth, and then forcefully exhales. With the open circuit method, there is no display of inspiration and the subject can lose volume from full inspiration, prior to placement of the mouthpiece, without detection by the technician. Also, placement of the mouthpiece while holding at full inspiration is cumbersome and contributes to the systematic differences observed with these procedures [18]. Some instrumentation can also confound the procedural variability by employing the closed circuit method without displaying inspiratory volume or flow. Although the use of nose clips may not appreciably influence the forced vital capacity performed using the open circuit technique, some subjects breathe through the nose during the test when a closed circuit technique is used [14,18]. Also, adult subjects may be studied either sitting or standing [19], while for children under the age of 12 years the position should be indicated [14]. In any case, nose clips are recommended, and the same procedure (open or closed) and position should be used on repeat testing of the same subject.

VI. Importance of Technician Training

Perhaps the most difficult factor to control in the administration of pulmonary function testing is the technician's influence on the subject's performance. The FVC maneuver demands cooperation, and the subject must completely understand what is required. This responsibility rests totally with the technician, who must be aware of all pulmonary and nonpulmonary factors affecting the test. If a satisfactory series of tests cannot be obtained, the technician must report that the data are submaximal.

Adequate technician training and perhaps certification is an essential first step toward obtaining good quality pulmonary function data. Technicians must also be continuously evaluated to ensure that they continue to obtain the best possible performance from a subject. It is not unusual for some technicians to be incapable of mastering the art of coaching subjects properly on a continuing basis.

The pulmonary function technician should receive at least 16 hr of formal instruction followed by a period of monitoring either by direct observation or by review of time-volume or flow-volume tracings which they have collected. The formal instruction should consist of at least 6 hr of lectures and 10 hr of practical application. Due to the wide variety of instruments, it is important that the technician receive instruction on the type of spirometer which he or she will be using. The following topics should be included in the formal instruction.

Basic physiology of the forced vital capacity maneuver and the determinants of airflow limitation with emphasis on the reproducibility of results: Instruction in basic physiology is needed for the technician to understand why the forced expiratory volume maneuver is reproducible and why in a few subjects it may not be reproducible.

Instrumentation requirements, including calibration procedures, sources of error, and their correction: The technician should know how to check the spirometer system for accuracy and proper operation. If this training is lacking, then a large amount of inaccurate data could be collected without being detected.

Performance of the testing, including subject coaching, recognition of improperly performed maneuvers, and corrective action: If the test is invalid, the technician should be capable of coaching the subject to give a more acceptable test result. Coaching of a subject must often be modified to accommodate the subject.

Data quality, with emphasis on reproducibility: The technician should understand all the criteria listed above for judging test acceptability.

Measurement of tracings and calculations of results: The technician should understand the BTPS correction factor and be capable of measuring the FVC, FEV_1, and FEV_{25-75} by hand from a volume-time tracing using the back-extrapolation technique. The technician should also be taught to obtain predicted values and express the results as a percentage of predicted.

Due to the Cotton Dust Standard requirements for technician certification, the National Institute of Occupational Safety and Health has applied these basic guidelines in order to approve qualified training courses. At this time, several approved coarses are available throughout the United States.

VII. Standardization of Measurement and Computation

Measurements of the spirogram should be made from a series of at least three acceptable forced expiratory curves [14]. The maximal FVC and the maximal FEV_1 recorded should be obtained after examining the data from *all* the acceptable curves even if the maximum FVC and the maximum FEV_1 do not come from the same curve. The beginning of time for the FEV_1 should be obtained by the method of back extrapolation. If the FEF_{25-75} and/or instantaneous maximal expiratory flows are to be obtained, they should be measured from the single acceptable test which yields the greatest sum of FEV_1 and FVC. This is defined as the "best" curve.

Best efforts cannot be determined by simple inspection of a spirogram. Measurement and computation are required to determine the largest values. There is little difference between the largest values and the mean values if data are properly collected. However, independently selecting the largest value for FVC and FEV_1 accounts for an occasional influence of learning and possible deterioration in performance due to fatigue or induced bronchospasm. There is no need to discard the best FEV_1 value even if a maneuver is prematurely terminated.

The discriminating quality of spirometry is greatly influenced by the time duration of the forced expiratory spirogram for obstructive subjects. If a severely obstructed subject performs an FVC maneuver with flow continuing for 10 sec, the subject may produce a relatively normal FVC while abnormal values of FEV_1/FVC, FEF_{25-75} and $\dot{V}_{\%\ FVC}$ would be observed. If this same subject's spirogram were terminated after 6 sec, the FVC would be reduced, while the other parameters would be substantially increased. Though the discriminating quality of the 10 sec FVC is advantageous, it may be difficult for an obstructed subject to repeat the maneuver several times with equally sustained effort. Therefore, the FVC and those parameters influenced by it are extremely effort dependent as the subject approaches full expiration. One could conduct an FEV_6 or FEV_7 and base all other parameters on this volume. Though variability would be reduced, some of the discrimination between obstructive and restrictive disease is lost. This tradeoff is constantly encountered in epidemiological investigations where test repeatability and sensitivity must be optimized. However, if one decides to base these parameters on an FEV_6 or FEV_7, the maneuver should be labeled as such and not be considered a forced vital capacity.

One facet of measurement and computation which is often overlooked is the correction of volumes and flows to body temperature and pressure saturated with water vapor (BTPS). Approximately a 1% change in volume or flow (equivalent to the yearly predicted decline for some parameters) is introduced for every 2°change in temperature or 200 ml of mercury change in barometric pressure. Therefore, temperature and pressure should be monitored in order to make correct measurements. However, since the correction factors from ATPS to BTPS at 22°C are 1.0904, 1.0910, and 1.0915 for barometric pressures of 770, 760, and 750 mmHg, respectively, it is unnecessary to correct for small deviations from standard barometric pressure. Some instruments display the data on a graph which has two volume grids, one in ATPS (ambient temperatures and pressures saturated with water vapor) and the other in BTPS. It is important to note that the values in BTPS on these graphs are corrected only for one specific temperature and pressure, usually 25°C and 760 mmHg. Therefore, if the actual spirometer temperature or pressure is different, this BTPS output will be incorrect.

Manufacturers of mass flow meters (hot wires) often indicate that their instruments are not affected by temperature and therefore a correction to BTPS is not necessary. However, it is important to note that these instruments are significantly affected by differences in water vapor. For such instruments, calibration with a syringe of dry air will yield significantly different results than with a syringe containing air saturated with water vapor. Therefore, correction factors should be obtained from these manufacturers.

VIII. Data Interpretation

Once some measurement of ventilatory function has been obtained using adequate equipment and procedures, the next step is to interpret the results. Because measures of ventilatory function are dependent on age, height, sex, race, and many other factors, care must be taken to consider these factors in interpreting any measurements. There are two basic approaches to evaluating ventilatory tests. One approach is to use the subject as his or her own control and follow changes in ventilatory function with time. The second, more common method is to compare the measured values with "normal values" through the use of prediction equations. The sensitivity of any test of ventilatory function is dependent to a large extent on how well these various factors, such as age and height, can be removed from the inherent variability of the parameter both for a given subject and within a normal population, the latter being greater. For example, the within-subject coefficient of variation is approximately 3% for the FVC compared to approximately 14% within a population [20-22].

Using a subject as his or her own control and obtaining repeated measurements is considered by many as the preferred method; however, this is often impractical. The normal yearly decrement in ventilatory function is small (approximately 25 ml/year [23] for the FVC); however, the inherent variability of the parameter requires that an abnormality can only be detected if the observed changes are large or if the subject is followed over an extended period of time. In addition, while there have been many cross-sectional studies of ventilatory function of "normal" populations, which provide a reasonable estimate of the decrements of ventilatory function for age, there have been relatively few longitudinal studies to provide an estimate of the variability of this decrement within a given subject. Until more data are gathered by longitudinal studies, comparison of a subject's observed values with some "normal" or expected values will continue to be necessary.

Since age and height are strongly related to ventilatory function, most prediction equations include these parameters in their estimate of ventilatory function. Ideally, the prediction equations should be derived from a study of healthy, normal, nonsmoking individuals using procedures and equipment which conform to the requirements presented here. Many of the published predicted normal standards or equations have included nonsmokers, smokers, and former smokers. Since cigarette smoking has been shown to adversely affect pulmonary function, any population which includes smokers and former smokers could hardly be considered "normal." In addition, many studies have not considered or critically examined other important factors such as previous history of respiratory disease and exposure to occupational or environmental agents which may affect the respiratory system.

One study which attempted to use a healthy nonsmoking population was conducted by Morris and associates [23]. They tested 998 healthy nonsmokers who lived near Portland, Oregon, and were members of the Church of Jesus Christ of Latter-day Saints. In addition, Morris used a Stead-Wells spirometer which has been shown to meet the ATS instrumentation recommendations [14,17].

Although the Morris study provided some of the best predicted standards, there are still potential problems with adopting them. First, the methods of calculation were those of Kory and associates [24], and therefore their method of calculating the FEV_1 did not conform with the method of back extrapolation. Second, a single best effort was always selected for determination of the FVC, FEV_1, etc., which does not conform with the recommended method of using the largest FVC and FEV_1, regardless of the curve(s) on which they occur. Also, the FEF_{25-75} should be measured from the curve with the largest sum of FVC plus FEV_1. Finally, some question remains as to whether the population used by Morris adequately represents an average normal healthy population.

Morris performed an interesting comparison of various prediction equations and demonstrated large differences between them. For example, he reported as much as an 820 ml difference between their observed mean FVC and the predicted mean FVC of a previous study [23].

In a more recent study, Knudson and associates [25] reported prediction equations for men and women obtained from 746 healthy nonsmoking subjects who live in Tucson, Arizona. While they used equipment and procedures which appear to meet the recommendation, the authors reported the FVC and FEV_1 obtained from averaging the best two of five values. This method of averaging does not conform with the ATS recommended use of the largest FVC and FEV_1 in deriving their equations. However, their comparison of the largest of the first three FVC and FEV_1 values with the average of the best two of five did not show any statistically significant differences.

An additional consideration in the comparison of a subject's observed value with a predicted value is the ethnic background. For example, several studies [26-28] have shown that male blacks have a predicted FVC from 10 to 15% lower than their white counterparts of the same age and height. These reports have recommended multiplying the predicted value obtained from a white population by approximately 0.85. Obviously, a more desirable approach would be to develop prediction equations for every ethnic group. Only by using this approach will it be possible to fully compensate for ethnic differences in the relationship between ventilatory function, age, and height.

After selecting appropriate predicted values, one can determine whether the observed values are significantly different from normal. Measurements of ventilatory function with large standard errors (SE) and poor correlation with age and height must have a corresponding large departure from the predicted value in order to be significant. Morris and associates [23] found that males aged 30-39 years had a mean FVC of 5.38 liters with a standard deviation of

0.89 liters. Therefore, 16% of the normal individuals studied would have an FVC of 5.38 − 0.89 = 4.49 liters or less, and 2.5% of the normal individuals would have an FVC of 5.38 − 1.78 = 3.60 liters or less. If the observed values are expressed as a percentage of predicted, 2.5% of the normal individuals studied would have an observed value less than 67%, 69%, and 47% of predicted for FVC, FEV_1, and FEF_{25-75}, respectively. In a similar type of analysis, Knudson and associates [29] determined the percent of predicted value above which 95% of asymptomatic nonsmokers fell. They found that 95% of the males aged 16-35 years had an FEV_1 of 81.8% of predicted or greater and a $\dot{V}_{max_{50}}$ of 66.1% of predicted or greater. The lower percentage of prediction for the $\dot{V}_{max_{50}}$ is a result of its larger variability. Therefore, a patient must have observed values for the FEF_{25-75} and instantaneous flow rates considerably less than 80% of predicted to indicate significant abnormality.

It has been proposed that a good method of ensuring that the patient is giving the best possible effort is to compare the test results with some predicted value while the test is being conducted. If the subject's observed value is below the predicted, then the technician is encouraged to coach the subject to expend more effect. While on the surface this technique seems reasonable, there are potential problems with this approach. If coaching is dependent on the prediction equations used, the test results obtained will be biased toward these predicted values. Subjects with ventilatory function values above normal will not be encouraged to try harder, in contrast to the abnormal subject who will receive considerably more coaching. A better approach is to use criteria which depend on the reproducibility of the test results, and only after testing of the subject is completed should the observed values be compared with predicted values.

In many epidemiological studies, lung function is used to determine if a particular harmful agent has a detrimental effect on respiratory health. To detect these effects, mean function values in the exposed population are compared to expected values of a nonexposed group. Since it is often difficult and expensive to obtain values on a nonexposed group, the observed mean values are sometimes compared to published normal values. The observed values for each subject can be divided by the corresponding predicted value for every subject, and results are expressed as an average observed/predicted percentage. Considerable care must be taken in interpreting the results of these types of analyses. For reasons discussed previously, the results obtained by a study may not be directly comparable to a published predicted equation obtained using different equipment, procedures, and analysis. In addition, many normal studies have excluded smokers, exsmokers, and symptomatic subjects, and therefore the normal population may be considerably more healthy than an appropriate nonexposed or control group. Symptom status may be compared by using the Medical Research Council questionnaire commonly employed in epidemiological surveys [30].

Ideally, when any exposed group is studied, a matched nonexposed control group should be studied at the same time using the same equipment, procedures, and technicians. Taking care to match the two populations with respect to age, height, sex, ethnic group, history, and smoking status should allow direct comparison of population mean values. Depending on how well the populations are matched, it is possible to attach significance to even small differences in population mean values and thereby increase the sensitivity of the study. Although prediction equations or covariance analysis can be used to compensate for imperfect matching of populations, these techniques require several assumptions which complicate interpretation of the study results.

IX. Special Problems of Field Studies

It is often advantageous to conduct pulmonary function tests at the industrial site. Time away from the job is reduced, and lung function can be assessed in conjunction with estimates of industrial exposure. In addition, on-site testing is required if an acute response is to be detected by pre- and postshift studies. Since rapid testing of large populations is often desirable, it becomes necessary to employ an automated data collection system. A completely automated system will reduce testing and data turnaround time by eliminating data transcription, computation, and reduction by the technician; however, it can pose serious problems in transport and setup in the industrial environment. One solution to this problem is the self-contained mobile laboratory. Testing equipment, calibration equipment, and any test gas cylinders required for the investigation remain together, avoiding loss or damage during shipment. At the site, the mobile laboratory provides adequate working space and a controlled environment. The success of a mobile laboratory requires careful installation of the test equipment. All equipment should be shock-mounted and shielded from spurious electrical inputs. An adequate electrical system must also facilitate the large capacity heating and cooling units essential for a controlled laboratory environment. Extreme temperatures are not only uncomfortable for personnel and subjects, but may adversely affect test equipment. Service access to the rear of equipment should be provided by the addition of doors or hatches to the vehicle. The location of equipment should facilitate testing and provide good balance for driving safety. Even the most sophisticated equipment can be suitably housed in a mobile unit. The laboratory currently employed in field studies nationwide by Tulane University School of Medicine is displayed in Figures 1 and 2 [31].* A Winnebago motor home houses a pulmonary laboratory, a computer interface for data transmission, a CRT (cathode ray tube) for display of data, four diskette drives for magnetic data storage, and a printer. The laboratory's capabilities include measuring both timed volumes and flow

*Design engineering by Henry Glindmeyer, D. Eng. Installation of equipment by Biomedical Associates, Inc.

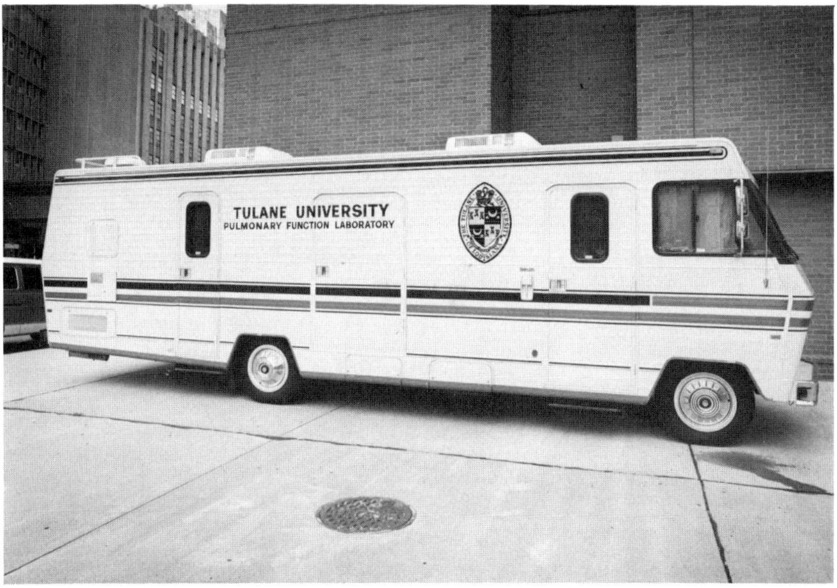

Figure 1 Exterior of mobile laboratory displays several access hatches and electronic leveling jacks. Test tanks are mounted on roll-out storage trays (not shown).

rates from the forced vital capacity maneuver, lung volumes and capacities, single-breath diffusing capacity, and parameters from the He-O_2 flow-volume maneuver. In addition, data reduced from pre- and postshift studies include across-shift isovolume-determined flow rates. All data are first displayed on the CRT for technician acceptance, and are then stored on IBM compatible diskettes and finally printed.

Because of the advantage of the automated system, many investigators are beginning to switch to more sophisticated equipment. The most important aspect of a transition is maintaining compatibility, or at least documenting the variability between past methods of data collection and those introduced by the new system. Subtle differences, e.g., computer initiation thresholds, data transmission resolutions, data reduction methods, can pose significant problems, especially if a new system is introduced during the course of a longitudinal study. Defining past operational procedures is a necessary first step in documenting the requirements of a new system.

Those who undertake to equip and operate a mobile laboratory will face a number of problems, some will be of a general nature; however, others will be unique to the equipment and vehicle chosen. Experience points to the need for good engineering support in the planning, establishment, and operation of a mobile laboratory.

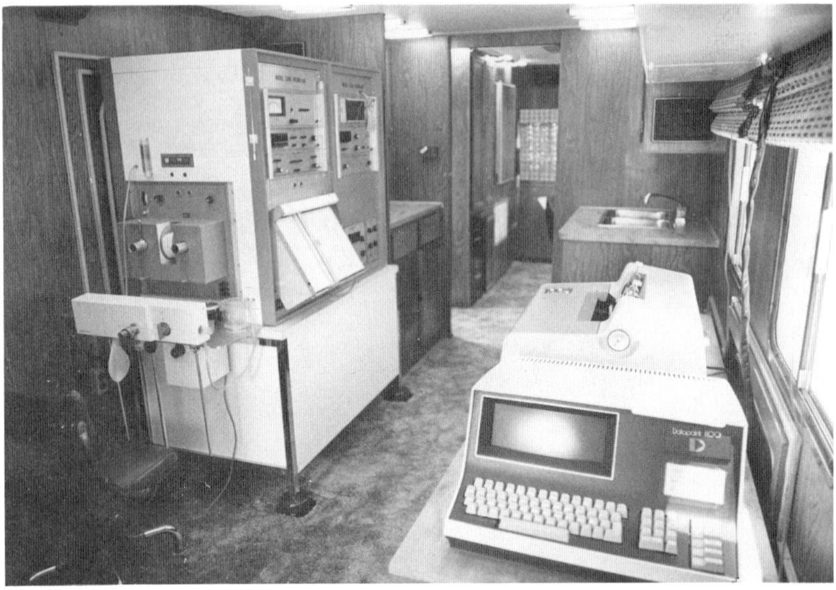

Figure 2 View toward rear of laboratory displays Pulmolab, CRT, and printer. Compartment behind Pulmolab can be used for exercise testing equipment or plethysmography. Rear of unit contains generator, refrigerator, head, water storage, filing cabinet, and voltage regulator. Driving area is used for administering the questionnaires.

X. Conclusion

Spirometry has become a cornerstone of epidemiological studies of occupational lung disease. Progress is being made to resolve the six special problems outlined in the introduction. Many of these problems are being met by developing recommendations and standards for instrumentation, test procedures, measurements and calculation, and interpretation. Great care has been and should be taken when standards are developed to allow for reasonable flexibility and innovation. Therefore, the standards outlined in this chapter should be considered a starting point, not final and inflexible.

Development of recommendations for spirometry can serve as a model for development of other lung function testing techniques. However, as new techniques develop, opportunity for standardization should be taken sooner than it was with spirometry. The principal research laboratories using new methods should discuss uniformity of testing techniques, measurement, and interpretation, so that research data will be comparable, and implementation of the techniques in occupational health research can be more rapid.

References

1. Morgan, W. K. C., and N. L. Lapp, Respiratory disease in coal mines, *Am. Rev. Respir. Dis.*, **113**:531 (1976).
2. Ziskind, M., D. B. Ellithorpe, and H. Weill, State of the art–silicosis, *Am. Rev. Respir. Dis.*, **113**:643 (1976).
3. Jones, R. N., J. Carr, H. Glindmeyer, J. Diem, and H. Weill, Respiratory health and dust levels in cottonseed mills, *Thorax*, **32**:281–286 (1977).
4. Jones, R. N., and H. Weill, Occupational lung diseases, *Basic of RD*, Vol. 6, No. 3 (1978).
5. Becklake, M. R., Asbestos-related diseases of the lungs and other organs: Their epidemiology and implications for clinical practice, *Am. Rev. Respir. Dis.*, **114**:187 (1976).
6. Leith, D. C., and J. Mead, *Principles of Body Plethysmography*. National Heart and Lung Institute, Division of Lung Diseases, November, 1974.
7. Macklem, P. T., *Procedures for Standardized Measurement of Lung Mechanics*. National Heart and Lung Institute, Division of Lung Diseases, November, 1974.
8. See Chapter 5 (pages 87–98) in this monograph.
9. Fry, D. L., and R. E. Hyatt, Pulmonary mechanics, *Am. J. Med.*, **29**: 672–689 (1960).
10. Mead, J., J. M. Turner, P. T. Macklem, and J. B. Little, Significance of the relationship between lung recoil and maximum expiratory flow, *J. Appl. Physiol.*, **22**:95–108 (1967).
11. Weill, H., Pulmonary function testing in industry, *J. Occup. Med.*, **15**: 693–699 (1973).
12. Fitzgerald, M. X., A. A. Smith, and E. A. Gaensler, Evaluation of "electronic" spirometers, *N. Engl. J. Med.*, **289**:1283–1288 (1973).
13. Gardner, R. M. (Chairman), American Thoracic Society–Report of Snowbird workshop on standardization of spirometry, *ATS News*, **3**:20–24 (Summer 1977).
14. Gardner, R. M. (Chairman), ATS statement–Snowbird workshop on standardization of spirometry, *Am. Rev. Respir. Dis.*, **119**:831–838 (1978).
15. Hankinson, J. L., and M. R. Peterson, Data analysis for spirometry instrument standards (abstract), *Am. Rev. Respir. Dis.*, **115**(supplement):116 (1977).
16. Cochrane, G. M., F. Prieto, and T. J. H. Clark, Intra-subject variables of maximum expiratory flow volume curve, *Thorax*, **32**:171 (1977).
17. Gardner, R. M., J. L. Hankinson, and B. J. West, Evaluating commercially available spirometers, *Am. Rev. Respir. Dis.*, **121**:73–82 (1980).
18. Glindmeyer, H. W., S. T. Anderson, J. E. Diem, and H. Weill, A comparison of the Jones and Stead-Wells spirometers, *Chest*, **73**:596–602 (1978).
19. Pierson, D. J., H. P. Dick, and T. L. Petty, A comparison of spirometric values with subjects in standing and sitting positions, *Chest*, **70**:17 (1976).
20. McCarthy, D. S., D. B. Craig, and R. M. Cherniack, Intraindividual variability in maximal expiratory flow volume and closing volume in asymptomatic subjects, *Am. Rev. Respir. Dis.*, **112**:407–411 (1975).

21. Dawson, A., Reproducibility of spirometric measurements in normal subjects, *Am. Rev. Respir. Dis.*, **93**:264–268 (1966).
22. Black, L. F., K. Offord, and R. E. Hyatt, Variability in the maximal expiratory flow volume curve in asymptomatic smokers and in nonsmokers, *Am. Rev. Respir. Dis.*, **110**:282–292 (1974).
23. Morris, J. F., A. Kiski, and L. C. Johnson, Spirometric standards for healthy nonsmoking adults, *Am. Rev. Respir. Dis.*, **103**:57 (1971).
24. Kory, R. C., R. Callahan, H. G. Boren, and J. C. Syner, The Veterans Administration-Army cooperative study of pulmonary function. I. Clinical spirometry in normal men, *Am. J. Med.*, **30**:243 (1961).
25. Knudson, R. J., R. C. Slatin, M. D. Lebowitz, and B. Burrows, The maximal expiratory flow-volume curve: Normal standards, variability and effects of age, *Am. Rev. Respir. Dis.*, **113**:587 (1976).
26. Rossiter, C. E., and H. Weill, Ethnic differences in lung function: Evidence for proportional differences, *Int. J. Epidemiol.*, **3**:55 (1974).
27. Lapp, N. L., H. E. Amandus, R. Hall, and W. K. C. Morgan, Lung volumes and flow rates in black and white subjects, *Thorax*, **29**:185 (1974).
28. Damon, A., Negro-white differences in pulmonary function (vital capacity, timed vital capacity, and expiratory flow rates), *Hum. Biol.*, **38**:380 (1966).
29. Knudson, R. J., B. Burrows, and M. D. Lebowitz, The maximum flow volume curve: Its use in the detection of ventilatory abnormalities in a population study, *Am. Rev. Respir. Dis.*, **114**:871–879 (1976).
30. Ferris, B. G., Epidemiology Standardization Project II, recommended respiratory disease questionnaires for use with adults and children in epidemiologic research, *Am. Rev. Respir. Dis.*, **118**(supplement):7–53 (1978).
31. Glindmeyer, H. W., H. Weill, R. Jones, and M. Ziskind, Design and operation of a mobile pulmonary function laboratory, *J. Occup. Med.*, **16**:584–588 (1974).
32. Despar, P. J., M. Leroux, and P. T. Macklem, Site of airway obstruction in asthma determined by measuring maximal expiratory flow breathing air and helium-oxygen mixture, *J. Clin. Invest.*, **51**:3235–3243 (1972).
33. Schilden, D. P., A. Robert, and D. L. Fry, Effect of gas density and viscosity on the maximal expiratory flow-volume relationship, *J. Clin. Invest.*, **42**:1705–1713 (1963).
34. Cosio, M., H. Ghezzo, J. C. Hogg, R. Corbin, M. Loveland, J. Dosman, and P. T. Macklem, The relationship between structural changes in small airways and pulmonary function tests, *N. Engl. J. Med.*, **298**:1277–1281 (1977).
35. Fairman, R. D., J. Hankinson, H. Imbus, N. L. Lapp, and W. K. C. Morgan, Pilot study of closing volume in byssinosis, *Br. J. Ind. Med.*, **32**:235–238 (1975).
36. Cotes, J. E., *Lung Function,* 3d Ed. Blackwell Scientific Publications, London, 1975, pp. 238–259.

37. Bouhuys, A., *Breathing*. Grune & Stratton, New York, 1974.
38. Bouhuys, A., *Airways Dynamics*, Charles C. Thomas, Springfield, Illinois, 1970.
39. DuBois, A. B., A. W. Brody, P. H. Lewis, and B. F. Burgess, Jr., Oscillation mechanics of lungs and chest in man, *J. Appl. Physiol.*, **8**:587–594 (1956).
40. Fischer, A. B., A. B. DuBois, and R. W. Hyde, Evaluation of the forced oscillation technique for the determination of resistance to breathing, *J. Clin. Invest.*, **47**:2045–2057 (1968).
41. Frank, N. R., J. Mead, and J. L. Whittenberger, Comparative sensitivity of four methods for measuring changes in respiratory flow resistance in man, *J. Appl. Physiol.*, **31**:934–938 (1971).

5

Physiologic Measurements Providing Enhanced Sensitivity in Detecting Early Effects of Inhalants

ROLAND H. INGRAM, JR. and E. R. MC FADDEN, JR.

Peter Bent Brigham Hospital
Harvard Medical School
Boston, Massachusetts

I. Introduction

Occupational pulmonary diseases have been recognized for hundreds of years. In 1662, Van Helmont described the development of dyspnea in a monk whose job was to care for old manuscripts [1]. In 1700, Ramazzini [2], in the preface to De Morbis Artificum, implored his readers to add another question to the list put forth by Hippocrates in his work "Affections."

> What occupation does the patient follow? Though this question may be concerned with the exciting causes, yet I regard it as well-timed or rather indispensable, and it should be particularly kept in mind when the patient to be treated belongs to the common people. In medical practice, however, I find that attention is hardly ever

---

Supported in part by grants HL 16463 and HL 17873 and Research Center Development Award HL 00013 (E.R.McF) from the National Heart, Lung, and Blood Institute, National Institutes of Health, Bethesda, Maryland.

> payed to this matter, or if the doctor in attendance knows it without asking, he gives little heed to it, though for effective treatment evidence of this sort has the utmost weight. . .

Seventy years later, these words were taken quite literally by Morgagni [3] as he attempted to seek proof of the possible association between work environment and pulmonary disease by searching at autopsy for hemp and feather particles in the "air vesicles" of the lungs of patients with asthma, whose business it was to make the "fibers for ropes" and "to dress and cleanse feathers with which beds are fluff'd."

It is apparent that at this stage of technological development, the initial detection of work-related pulmonary disorders was based upon there being either intermittently acute or severe chronic symptoms in association with specific employment. In the latter instance, the enormous functional reserve of the lungs and airways must have been depleted and seriously encroached upon before such severe symptoms could have occurred. Clearly, if chronic, this is a stage of disease beyond which any preventive measures could be expected to be effective for an individual worker.

In more recent times, chest radiography and spirometry have been performed in order to make an earlier diagnosis and to document the chronic effects of occupational exposure on individuals and on groups of workers. With the use of these techniques, detection at an earlier stage and identification of newer occupational hazards have occurred. Multiplication of the varieties of occupations with new technologies and agents to which workers are exposed and increasing awareness by the labor unions, management, legislators, and the public of both the health hazards of certain occupations and the financial costs of illness have led to more comprehensive programs designed to improve working environments, to improve detection, and, it is hoped, to prevent occupational lung diseases.

It has become apparent in the past few years that both chest radiography and spirometry may be inadequate tools for screening. The reason is that both may be quite normal at a time when there is considerable obstruction in the small airways, whether due to intrinsic disease or secondary to a parenchymal process. Several techniques, such as use of the single-breath nitrogen test, frequency-dependent behavior, and isovolumetric comparisons of maximal expiratory flow with gases of different densities, that are purported to correlate with subtle changes, have been developed and tested to a limited extent. Whether the demonstration of such subtle changes in lung function serves to identify those persons at greater risk to develop chronic disease is uncertain. However, implicit in the designation of "early effects of inhalants" is that these do, indeed, represent the initial abnormality in an often silent, yet inexorable march toward severe and irreversible lung disease. If this implication represented established fact, then development of yet newer and more sensitive techniques would be not only justifiable but desirable, and the application of known, recent techniques would be mandatory. Data are insufficient at present to support the desire or to justify a mandate. However, preliminary data are sufficiently encouraging that some of the more current measurements should and will be applied to the assessment of the tests themselves, in addition to the pulmonary effects of various occupational exposures.

Rather than deal with those exposures leading to fibrotic parenchymal diseases, we shall focus upon those associated with airway and destructive parenchymal lesions. Our purpose is to utilize the information available concerning the chronic effects of cigarette smoke on airways as a pathophysiological paradigm, since there has been relatively limited application of these newer techniques to the problem of occupational lung disease.

Before exploring the physiology and background for the newer tests, it is worthwhile to consider the present standard physiologic technique for the assessment of occupational lung dysfunction, the forced expiratory spirogram. From this maneuver, the forced expired volume in one second (FEV) has been the most often tabulated because of its relatively low coefficient of variation. For acute changes during a work shift, an individual serves as his or her own control, and the data are useful in detecting those who react to the inhalant. Hence, the exposure can be avoided or modified and the acute response prevented. Although this is an apparently straightforward approach, the true health implications of acute responses are far from being clear [4]. If, however, it is assumed that acute obstructive responses are nefarious, there are compelling data that show that there are acute effects that will be missed using this time-honored technique [5,6]. The chronic effects of exposure present a different problem. Although the FEV has been extremely useful for detection and for determining the magnitude of a given problem in both horizontal and longitudinal studies, the data appear to be less than ideal in serving the goal of prevention. With most chronic exposures, once the FEV becomes frankly abnormal, there is little chance for recovery of normal function. It would appear that the damage has been done and the only two concurrent courses of action available are to remove the victim from the offending exposure, thereby decreasing the rate of decline, and to improve the environment for those who might otherwise follow the same path to irreversible obstructive disease.

Implicit in our discussion to this point is that prior to development of an abnormal FEV, more subtle changes are detectable by the application of more sensitive techniques. All the newer tests are based upon one or both of two principles. The first is that small airways, because of their large total cross-sectional area, contribute only a small percentage to the total airway resistance [7], such that significant obstruction can be present in them without being detectable by measurement of FEV. The second is that inhalation to total lung capacity, which is necessary for performing a forced expiratory spirogram, can either totally or partially obscure airway obstruction ordinarily present in the breathing range either by stretching individual airways or by recruiting previously closed ones [8]. Hence, by the first principle, what is present may not be detected; by the second principle, what is there may be modified by the very maneuver designed to detect it.

First, let us explore the first principle, i.e., the feasibility of physiologically sounding out the silent zone [9] of the lung represented by small airways. In order to attribute to small airways any abnormalities in the tests purported to indicate relatively isolated obstruction of these airways, the elastic recoil properties of the lung should also be normal, indicating an intact parenchyma, and the overall airway resistance should be normal, indicating relative patency of the larger central airways that normally account for most of the resistance. Certainly, this is frequently the case with chronic cigarette smoking and, by analogy, should be the situation with chronic exposure to occupational factors that influence airways. It should be pointed out that airway resistance, FEV_1, and elastic recoil properties of the lung may well change in any individual with exposure to an inhalant or may be significantly more impaired in a population chronically exposed to a hostile environment as compared with one not exposed, yet they may still be within the range of normal. It is at such an early stage before symptoms appear and when ordinarily performed lung function tests are within the normal range that abnormalities can be detected, which indicate the presence of obstructive disease in small airways. Recently, structural abnormalities, consisting of inflammatory changes in small airways, have been shown to correlate with abnormalities in the tests to be described [10]. From a preventive standpoint, it is important to note that cessation of exposure is associated with return of these subtle abnormalities to normal [11,12] and, by inference, regression of the pathological findings.

The three tests listed above and now to be described have recently been modified, reinterpreted, or developed for the detection of small airway obstruction. These are (1) The single-breath nitrogen test, modified by Anthonisen et al. [13] from the original described by Comroe and Fowler [14]; (2) frequency dependence of compliance, resistance, or nitrogen washout, reinterpreted by Woolcock et al. [15], based upon the original time constant concept of Otis and co-workers [16]; and (3) isovolumetric comparison of maximal expiratory flow rates ($\dot{V}_{max}$) with air and after the lungs have been filled with a gas mixture containing 80% helium and 20% oxygen as developed by Despas et al. [17], and by Dosman and colleagues [18], extending the original observations of Schilder et al. [19].

In discussing these three tests, we shall consider what each measures, explore the identifiable performance and technical factors that influence the measurements, examine their within- and between-subject variation, and assess the ease with which they might be applied to the study of airway obstruction in an occupational setting. It is worth reiterating at this point that abnormalities in these tests, rather than indicating obstruction of small airways, reflect the combined derangement of all airways and parenchyma, *unless* the patency of central airways is reasonably assured and the integrity of the parenchyma is intact. If the FEV_1 or FEV_1/FVC (forced vital capacity) ratio is abnormal, it is difficult to justify the application of any of the tests to be discussed if the purpose is to provide an early diagnosis. In that case, the diagnosis will, in fact, have already been made a bit later than hoped for.

II. Single-Breath Nitrogen Test

The single-breath nitrogen test gives indices of both intraregional (within lobes) and interregional (between lobes) nonhomogeneity of the distribution of inspired gas [20]. The major intraregional index is the slope of phase III, or alveolar plateau; and the main interregional index is the volume at which phase IV, or airway closure, occurs. The slope of phase III is profoundly influenced by the rate of exhalation [21] and the time of breath holding [14]. The slope is decreased by both increasing flow rates and breath-holding time. Even when these two factors are standardized, the between- and within-subject variances are still large, giving a relatively poor signal-to-noise ratio [22].

Phase IV measurements as an indicator of the lung volume at the onset of basilar airway closure can be increased by loss of parenchymal support of airways closure can be increased by loss of parenchymal support of airways or intrinsic instability of diseased airways. The former factor is thought to account for systematic increases with age [13], whereas in young smokers the latter seems more likely [23]. Of the technical aspects that can influence this measurement, expiratory flow rates within a reasonable range have relatively little influence [24]. Even when procedures are highly standardized, closing volume measurements also have a high degree of variability due to various combinations of reader error, differences in the exhaled vital capacity due to incomplete filling and/or emptying of the lungs, and, possibly, inherent variations in the volume at which airway closure actually occurs. Differences do not seem to be due to subject factors such as diurnal or between-day variations or to a training effect [25]. Becklake and co-workers found that the between-subject variance exceeds that seen within subjects, giving a reasonable signal-to-noise ratio if the mean of three independently analyzed tests is used [22]. Despite the possible limitations of values derived from the single-breath test, large horizontal studies on cigarette smokers have demonstrated a significant number of abnormalities in excess of those found with spirometry [26].

As concerns the ease of application of this test to workers in an occupational setting, the test is noninvasive, yet it requires more time to perform three of them sequentially than an equivalent number of forced exhalations. Also, it requires an oxygen supply, a nitrogen analyzer, and an x-y recorder. Whether the extra time and equipment will be justified by an increased yield of abnormalities has yet to be determined [27].

III. Frequency-Dependent Tests

These tests make use of the fact that normal lungs behave as if all of the millions of alveoli fill and empty in relative unison, even at quite rapid breathing frequencies. Asynchronous behavior, if the application of force at the surface of the lung is uniform, indicates that there is nonuniformity of the time constants (resistance times compliance) of the lung units and is reflected by a decrease in dynamic compliance and resistance with increasing breathing frequency [15]. Frequency-dependent behavior correlates well with changes in the distribution of inspired gas [28]; hence, these tests are also, like the single-breath maneuver, indicators of nonhomogeneity of inspired gas which is mostly due to intraregional rather than interregional disparities [20]. The assumption is often made that normal overall lung pressure-volume relationships indicate normal regional compliances and that frequency-dependent behavior, under those circumstances, indicates inequality of time constants due to regional variations in resistance. The most often used test in this category has been frequency dependence of compliance, which has been considered by some as the "gold standard" for making the diagnosis of small airway obstruction. Recent studies have focused upon within-subject variance that might impair the interpretability of results [29], but, more importantly, the burden of precisely tuned instrumentation, the invasive need for swallowing an esophageal balloon, and the necessity of maintaining a constant end-expired lung volume and tidal volume make the test an impractical one to use in any large-scale study, especially in field testing.

Dependent upon identical principles is frequency dependence of total respiratory resistance. This test examines the transthoracic pressure in phase with flow during forced oscillations at the mouth. The advantage of this test is that it is simpler to perform and noninvasive and has correlated well with frequency dependence of compliance in a small series of subjects [30]. However, the within- and between-subject variation has not, as yet, been tested. There is good reason to suspect that variations in glottic aperture occur that would profoundly affect results [31]. Although it is possible that frequency dependence of total respiratory resistance may find a place in the large-scale evaluation of early airway obstruction, sufficient experience and data are not available to make a realistic assessment of its utility.

Again utilizing the same principles, the use of frequency dependence of nitrogen washout has been proposed as a noninvasive alternative to frequency dependence of compliance [32] since it correlates well with abnormalities in the latter [28]. However, not only are there performance and variability factors in common with frequency dependence of compliance, there is the need for the same expensive and delicate equipment required for the single-breath test. Furthermore, the added necessity for additional subject time and for corrections for the longer lag plus rise time of the nitrogen signal in comparison to the volume signal make this test too demanding for practical use in the setting of field testing.

To sum up our opinion, the frequency-dependent tests will remain as research tools to be utilized only in a rigorous research laboratory setting on small numbers of subjects for exploration of pathophysiologic mechanisms rather than for practical and meaningful surveys of large populations.

IV. Isovolumetric Comparisons of Maximal Expiratory Flow ($\dot{V}_{max}$) with Gases of Different Density

Schilder and co-workers demonstrated that $\dot{V}_{max}$ varies inversely with gas density in normal subjects [19]. With 80% helium and 20% oxygen (HeO_2), a gas mixture one-third as dense as air, $\dot{V}_{max}$ was found to be approximately 50% greater than with air in the midvital capacity range and fell much closer to and eventually below air values as residual volume was approached. These two observations were later applied to the study of early airway obstruction in smokers. The basic idea is that the relative contribution of large airways to flow limitation is great in normal subjects and it is in these airways, whose total cross-sectional area is small, that the highly density-dependent flow regimes of turbulence and convective acceleration predominate. With the development of small airway obstruction, the flow-limiting portion of the airways shortens and moves into the periphery of the lung. Here the total cross-sectional area, although compromised, remains large and density insensitive, and laminar flow predominates [17]. The result of these changes would be relative preservation of airflow due to shortening of the flow-limiting airways and a disproportionate decrease in HeO_2 flow. Hutcheon and colleagues were impressed that the volume at which HeO_2 and air values were the same (i.e., the volume of the isoflow—$V_{iso}\dot{V}$) was higher in smokers than in nonsmokers [33]. Dosman et al. pointed out that $V_{iso}\dot{V}$ was greatly influenced by the elastic recoil of the lung and increased as elastic recoil diminished with age [18]. In contrast to the age effect on $V_{iso}\dot{V}$, the increase in flow with HeO_2 at 50% of the vital capacity (so-called $\Delta\dot{V}_{max_{50}}$) was independent of elastic recoil pressure and age in nonsmokers. Thus, these workers interpreted the lower $\Delta\dot{V}_{max_{50}}$ in smokers as representing small airway obstruction rather than parenchymal abnormalities. For practical application, rather than requiring a complete washin of HeO_2, the test has been standardized to examine HeO_2 $\dot{V}_{max}$ after taking three full vital capacities of this mixture. If washin were less than complete in smokers due to intraregional nonhomogeneity, the

$\Delta\dot{V}_{max_{50}}$ value would be a hybrid test of both inspired gas distribution and density effects on the determinants of $\dot{V}_{max}$. Since these initial observations were made using a plethysmograph, the potential effects of intrathoracic gas compression on obscuring the relationship between lung volume and $\dot{V}_{max}$ need to be considered if a spirometer is to be used. During forced exhalations, when high intrathoracic pressures are generated, the instantaneous change in lung volume exceeds the volume displaced at the mouth due to compression of thoracic gas [34]. If the pressures generated with air were different than those with HeO_2, there would be a great deal of variation in results. Although the degree of variability with spirometric comparisons is potentially large, Dosman (personal communication) has found essentially identical $\Delta\dot{V}_{max_{50}}$ results with spirometric and plethysmographic methods. While the within- and between-subject variances of this value have not been systematically assessed, the additional need only for a gas cylinder containing HeO_2 and the additional time requirement only for three vital capacities of washin plus three additional forced exhalations, maneuvers to which the subjects are already accustomed, make the comparison of $\dot{V}_{max}HeO_2$ to that of air a potentially useful, simple, rapid, and valuable addition to physiologic testing in a field setting. Perhaps as more data are collected on gas density effects on forced expiratory spirograms, it will turn out that simple ratios of FEV_1 on the two gases will be a sensitive index of early airway obstruction. Although the FEV_1 includes emptying of the lung at large volumes at which flow is dependent upon the degree of effort in addition to the mechanical properties of the lungs and airways, it might be supposed that such a ratio would be more variable than would comparisons made over the effort-independent portion of the forced vital capacity. However, the value of the FEV_1 continues to be its relatively low coefficient of variation as compared to other values derived from the forced expiratory spirogram. Hence, it would not be too farfetched to expect the ratio of FEV_1 on air to that on HeO_2 to provide additional information, and it would be pleasing to have the value of the FEV_1 increased further by establishing its usefulness as an assessment of early airway obstruction.

Certainly, more data are needed before any firmly based recommendation can be made as to the role of spirograms before and after HeO_2 in the study of occupational lung diseases. Nonetheless, simplicity of techniques, soundness of principles, and encouraging preliminary data engender in us a sufficient sense of optimism that we consider this a reasonable method to apply to research on an occupational exposure anticipated to result in airway disease.

The second principle, concerning the volume history effect of going to total lung capacity, not only presents the problem of interfering with the detection of obstruction that may have been present before full inhalation, but also presents the possibility of preferentially reversing small airway obstruction. There are three related mechanisms by which full inflation could ameliorate obstruction present at lung volume in the breathing range. First, airways can be closed at volumes above functional residual capacity [35] and might not close during rapid deflation if airway hysteresis exceeds parenchymal hysteresis. Second, without airway closure having been present, if airway hysteresis exceeds parenchymal hysteresis, airways will be larger at any lung volume when reached during deflation from total lung capacity [36]. Third, the inflation itself might reverse resting zone or induced constriction of airways for several seconds [8]. Most of the volume history effects are thought to be due to smooth muscle tone [37,38]. The assessment of airway caliber even without bronchoconstrictor challenges by forced exhalations begun at or near functional residual capacity (so-called partial expiratory flow-volume curve, PEFV) consistently reveals lower flow rates than on maximal expiratory flow-volume curves (MEFV) at the same lung volume [5]. The isovolumetric flow differences between partial and maximal maneuvers are even more striking after bronchoconstrictor challenges. Hence, the combination of a PEFV and an MEFV maneuver in sequence should give a reasonable assessment of the immediately reversible airway constrictive component.

By utilizing HeO_2 and air for PEFV and MEFV maneuvers, cigarette smokers without other demonstrable abnormalities can be shown to have small airway obstruction that is reversed by going to total lung capacity [6], demonstrating that combinations of volume history considerations and gases of various density during $\dot{V}_{max}$ can give information on sites of airway obstruction. Although of great physiologic significance and of potential value in the assessment of early airway effects, this technique is difficult to standardize in terms of matching lung volumes on the partial and maximal maneuvers, and the within- and between-individual variation has not been established.

Although, as discussed in detail elsewhere in this series, the role of intermittently acute airway responses in the pathogenesis of chronic airway disease is not at all clear [4], the degree of acute responsiveness both in terms of airway site and overall magnitude represents an area in which research is needed. For this purpose, the techniques described herein offer some promise.

V. Conclusions

It is now apparent that a series of tests can be performed that will, in a chronic situation, reveal functional abnormalities well before the simple forced expiratory spirogram becomes abnormal; and, in an acute situation, disclose functional changes not detectable by use of ordinary techniques. It is not clear, however, that such subtle changes, either acutely or chronically, occur predominantly in those individuals at greater risk to develop chronic obstructive airway disease. The acceptance of any of these tests as routine adjuncts to the ordinary forced expiratory spirogram in occupation surveys should await the demonstration of their reproducibility, ease of performance, and increased yield.

Hence, investigation over the next several years need be concerned as much with the evaluation of tests as with the assessment of occupational lung diseases. In fact, it is possible that evaluation and validation of these tests might be a *consequence* of their use in an occupational setting in which dose-response relationships might or might not show their superiority in detecting early effects of exposure.

References

1. Van Helmont, L. B., *Oriatrike, or Physick Refined.* London, Lodowick Loyd, 1662.
2. Ramazzini, B., De Morbis Artificum. In *Opera Omnia Medica et Physica.* London, Paul and Isaac Vaillant, 1717.
3. Morgagni, J., The seats and causes of disease investigated by anatomy. Translated by B. Alexander. London, A. Miller, Vol. 1, letter XV, articles 3–26, 1796.
4. Ingram, R. H., Jr., and E. R. McFadden, Jr., Acute responsiveness of the airways in the transition between health and disease. In *The Lung in the Transition between Health and Disease,* Vol. 12 of Lung Biology in Health and Disease. Edited by P. T. Macklem and S. Permutt. New York, Marcel Dekker, Inc., 1979.
5. Bouhuys, A., V. R. Hunt, B. M. Kim, and A. Zapletal, Maximal expiratory flow rates in induced bronchoconstriction in man, *J. Clin. Invest.,* **48**: 1159–1168 (1969).
6. Brown, N. E., E. R. McFadden, Jr., and R. H. Ingram, Jr., Airway responses to inhaled histamine in asymptomatic smokers and non-smokers, *J. Appl. Physiol.,* **42**:508–513 (1977).
7. Macklem, P. T., and J. Mead, Resistance of central and peripheral airways as measured by a retrograde catheter, *J. Appl. Physiol.,* **22**:395–401 (1967).
8. Nadel, J. A., and D. F. Tierney, Effect of a previous deep inspiration on airways resistance in man, *J. Appl. Physiol.,* **16**:717–719 (1961).
9. Mead, J., The lung's quiet zone, *N. Engl. J. Med.,* **282**:1318–1319 (1970).
10. Cosio, M., H. Ghezzo, J. C. Hogg, R. Corbin, M. Loveland, J. Dosman, and P. T. Macklem, The relations between structural changes in small airways and pulmonary function tests, *N. Engl. J. Med.,* **298**:1277–1281 (1978).
11. McFadden, E. R., Jr., and D. A. Linden, A reduction in maximum midexpiratory flow rate: A spirographic manifestation of small airway disease, *Am. J. Med.,* **52**:725–737 (1972).
12. Ingram, R. H., Jr., and C. F. O'Cain, Frequency dependence of compliance in apparently healthy smokers versus non-smokers, *Bull. Physiopathol. Respir. (Nancy),* **7**:195–210 (1971).
13. Anthonisen, N. R., J. Danson, P. C. Robertson, and W. R. D. Ross, Airway closure as a function of age, *Respir. Physiol.,* **8**:58–65 (1969–70).

14. Comroe, J. H., and W. S. Fowler, Lung function studies. VI. Detection of uneven alveolar ventilation during a single breath of oxygen, *Am. J. Med.*, **10**:408 (1951).
15. Woolcock, A. J., N. J. Vincent, and P. T. Macklem, Frequency dependence of compliance as a test for obstruction in small airways, *J. Clin. Invest.*, **48**:1097–1106 (1969).
16. Otis, A. B., C. B. McKerrow, R. A. Bartlett, J. Mead, M. B. McIlroy, N. J. Selversone, and E. P. Radford, Mechanical factors in distribution of pulmonary ventilation, *J. Appl. Physiol.*, **8**:427–443 (1956).
17. Despas, P. J., M. Leroux, and P. T. Macklem, Site of airway obstruction in asthma as determined by measuring maximal expiratory flow breathing air and a helium-oxygen mixture, *J. Clin. Invest.*, **51**:3235–3243 (1972).
18. Dosman, J., F. Bode, J. Urbanetti, R. Martin, and P. T. Macklem, The use of a helium-oxygen mixture during maximum expiratory flow to demonstrate obstruction in small airways in smokers, *J. Clin. Invest.*, **55**:1090–1099 (1975).
19. Schilder, D. P., A. Roberts, and D. L. Fry, Effect of gas density and viscosity on the maximal expiratory flow-volume relationship, *J. Clin. Invest.*, **42**:1705–1713 (1963).
20. Engel, L. A., and P. T. Macklem, Gas mixing and distribution in the lung. In *International Review of Physiology, Respiration Physiology* II, Vol. 14. Edited by J. G. Widdicombe. Baltimore, University Park Press, 1977, pp. 37–82.
21. Bashoff, M. A., R. H. Ingram, Jr., and D. P. Schilder, Effect of expiratory flow on the nitrogen concentration versus volume relationship, *J. Appl. Physiol.*, **23**:895–901 (1967).
22. Becklake, M. R., M. Leclerc, H. Strobach, and J. Swift, The N_2 closing volume test in population studies: Sources of variation and reproducibility, *Am. Rev. Respir. Dis.*, **111**:141–147 (1975).
23. Ingram, R. H., Jr., C. F. O'Cain, and W. W. Fridy, Jr., Simultaneous quasi-static lung pressure-volume curves and "closing volume" measurements, *J. Appl. Physiol.*, **36**:135–141 (1974).
24. Travis, D. M., M. Green, and H. Don, Expiratory flow rate and closing volumes, *J. Appl. Physiol.*, **35**:626–630 (1973).
25. McFadden, E. R., Jr., B. Holmes, and R. Kiker, Variability of closing volume measurements in normal man, *Am. Rev. Respir. Dis.*, **111**:135–140 (1975).
26. Buist, A. S., D. L. Van Fleet, and B. B. Ross, A comparison of conventional spirometric tests and the test of closing volume in an emphysema screening center, *Am. Rev. Respir. Dis.*, **107**:735–743 (1973).
27. Ingram, R. H., Jr., and E. R. McFadden, Jr., Closing volume and the natural history of chronic airway obstruction, *Am. Rev. Respir. Dis.*, **116**:973–975 (1977).
28. Ingram, R. H., Jr., and D. P. Schilder, Association of a decrease in dynamic compliance with a change in gas distribution, *J. Appl. Physiol.*, **23**:911–916 (1967).

29. Guyatt, A. R., J. A. Siddorn, H. M. Brash, and D. C. Flenley, Reproducibility of dynamic compliance and flow-volume curves in man, *J. Appl. Physiol.,* **39**:341–348 (1975).
30. Kjelgaard, J. M., R. W. Hyde, D. M. Speers, and W. W. Reichert, Frequency dependence of total respiratory resistance in early airway disease, *Am. Rev. Respir. Dis.,* **114**:501–508 (1976).
31. Jackson, A. C., P. J. Gulesian, Jr., and J. Mead, Glottic aperture during panting with voluntary limitation of tidal volume, *J. Appl. Physiol.,* **39**: 834–836 (1975).
32. Wanner, A., S. Zarzecki, N. Atkins, A. Zapata, and M. A. Sackner, Relationship between frequency dependence of lung compliance and distribution of ventilation, *J. Clin. Invest.,* **54**:1200–1213 (1974).
33. Hutcheon, M., P. Griffin, H. Levison, and N. Zamel, Volume of isoflow: A new test in detection of mild abnormalities of lung mechanics, *Am. Rev. Respir. Dis.,* **110**:458–465 (1974).
34. Ingram, R. H., Jr., and D. P. Schilder, Effect of gas compression on the flow-volume curve of the forced vital capacity, *Am. Rev. Respir. Dis.,* **94**: 56–63 (1966).
35. Leblanc, P., F. Ruff, and J. Milic-Emili, Effects of age and body position on airway closure in man, *J. Appl. Physiol.,* **28**:448–451 (1970).
36. Froeb, H. F., and J. Mead, Relative hysteresis of the dead space and lung in vivo, *J. Appl. Physiol.,* **25**:244–248 (1968).
37. Vincent, N. J., R. Knudson, D. E. Leith, P. T. Macklem, and J. Mead, Factors influencing pulmonary resistance, *J. Appl. Physiol.,* **29**:236–243 (1970).
38. Green, M., and J. Mead, Time dependence of flow-volume curves, *J. Appl. Physiol.,* **37**:793–797 (1974).

6

Exercise Testing

J. E. COTES

The University of Newcastle upon Tyne
Newcastle upon Tyne, England

I. Introduction

Any disease process affecting the lungs inevitably impairs its function as an organ of ventilation and gas exchange. These attributes may be assessed in isolation using the tests described in other chapters. Their overall effect upon performance is assessed by eliciting the symptom of breathlessness on exertion and by measuring the ventilation in circumstances when the demand on the respiratory apparatus is increased. The test stimulus is then usually exercise, but possibly more attention should be paid to other stimuli including speech and hypoxia. Speech is normally not a cause of breathlessness except in the presence of gross respiratory impairment but with mild impairment it may become so in combination with exercise. However, the stimulus is then difficult to standardize and the response not easy to measure. Exercise has the advantages that it may be applied at all levels of intensity, does not interfere with measurement, and is usually without risk, but has the possible disadvantage that the mode of exercise will influence the result.

The determinants of the normal response include the size of the muscles which contribute to the exercise, their distribution within the body, the tension as a proportion of maximum which is developed and whether isometric or isotonic, the mass of the parts which are moved, and if the exercise is habitual, occasional, or being performed for the first time. The state of general physical training of the subject also influences the result.

The exercise test will provide information on the cardiorespiratory response to exercise including the uptake of oxygen and output of carbon dioxide, ventilation, its distribution as between tidal volume and respiratory frequency, the cardiac frequency, and, if required, other variables including the cardiac output, the arterial blood gases, and aspects of lung mechanics. These measurements throw light on the physiological responses including the type and extent of any abnormality. In addition, the exercise test may be used to assess the capacity for exercise including the mode of limitation which may be primarily circulatory, ventilatory, or due to cough, phlegm, pain, or another symptom. Thus the test provides a unique insight into the subject's personality and attributes difficult to obtain in other ways. For this reason, if not on account of the requirements for medical surveillance, the exercise test should, where possible, be conducted by the physician in charge of the case; the report should include a description summarizing the clinical aspects of the response.

In the context of occupational medicine the exercise test is an essential component of the overall assessment of respiratory function [1]. The results will be of use for the assessment of physical condition, diagnosis of occupational lung disease, assessment of disability, management of the chronic stage of the condition including rehabilitation and in relation to reemployment. This article describes how the exercise test may be performed and the ways in which the information may be used.

II. Basic Information

For abbreviations, symbols, and units, see Appendix, page 121.

A. Ventilation

In relation to disorders of the respiratory system, the ventilatory response to exercise is of the highest importance. The measurement is usually made by collection and analysis of expired gas, but measurement of the volume of inspired gas is often preferable. The gas is entrained through a mask or breathing valve but these devices themselves influence the ventilation by their deadspace and resistance. Alternatively the chest wall movement is measured with an inductance plethysmograph but the accuracy is less. A deadspace mask of 15 ml is achieved by using a divider in the mouthpiece separating the inspiratory and expiratory pathways, but is seldom used. However, most breathing valves have a deadspace of the order of 30–50 ml which is acceptable. An auronasal mask may have a deadspace of 150 ml while an even larger deadspace may all too easily be acquired by the injudicious accumulation of taps, pneumotachographs, and other devices which abound in a respiratory laboratory. For use during submaximal exercise the inspiratory resistance to flow expressed as the suction developed at the mouthpiece at a flow rate of 100 liters/min should not exceed 15 kPa (1.5 cmH_2O) or for maximal exercise 0.1 kPa (1 cmH_2O). The expiratory back-pressure should not exceed twice these amounts. The volume-measuring device may be a spirometer, a gas meter, or a pneumotachograph. The spirometer is usually of the Tissot type when it has the disadvantage of a high inertia sometimes leading to overshoot; the alternative of a small bellows or servospirometer which empties between breaths is attractive but not usually attained. Portable gas meters are used during occupational surveys (e.g., Max Plank) but have a high resistance to airflow, while the large low-resistance domestic gas meter formerly the mainstay of many exercise laboratories (Parkinson and Cowan CD4) is now no longer available in its original form. At the present time the choice for most laboratories is between a modified respiratory anemometer (Wright) for studies on ambulant subjects and a pneumotachograph and integrator which should preferably reset automatically between breaths in order to compensate for drift. The pneumotachograph is mounted proximal to the inspiratory valve as in this position the deadspace is of no consequence and condensation of water vapor does not occur. For the registration of duration of inspiration, there is a need to decide on criteria for the start and end of the breath. The system should be calibrated with fluctuating flows using a pump to mimic normal breathing as well as with steady flows using a calibrated rotameter. Biological calibration of a pneumotachograph and integrator should be undertaken by comparing the volume recorded over a whole number of breaths with that obtained using a Douglas bag and calibrated wet gas meter. The bag should have tubing of diameter at least 3 cm and be suspended vertically; the gas should be expelled through the gas meter at a constant rate. Gas volumes are converted to body temperatures saturated with water vapor (BTPS). An equation for making the correction is given in Table 1. For obtaining the relationship of the ventilation to the consumption of oxygen it should also be corrected for the instrumental deadspace ($\dot{V}D_i$) which as a first approximation exerts an additive effect, i.e., $\dot{V}E_{corr} = \dot{V}E_{obs} - VD_i \times fR$.

B. Gas Exchange

The measurement of uptake of oxygen and evolution of carbon dioxide entails analysis of the mixed expired gas for these two gases and registration of ventilation in the mode described above. The mixing of the expired gas is usually performed by having the gas pass through a chamber containing baffles and of

Table 1 Conversion of Gas Volumes from Ambient Temperature and Pressure (ATP) to Body Temperature Saturated with Water Vapor (BTPS)

$$\dot{V}_{BTPS} = V_{ATP} \times \frac{310}{273 + t} \times \frac{P_B - P_{H_2Ot}}{P_B - P_{H_2O(37)}}$$

where P_B is barometric pressure, t is ambient temperature, and P_{H_2O} is aqueous vapor pressure. At 37°C this is 6.3 kPa (47 mmHg) and at t °C, is given by $P_{H_2Ot} = 0.1333\,(9.993 - 0.3952t + 0.03775t^2)$ where 0.1333 converts from mmHg to kPa.

Source: Data from Ref. 3.

capacity approximately 4 liters; a stirrer in the chamber is an additional refinement. The concentration of oxygen is usually measured using a paramagnetic oxygen meter but a polarograph or mass spectrometer may also be used; except in the last instance the carbon dioxide concentration is measured by an infrared analyzer. When collating the dial readings or output signals from the analyzers allowance should be made for any differences in the response times for oxygen and carbon dioxide or between them and the volume recorder. The analyzers are calibrated over the appropriate range of concentrations using gas mixtures which are either made up in cylinders and after mixing are analyzed on a Lloyd Haldane apparatus or are prepared using a Wösthoff pump. The results should now be expressed as millimoles of gas absorbed or evolved per minute but the traditional units (1 STPD min^{-1}) are still acceptable. The calculations are given in Table 2.

C. Cardiac Frequency

This is obtained from the electrocardiogram which is also used for monitoring the condition of the subject during the exercise. The electrodes are applied as for the chest lead V5 with two over the sternum and one over the cardiac apex and the signal is filtered to minimize electrical noise generated by contraction of skeletal muscles during the exercise. For inspection during the test the ECG is displayed on an oscilloscope and for counting the frequency or for checking the heart rate meter it is also registered on an appropriate recorder.

D. Cardiac Output

This is usually measured by a carbon dioxide rebreathing method, preferably that due to Farhi and his colleagues [2] which avoids error on account of gas passing into or out of solution in the tissue of the lung during the period of rebreathing.

Table 2 Calculation of Uptake of Oxygen and Respiratory Exchange Ratio (R) from the Ventilation Minute Volume (liters/min) and the Fractional Concentrations (F) of O_2, CO_2, and N_2 in the Mixed Expired Gas[a]

$$O_2 \text{ uptake} = a\, \dot{V}_{E,BTPS} \times (0.2648\, F_{E_{N_2}} - F_{E_{O_2}})$$

where a for $\dot{N}O_2$ (mmol/min) is 36.9

and for $\dot{V}O_2$ (litersSTPD min^{-1}) is 0.836

$$R = F_{E_{CO_2}}/(0.2648\, F_{E_{N_2}} - F_{E_{O_2}})$$

[a]See also Table 1.
Source: Data from Ref. 3.

E. Arterial Blood Gases

These are best obtained by sampling from a catheter in the brachial artery which also permits collection of blood samples for the measurement of cardiac output by an indicator dilution method. The use of these procedures is best confined to the hospital lung function laboratory. In other circumstances blood may be obtained from the lobe of the ear, after application of a topical vasodilator ointment, by puncture with a needle through to a sterile cork.

F. Indices of Respiratory Drive

In the context of exercise testing the ventilatory response to exercise provides an index of respiratory drive. It is the result of many factors including the intensity of the stimulus, the sensitivity of the respiratory center to the several components of the stimulus, the integrity of the neuromuscular system of the thorax, and the compliance and resistance of the lungs and chest wall. The sensitivity to carbon dioxide may be assessed by the rebreathing method of Read in which the subject rebreathes from a bag which initially contains between 3 and 5 liters of a gas mixture comprising 5% CO_2 in oxygen. The ventilation is recorded by enclosing the bag in a box which is connected via valves to a suitable ventilation meter (Sec. II.A). The tension of carbon dioxide in the bag is recorded continuously by sampling into an infrared gas analyzer and the sensitivity is the slope of the relationship of the ventilation on the tension of carbon dioxide. It has the units 1 min^{-1} kPa^{-1} (or 1 min^{-1} $mmHg^{-1}$) and should be standardized for body size usually by relating the result to the vital capacity of the subject (Table 3).

The sensitivity to CO_2 reflects the neural drive to the respiratory muscles, their mechanical efficiency, and the work which needs to be done to ventilate the thorax. The former two components may be assessed separately from the third by measuring the pressure which develops at the lips during inspiration

Table 3 Reference Values for the Physiological Response to Exercise and Respiratory Sensitivity in Adults[a]

Index	Equation	Standard deviation
$\dot{V}E_{submax}$ (liters/min)	22 [÷ 44.6] $\dot{N}O_2$ + 2	5.4
Vt_{30} (liters)	0.1 (VC + 0.87)	0.22
Vt_{max} (liters)	0.65 (VC − 1)	0.21
$\dot{N}O_2$ [cycling(mmol/min)]	44.6 [0.0 118 W + 0.00 68 M − 0.09]	0.09
$\dot{N}O_2$ [walking(mmol/min)]	44.6 [0.006 M + 0.00036 MV^2]	0.16
$\dot{N}O_2$ [stepping(mmol/min)]	44.6 [0.15 W + 0.16]	15
fC_{submax} (min^{-1})	34 + 1590 FFM^{-1} + 2590 [÷ 44.6] FFM^{-1} $\dot{N}O_2$	15
fC_{max} (min^{-1})	210 − 0.65 age (years)	19
$\dot{Q}t_{submax}$ liters(min)	6.4 [÷ 44.6] $\dot{N}O_2$ + 3.4	0.9
SCO_2 (liters min^{-1} kPa^{-1})	7.5 [(0.89 + 0.35 VC)]	0.58

[a]When oxygen uptake is reported as $\dot{V}O_2$ in liters per minute, the term 44.6 is omitted. When SCO_2 is reported in traditional units (liters min^{-1} $mmHg^{-1}$), the term 7.5 is omitted.
Source: Data from Ref. 3.

against a closed airway. Two indices are in regular use, the pressure 0.1 sec after the start of inspiration $P_{0.1}$ and the maximal rate of rise of pressure at the start of inspiration $[(dP/dt)_{max}]$. Their use is described elsewhere [3].

G. Anthropometry

The measurements of relevance for interpreting the cardiorespiratory response to exercise include the body mass, the fat-free mass, the volume of the heart, and the dimensions of the legs, e.g., the leg length, the diameter and skinfold thickness of the thigh and calf, and the fat-free volume of the leg. Of these, the fat-free mass merits description here. The body surface area, while of historic interest, is not particularly useful; in addition it should be noted that when the area is derived from stature and body mass, the prediction equation should take into account the ethnic group. The fat-free mass is traditionally calculated from the body density which is obtained by underwater weighing; the erroneous assumption is then made that the density of this compartment is known and constant. However, for interpreting the cardiac frequency response to exercise the error is unimportant. The densitometry may be replaced by an estimate based on body mass and four skinfold thicknesses. These are measured using Harpenden skin calipers applied to the midpoints of the long axis of the left

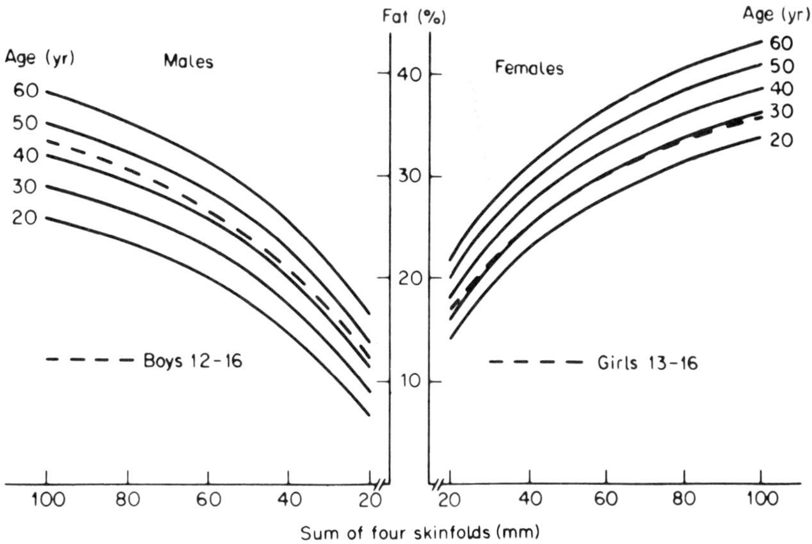

Figure 1 Approximate relationship of an index of skinfold thickness to the percentage of body mass which is fat. This may be used to estimate the fat-free mass as follows:

$$\text{FFM} = \text{body mass} \times (100 - \%\ \text{fat}) \div 100\ (\text{kg})$$

The coefficient of variation of the estimate is of the order of 6% [3].

upper arm in the midline anteriorly and posteriorly, to the skin below and medial to the tip of the left scapula, and to the anterior abdominal wall above the anterior superior iliac crest. The sum of the four skinfold thicknesses reflects the percentage of body mass which is fat (Fig. 1).

III. Manipulation of the Basic Information

The indices which have been described in Section II may be used without further manipulation as when they relate to a steady setting of the ergometer or to maximal exercise. More often they are used to derive secondary indices including those which are based on the relationships of the ventilation minute volume and of the cardiac frequency to the uptake of oxygen, of the minute volume to the tidal volume (Hey plot), and of the tidal volume to the durations of inspiration and expiration (von Euler plot). In addition, the tidal volume may be divided by the times of inspiration and of expiration to yield, respectively, the mean inspiratory and expiratory flow rates. The relationships may be derived using

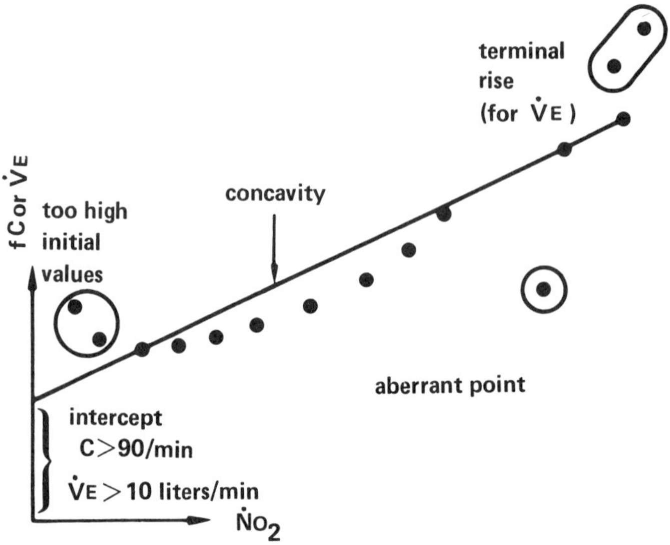

Figure 2 Some faults which can be detected by scrutiny of the intermediate results of a progressive exercise test. In most instances they constitute reasons for rejecting the measurement but it may be sufficient to exclude one or more points [3]. (See also Sec.V.)

information collected each breath or each minute or half minute. In the latter instance there may be an error due to the time interval not comprising a whole number of breaths. The relationships are usually best displayed graphically as this provides an indication of both the interval consistency, hence the reliability of the observations (Fig. 2), and the appropriateness of the derived indices for each individual (Fig. 3). The processing of the information may be carried out manually or using a microprocessor or small computer which may be on-line or be fed with appropriate data subsequently via a magnetic or paper tape.

IV. Varieties of Test Exercise

A. The Exercise Profile

The exercise may be of constant intensity (rectangular) as when it is intended to relate the physiological response to the rate of external work. Measurements made after the subject has been exercising for 5 min are then representative of the "steady state" except when the ambient temperature is high or the work rate is near to the capacity for exercise of the subject. Several periods of rectangular

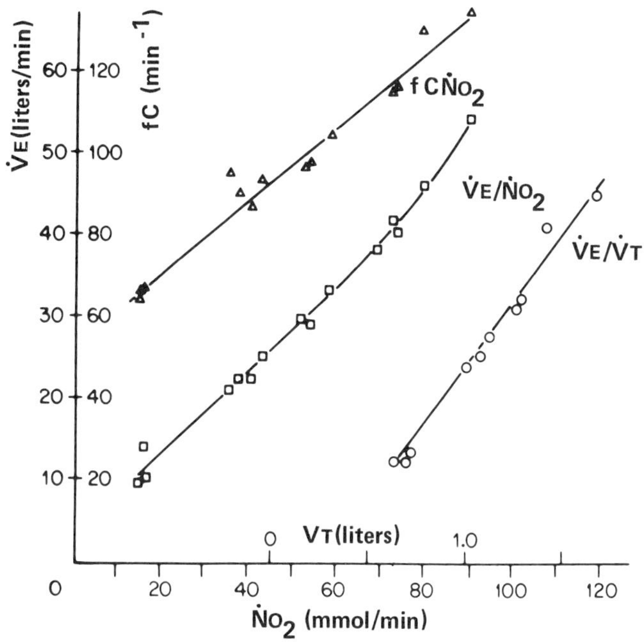

Figure 3 Relationships for a healthy subject of cardiac frequency (fC) and ventilation ($\dot{V}_E$) on oxygen uptake ($\dot{N}O_2$) and of ventilation on tidal volume ($\dot{V}_T$). The ventilation data plotted against oxygen uptake have been corrected for the deadspace of the apparatus [3].

exercise each of 6 min duration and of graded intensity may be performed consecutively.

Exercise of progressively increasing intensity provides information on the physiological response to a range of work levels. The load may be increased continuously (triangular) or in increments every 1 to 3 min (staircase); the physiological responses (Fig. 3) are then acceptably consistent with respect to each other but, except in the case of 3 min increments, are less than those to be expected for steady-state exercise at the same rate of external work.

B. Maximal Exercise

This is usually approached gradually being preceded by triangular or staircase exercise or by steady-state exercises of increasing intensity. It is usually described in terms of the maximal oxygen consumption (aerobic capacity) which in subjects with normal cardiorespiratory systems is easier to interpret than is

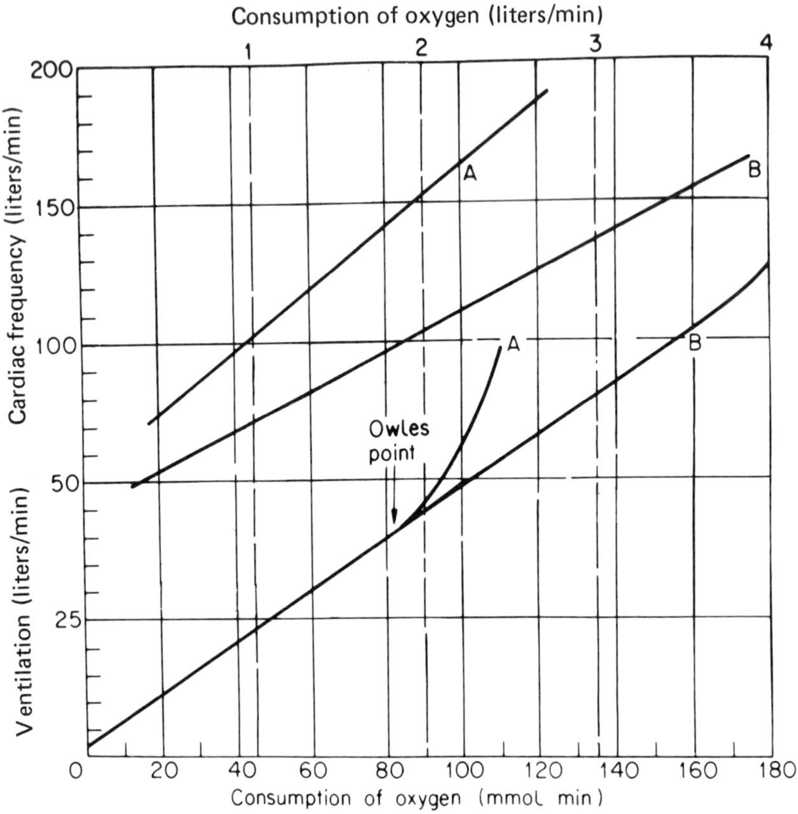

Figure 4 The relationships of the ventilation and the cardiac frequency to the consumption of oxygen at rest and during exercise. When the measurements were made, subject A was untrained and had a small capacity for exercise. Subject B was a world-class athlete. During moderate exercise while breathing air the values for ventilation are similar but the cardiac frequencies differ. During strenuous exercise all the values diverge. The maximal oxygen uptake may be estimated indirectly from the regression line of cardiac frequency on consumption of oxygen during submaximal exercise. For this purpose the line is extrapolated to an assumed maximal cardiac frequency (Table 3) and the corresponding consumption of oxygen is then read off the diagram [3].

the maximal work rate. It may be said to have been attained when a further increment in the rate of work fails to elicit a measurable increase in the consumption of oxygen. The safety precautions which should be adopted are summarized in Section IV.F. However, the procedure should only be applied where it is both necessary and appropriate including that the subject is fully prepared to undertake it. In most circumstances a submaximal procedure may be used instead [4]. Alternatively, the maximal oxygen uptake may be deduced by extrapolation up to the estimated maximal cardiac frequency for the subject of the relationship of the exercise cardiac frequency to the uptake of oxygen. The maximal frequency is given in Table 3; the procedure and the related changes in ventilation are illustrated in Figure 4. In subjects with pulmonary disease the exercise is usually limited by inability to further increase the ventilation minute volume. In these circumstances the exercise cardiac frequency does not approach the biological maximum and the indirect procedure is invalid.

C. Stepping Exercise

Stepping on and off a box provides the simplest form of ergometry. The essential requirements are that the subject raises the center of gravity of the body through the full height of the step in time with a metronome and, except for the Harvard pack test, does not obtain help from the arms. With a fixed step height and frequency the energy expenditure is nearly proportional to the body weight of the subject; hence for subjects using the same exercise settings the energy expenditure on average comprises a fairly constant proportion of their respective maxima. The 1 min step test of Baldwin et al. (step height 0.2 m and frequency 30 min^{-1}) [5] is of this form. Alternatively the step height h and frequency f may be adjusted in the light of the body mass of the subject m, so that each performs the same amount of vertical work against gravity, i.e.,

$$\text{Work rate (W)} = h\,(\text{m}) \times f\,(\text{min}^{-1}) \times M\,(\text{kg}) \times 0.163 \tag{1}$$

The step test of Hugh-Jones [6] employs a work rate of 57 W for which the average ventilation minute volume is 33 liters/min and the uptake of oxygen 62 mmol/min; however, the latter varies somewhat with the body mass of the subject. The measurement of ventilation during the test provides a simple means of assessing whether the ventilatory cost of activities is increased (see Fig. 7). An ability to complete the test is also evidence that any ventilatory impairment which the subject may have is insufficient to preclude employment. Other step tests include the Harvard pack test for physical fitness (40 cm step, 30 times per minute plus pack) [7] and the motorized step test of Nagle et al. [8] in which the height of the step is raised progressively during the test; this permits the performance of triangular exercise. Stepping exercise is used for the Masters test for coronary insufficiency (two steps each of 23 cm ascended 5 to 25 times per minute). The ability to climb stairs also provides a useful guide to the capacity for exercise.

D. Cycle Ergometry

This form of exercise lends itself to the performance of triangular or staircase exercise over a wide range of intensities in a short time. Rates of increase of 10 to 25 W/min may be used for this purpose. In addition, at any rate of external work the uptake of oxygen, while not independent of the body mass of the subject, is confined within narrow limits. The equipment is compact and fairly cheap and on account of the subject being seated it is very safe to use. However, it has the disadvantage that in many developed countries few people cycle, the cardiac frequency relative to the uptake of oxygen is higher than for walking, and, partly on this account, the maximal oxygen uptake is less than for other types of ergometry. The cycle ergometer was adopted as standard for studies in human adaptability undertaken as part of the International Biological Programme [9] ; it was at one time the only form of ergometry used for study of occupational lung disease within the European Economic Community.

E. Walking

This is the most natural form of exercise and is the basis of the clinical grades of breathlessness of Fletcher [10] (see also Sect. VI). The maximal distance which the subject can walk in 12 min is also a good guide to the capacity for exercise [11] . However, the motorized treadmill provides the best available means for measuring the capacity for exercise and it may be used submaximally to provide triangular or staircase exercise. For this purpose the speed is usually set at 80 or 67 m min^{-1} (3.0 or 2.5 mph) and the incline raised progressively from zero to 7° or 15°. However, for respiratory cripples, lower speeds down to 7 m min^{-1} (0.25 mph) may be used, while for some track athletes 270 m min^{-1} (10 mph) may be appropriate. Alternatively, for cardiovascular studies especially, use may be made of the combination of speed and incline of Bruce [12] .

F. Safety Precautions

Any form of exercise inevitably carries a slight risk but this should not be exaggerated. Reasonable medical precautions include that the performance of test exercise is preceded by a medical interview and that in subjects in whom there is a risk of myocardial ischemia or of circulatory collapse the electrocardiogram is inspected continuously and the systemic blood pressure is recorded at intervals during the test. Consecutive ventricular ectopic beats or a failure of the blood pressure to rise are indications for abandoning the test. In addition, the subject should be advised to signal the occurrence of symptoms and to discontinue in the event of these becoming material, though the occurrence of an expected angina or other habitual symptom is not of itself a necessary indication for termination. The laboratory personnel should be trained in methods of resuscitation but this is more to assist each other in the event of their being involved in an accident than on account of any danger to which they are exposing the subject. In addition, experienced medical personnel should be on close call but, except for known risk cases, need not be in the laboratory.

Gymnastic precautions include that the subject is suitably clad and shod, and is within easy reach of sturdy support rails. In the case of a treadmill the subject should be able to slow or step off the belt and be constrained from over-riding by a strap or harness. A period of practice exercise should precede the study.

Technical precautions include that the equipment should be electrically safe and mechanically guarded and secure. There should be nonreturn and blow-off valves on the gas supply system which should operate at low pressure. All pipes, electrical leads, tubes, and moveable equipment should be stowed where they cannot impede the movement of personnel or become entangled with other items. These precautions should obtain in all laboratories and not be confined to exercise!

V. Physiological Response to Exercise

In the context of occupational medicine the ventilatory component of the response to exercise is important; it may be disturbed by the respiratory hazard (Sec. VIII.A), may be affected by the consequent disease, and may contribute to the associated breathlessness (Sec. VI).

At the start of rectangular exercise the ventilation rises abruptly due to increased central drive to respiration. This phase is followed by a progressive increase which the work of Matell [13] and of Diamond et al. [14] has shown to be related to the increased production of carbon dioxide. Subsequently during moderate exercise the ventilation levels off at the steady-state value; this is a linear function of the consumption of oxygen (Fig. 3). At higher rates of work the ventilation is further increased by acidemia; this is a consequence of increased production and diffusion into the blood of lactic acid relative to its utilization and may be due to insufficient delivery of oxygen to at least some fibers in the active muscles. The place on the graph relating ventilation to consumption of oxygen where the increase in ventilation occurs (Fig. 4) is sometimes called the anaerobic threshold; it is more appropriately called Owles point after its discoverer [15] as this is a courtesy and the inflection is not necessarily related to acidemia. The linear part of the curve is best defined by its coordinates or by the ventilation at specified levels of uptake of oxygen. It is described erroneously by the ventilation equivalent ($\dot{V}_E/\dot{V}O_2$) which implies a proportionality that does not exist and it is recommended that this term be abandoned. The maximal ventilation approaches or may sometimes exceed the maximal voluntary ventilation of the subject (Chap. 6). The relationship of the ventilation to the tidal volume and of the latter to the durations of inspiration and expiration have been recorded by Kay et al. [16], among others. The results show that except at high rates of work most of the increase in ventilation is due to an increase in the tidal volume. This is accompanied by an increase in the mean inspiratory and expiratory flow rates and a shortening of the duration of expiration. The duration of inspiration usually remains constant. The exercise tidal volume is a function of the vital capacity (Table 3).

The exercise cardiac frequency is a linear function of the consumption of oxygen and during exercise, but not during the transition from rest to exercise, this is also the case for the cardiac output. The relationships like those for ventilation are best described by their coordinates or by the frequency or output at specified levels of consumption of oxygen (e.g. 45 or 67 mmol/min, 1.0 or 1.5 liters/min). However, the use of the oxygen pulse ($\dot{V}O_2/fC$) is misleading in the same way as is the ventilation equivalent and should be abandoned. The cardiac frequency is less for subjects with large or muscular hearts than with small hearts, and the frequency, especially the maximal frequency, declines with age. Reference values for the physiological response to exercise are given in Table 3.

VI. Breathlessness

Breathlessness describes the state of a subject who experiences difficult, disordered, or unduly increased breathing. During near-maximal exercise the sensation frequently determines the breaking point and hence the capacity for exercise. It is contributed to by many factors including the rate of respiratory work, the forces developed by the respiratory muscles, the pattern of breathing with respect to respiratory frequency, flow rates, and tidal volume, the end-inspiratory expansion of the chest wall, the negative pressures developed within the thorax, the extent of respiratory drive by humoral agents, and the afferent nerve traffic from receptors in the lung. Thus it is not a specific symptom and any attempt at its assessment needs to take this into account.

A. Scores of Breathlessness and Ability to Take Exercise

The breathlessness may be graded subjectively using a descriptive or analog scale [17,18] or objectively according to what the subject can or cannot do; the latter in the form of the clinical grade of breathlessness of Fletcher (a disability score) [10] is used in the British MRC questionnaire on respiratory symptoms. The author's ability score based on these grades is given in Table 4 [19]. The ability

Table 4 Clinical Grades of Breathlessness of Fletcher and the Ability Scores Proposed by Cotes for Use in Assessment of Subjects with Chronic Nonspecific Lung Disease[a]

Description	Clinical grade	Ability score	$FEV_{1.0}$
Is living: needs help with feeding	–	8	0.3
With help can dress and sit out of bed	–	7	0.5
Can converse, walk 10 m, bath with help	–	6	0.7
Can walk 100 m, sing, climb 8 stairs	–	5	1.1
Can walk 400 m	4	4	1.6
Can walk unlimited distance at slow pace	3	3	2.1
Can walk at normal pace on level ground without becoming breathless	2	2	2.6
Can hurry on level ground and walk uphill without undue breathlessness	1	1	3.1

[a]The grades are assessed using the MRC Questionnaire on respiratory symptoms where comparison is made with a healthy man of the same age. The levels of forced expiratory volume are for men aged 50–75 years from Welsh mining valleys; they are approximate and the ranges are wide. The ability to take exercise is affected adversely by age and by increasing body mass.
Source: Data from Ref. 3.

may be assessed in greater detail by extending the range of activities which is included; one example is given in Figure 5.

B. Relation to Respiratory Function and Other Variables

The objective scoring of breathlessness is difficult when the causes are imperfectly understood and alter with circumstances. The score is usually based on a variable measured during exercise. This may be the rate of respiratory work, the peak inspiratory pressure, etc. Greatest success is achieved by relating the ventilation during exercise to that during maximal ventilation at rest. This was first attempted in the form of the dyspnoeic index (DI). Thus,

$$DI(\%) = 100\,(\dot{V}E_{ex}/MBC) \qquad (2)$$

where MBC is the maximal breathing capacity measured by maximal voluntary ventilation over 15 sec at rest or calculated from the forced expiratory volume [20]. The index rises to about 100% at the breaking point of exercise in athletes and most patients with lung disease; it is rather less in unfit but otherwise healthy people and may reach 125% in some respiratory cripples.

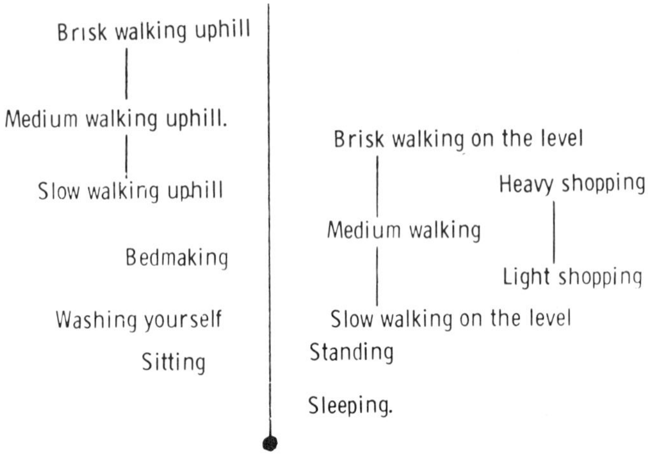

Figure 5 Oxygen-cost diagram of McGavin and colleagues [11]. The vertical line is normally 100 mm long, and the everyday activities listed are placed proportionately to their oxygen cost. Patients are asked to indicate the point above which they think their breathlessness would not let them go.

A more sophisticated version of the index may be derived from the maximal expiratory flow-volume curve. This curve defines the maximal flow rates which may be achieved during maximal ventilation at different lung volumes. In patients with disabling lung disease the resting respiratory level tends to rise during exercise; this has the effect that higher flow rates may be generated at the cost of a reduction in the tidal volume. The effect is usually beneficial, but the associated tachypnea increases the proportion of ventilation which is wasted in ventilating the physiological deadspace and this contributes to the limitation of exercise.

The relative success of the dyspneic index in quantifying breathlessness is greatest for healthy subjects and for patients with generalized diseases of the airways or the lung parenchyma. In the former patients the limitation is mainly due to the airway obstruction reducing the maximal breathing capacity while in the latter it is also due to the disease process leading to hypoxemia on exercise; this increases the chemoreceptor drive to ventilation and hence the level of ventilation during exercise. The dyspneic index is less informative in circumstances when the maximal breathing capacity changes between rest and exercise as in those patients with mitral stenosis who develop exertional pulmonary congestion. The maximal breathing capacity may also fall during exercise in asthmatics whose airway obstruction is exaggerated by exercise (exercise-induced asthma). Limitation of exercise by tachypnea in circumstances when this is probably due to stimulation of pulmonary J receptors is also poorly reflected in the dyspneic index. In coal miners with pneumoconiosis the grade of breathlessness is weakly correlated positively with the forced expiratory volume in one second (FEV_1) and negatively with the body mass (M) according to the following relationship.

$$\text{Grade} = 2.5 - 0.58\ FEV_1 + 0.025\ (M) \qquad (3)$$

Subjects whose grade of breathlessness increases have been observed in retrospect to have previously had a relatively low maximal oxygen uptake and $FEV_{1.0}$ and high exercise ventilation; the increase in breathlessness may be accompanied by a further fall in $FEV_{1.0}$, a gain in body weight, and aggravation of the score for bronchitis [21]. In these as in other respects the features resemble those in chronic lung disease with airflow obstruction.

C. Alleviation of Breathlessness

Relief of breathlessness may be effected by any means which reverses the underlying abnormality. Thus, correction of airflow obstruction by the use of bronchodilator drugs and abandoning smoking, a reduction in body weight, and an increase in the power of the respiratory muscles by appropriate training may all alleviate breathlessness and increase the capacity for exercise of the patient with occupational lung disease. In some patients including many with emphysema and with disease of the lung parenchyma the breathlessness during exercise may be reduced and the capacity for exercise increased by breathing oxygen-enriched air; away from the laboratory this may be provided by portable apparatus. However, not all patients benefit from portable oxygen, so a prior assessment should be carried out before its use is recommended. Assessment should take the form of a single- or double-blind trial in which the subject's capacity for exercise is assessed breathing air and oxygen. The assessment is best carried out using a treadmill at a rate of work which, when breathing air, the subject can only sustain for 2 min up to the onset of incapacitating breathlessness. A doubling of the walking time when breathing oxygen, together with a reduction in ventilation at 2 min compared with breathing air, is evidence of likely benefit from this form of treatment.

Exercise training is sometimes helpful for patients with lung disease but the criteria of suitability are less well established than in the case of patients with myocardial ischemia. The criteria include a grade of breathless which is out of proportion to the impairment of lung function, an exercise cardiac frequency which is high relative to the uptake of oxygen and fat-free mass of the subject, and an exercise tidal volume which is low relative to the vital capacity. Relative to the maximal breathing capacity a reduction in ability for sustained voluntary ventilation may also be an indication that the subject will benefit from training but this has still to be established by further research [22].

Summary of procedure for assessment of respiratory impairment

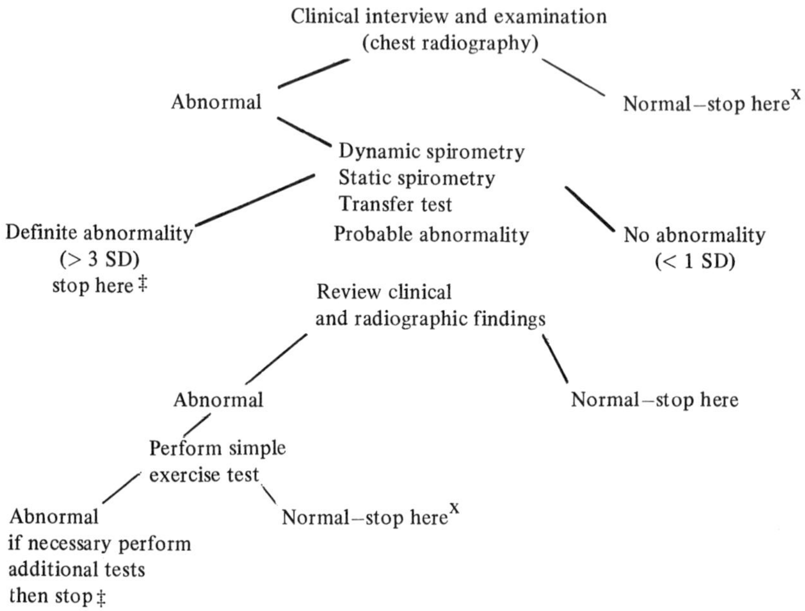

x no impairment: assessment may be repeated after 6 months
‡ decide on category of impairment

Figure 6 Schema for assessment of respiratory impairment [23].

VII. Disablement

A subject who has established lung disease of occupational origin may be disabled by the consequent changes in the lung or by the associated anxiety. The disability may be related to a claim for compensation. It may also be due to some other condition. Conversely, a subject with respiratory impairment may not be aware of disability though he or she is at risk on this account. Thus the level of insight and awareness is an important determinant which also puts a special responsibility on the investigator. Assessment of disablement is additionally difficult on account of the subject not always being prepared to collaborate wholeheartedly in the tests. In these circumstances the assessment of the capacity for exercise is seldom practical while even the measurement of the forced expiratory volume may not be reliable on account of the need for a maximal inspiratory effort preceding the forced expiration. Most subjects are willing to cooperate, especially in circumstances when the assessment may also be of value for prophylaxis or therapy. A schema for assessment is summarized in Figure 6.* Other subjects will usually cooperate and only fail to do so occasionally, a circumstance which is readily detectable. However, for a few subjects assessment is difficult because misleading results are obtained; in addition, their unreliability may not be detected. In these circumstances the tests of first choice include those which may be performed during regular breathing without respiratory gymnastics or maximal exercise. A progressive submaximal exercise test falls into this category. Criteria of reliability then include that the results are internally consistent (e.g., Fig. 2) and are compatible with the subject's ability to undertake voluntary exercise, for example in moving to or from the waiting room, laboratory, cafeteria, or parking lot. Given that the result is reliable, then an inability to double the oxygen uptake from its resting level is evidence for 100% disability [23]. Ability to develop an oxygen uptake of 60 mmol/min is evidence for ability to undertake light or moderate activity. A classification of activities in terms of their oxygen cost and ventilatory requirement is given in Fig. 7.

VIII. Exercise Performance in Occupational Lung Diseases

A. Acute Effects of Inhaling Dusts and Vapors

Small dust particles when they are inhaled stimulate mechanoreceptors in the large airways (the irritant receptors of Widdicombe [24] and in sufficient quantity cause a reflex bronchoconstriction on this account. Tobacco smoke exerts a similar effect. These agents probably also cause a reduction in the depth of breathing, but this action has not yet been studied adequately in humans. Irritants, including ammonia and CR gas, also influence exercise ventilation; low concentrations increase the depth while higher ones reduce the depth and increase the frequency of breathing. Both sets of changes are accompanied by a reduction in the ventilation minute volume relative to the consumption of oxygen [25]. A similar response probably occurs with other inhaled substances.

B. Pneumoconiosis of Coal Workers and Other Occupational Groups

Working in coal is associated with a reduced ventilatory capacity (FEV_1) and increased residual volume. The changes are due to obstruction to the lung air-

*A similar schema has been proposed by the American Lung Association/ American Thoracic Society Component Committee on disability criteria.

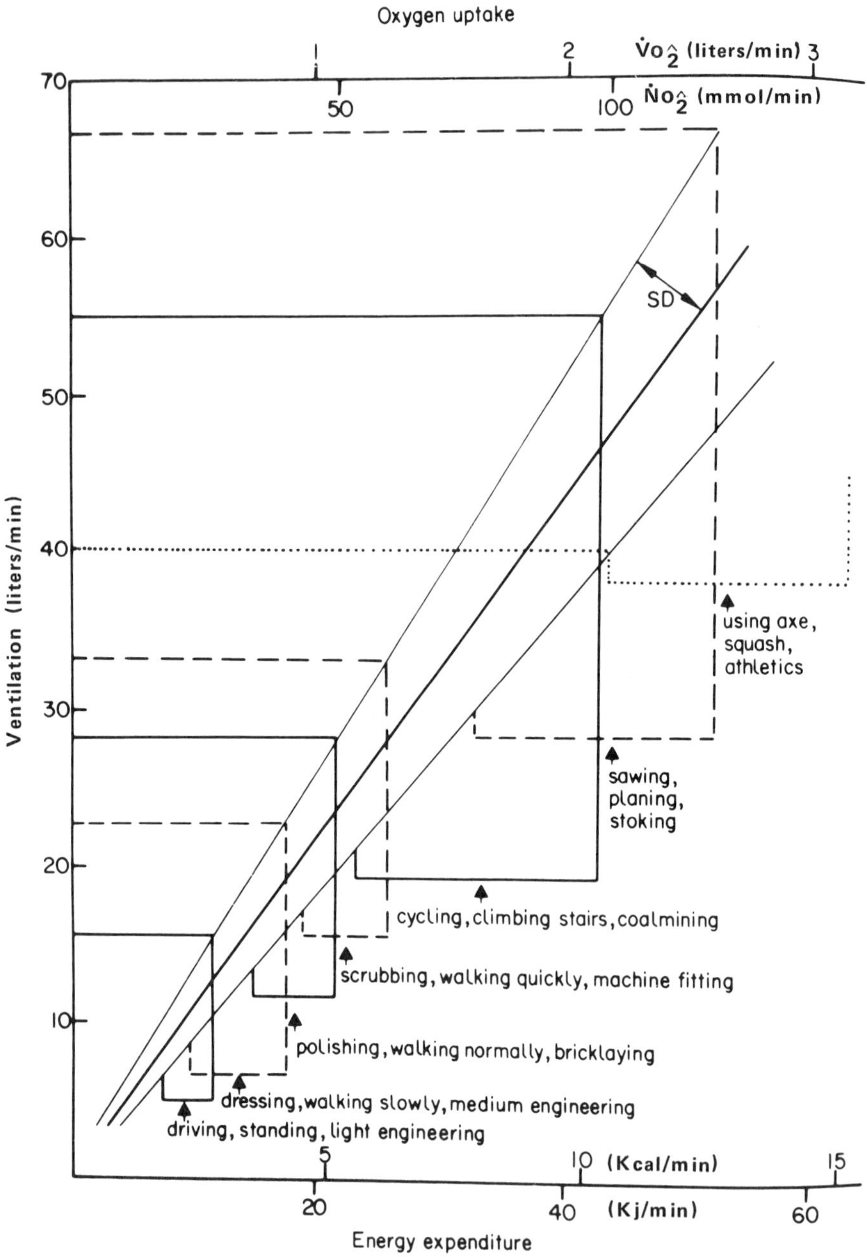

Figure 7 Average energy requirements and ventilation minute volumes of healthy men during activities of different intensity from the lightest to the most strenuous. The energy requirements of women performing the same tests are on average about 10% less but ventilatory costs are similar [3].

ways but their exact nature has not been determined. Simple pneumoconiosis usually exerts little additional effect, but some miners develop features of cystic lung with a further reduction in the ventilatory capacity, uneven distribution of ventilation and perfusion in the lung, and defective gas transfer. Progressive massive fibrosis contributes a space-occupying lesion and sometimes compensatory emphysema. The physiological response to exercise may be completely normal or there may be a reduction in the capacity for exercise. This may be accompanied by an increase in the ventilation relative to the consumption of oxygen. The increase is mainly due to enlargement of the physiological dead-space, but hypoxemia on exercise and/or functional over breathing may also contribute. The relationship of the breathing frequency to the tidal volume is usually that to be expected for the subject's vital capacity. With asbestosis a similar pattern of abnormality in the physiological response to exercise is usually observed; however, the increase in ventilation is often more marked and is linked with a transfer defect leading to progressive hypoxemia on exercise.

C. Disease of the Lung Parenchyma

In disease of the lung parenchyma, including farmer's lung and other causes of extrinsic allergic alveolitis, the changes in lung function include reductions in all subdivisions of the total lung capacity and in the transfer factor (diffusing capacity). The former change affects the exercise tidal volume which is nonetheless usually appropriate for the diminished vital capacity, while the latter is associated with progressive hypoxemia on exercise. This augments the ventilation minute volume which is then usually the principal cause of breathlessness. However, in some conditions, including beryllium disease [26] , the hyperventilation is accompanied by a greater reduction in the exercise tidal volume than would be predicted on the basis of the reduced vital capacity. This tachypnea may be due to stimulation of pulmonary J receptors. It leads to the development of symptoms in addition to breathlessness, for example anxiety which may be a consequence of the unusual pattern of breathing.

D. Physical Fitness Testing

An exercise test which is directed to the investigation of a respiratory hazard also yields information on the physical condition of the subject which may both be of use for diagnosis or treatment (see Sec. VI.C) and provide an additional reason for the exercise test being carried out. The information is contained mainly in the relationship of the cardiac frequency to the uptake of oxygen (Fig. 3) and in the maximal oxygen uptake which is normally dependent on it (Fig. 4). The physically active subject usually has a lower cardiac frequency relative to the uptake of oxygen than one who is inactive; in addition, the rate of rise of cardiac frequency at the start of exercise and the recovery afterward are more rapid. These differences form the basis for a number of tests of physical fitness, but it should be noted that in their interpretation there is a need to take into account the ambient temperature, the age, and the fat-free mass of the subjects [27,28]. In addition for subjects who habitually take exercise using the arms and back, the test exercise should preferably be of this type as the circulatory effect of training is fairly specific to the type of exercise which is performed.

The most widely used tests are of the recovery of heart rate after exercise (e.g., Harvard pack test). These tests are convenient in that apparently they only require a step and a stopwatch, but they have the disadvantage that the recovery varies with the type of exercise. In addition, the dictates of safety may require that the ECG is recorded during the test (Sec. IV.F). When this is done the procedure begins to resemble that described in Section IV.B with which it may be combined. The triangular or staircase profile of exercise is then appropriate. The cardiac frequency during the last minute of exercise is then closely correlated with the Harvard pack index [29]. The cardiac frequency at a specified oxygen uptake and standardized for fat-free mass is also a guide to the physical fitness, with the more active subjects having the lower values [30]. However, error in interpretation may arise from the subject having a medical condition which affects the cardiac frequency or being in recept of medication including steroids or β-blocking drugs.

IX. Comment

Despite its great relevance for the study of breathlessness, exercise testing is still the least used aspect of the assessment of lung function. There are a number of contributory reasons. The procedures have an undeserved reputation for being disagreeable if not dangerous, very dependent on subject cooperation, poorly reproducible, and compared with lung mechanics unsophisticated and difficult to interpret. In fact, in most respects the reverse is the case, though in the author's opinion the enthusiasm of some authorities for maximal exercise (e.g., Ref. 30) has diverted effort from developing the potential of submaximal tests; these lend themselves to serial measurements, but the tendency for cardiac frequency to be slightly higher on the first than on subsequent occasions needs to be taken into account, for example in epidemiological surveys. For these applications automatic equipment (e.g., P.K. Morgan Ltd.) now makes possible the "on-line" construction of the intermediate graphs shown in Figure 3 and the derivation of the indices of submaximal exercise which are described in this chapter. There is a strong case for using them both in the assessment of suspected occupational lung disease and with a view to learning more about the physiological responses to inhaled dust including the underlying control mechanisms in humans.

X. Appendix Abbreviations, Symbols, and Units

$\dot{V}I$, $\dot{V}E$	Inspiratory and expiratory ventilation per minute (liters/min)
$\dot{V}E_{45}$ or $\dot{V}E_{67}$	Ventilation at O_2 uptake of 45 or 67 mmol/min (1.0 or 1.5 liters/min)
VT, VD	Tidal volume and physiological dead space (liters)
VT_{30}	Tidal volume at $\dot{V}E$ = 30 liters/min
fR, fC	Respiratory and cardiac frequencies (min^{-1})
fC_{67}	Frequency at O_2 uptake of 67 mmol/min
t_I, t_E	Times of inspiration and expiration(s)
t_{tot}	Total breath durations
$\overline{\dot{V}I}$ and $\overline{\dot{V}E}$	Mean inspiratory and expiratory flow rates. For example: $\dot{V}I \div t_I$ or t_E (liters/min)
FI_{O_2} and FI_{CO_2}	Fractional concentrations of oxygen and carbon dioxide in inspired gas
FE_{O_2} and FE_{CO_2}	Fractional concentrations of oxygen and carbon dioxide in expired gas
$\dot{N}O_2$ and $\dot{N}CO_2$	Uptake of oxygen and evolution of carbon dioxide (mmol/min)
$\dot{V}O_2$ and $\dot{V}CO_2$	Uptake of oxygen and evolution of carbon dioxide (liters/min)
R	Respiratory exchange ratios ($\dot{N}CO_2/\dot{N}O_2$)
Q_t	Cardiac output (liters/min)
SV	Stroke volume (liters)
FFM	Fat free mass (kg)
M	Body mass (kg)
Fat(%)	Percentage of body mass which is fat.
SCO_2	Respiratory sensitivity to CO_2 (mmol min^{-1} kPa^{-1})
WR	Work rate (watts)
VC	Vital capacity

Acknowledgments

The author is indebted to Blackwell Scientific Publications, Oxford, for permission to reproduce from his book *Lung Function: Assessment and Application in Medicine,* 4th Ed., 1979, Figures 1, 2, 3, 4, and 7. The book is also the source of information given in Tables 1, 2, 3, and 4 and should be consulted for further details. Figure 5 is reproduced by kind permission of Dr. C. R. McGavin and the *British Medical Journal.*

References

1. International Labour Organisation, Respiratory function tests in pneumoconioses. Occupational Safety and Health Series No. 6, Geneva, 1966.
2. Farhi, L. E., M. S. Nesarajah, A. J. Olszowka, L. A. Metildi, and A. K. Ellis, Cardiac output determination by simple one-step rebreathing technique, *Respir. Physiol.,* **28**:141–159 (1976).
3. Cotes, J. E., *Lung Function: Assessment and Application in Medicine,* 4th ed. Blackwell Scientific, Oxford, 1979.
4. Cotes, J. E., Response to progressive exercise: A three-index test, *Br. J. Dis. Chest,* **66**:169–184 (1972).
5. Baldwin, E. deF., A. Cournand, and D. W. Richards, Jr., Pulmonary insufficiency. I. Physiological classification, clinical methods of analysis, standard values in normal subjects, *Medicine (Baltimore),* **27**:243–278 (1948).
6. Hugh-Jones, P., and A. V. Lambert, A simple standard exercise test and its use for measuring exertion dyspnoea, *Br. Med. J.,* **1**:65–71 (1952).
7. Sloan, A. W., The Harvard step test of dynamic fitness, *Triangle* (En.), **5**: 358–363 (1962).
8. Nagle, F. J., B. Balke, and J. P. Naughton, Gradational step tests for assessing work capacity, *J. Appl. Physiol.,* **20**:745–748 (1965).
9. Weiner, J. S., and J. A. Lourie, *Human Biology: A Guide to Field Methods.* Oxford, Blackwell Scientific, 1969.
10. Fletcher, C. M., The clinical diagnosis of pulmonary emphysema—an experimental study, *Proc. R. Soc. Med.,* **45**:577–584 (1952).
11. McGavin, C. R., M. Artvinli, H. Nade, and G. J. R. McHardy, Dyspnoea, disability, and distance walked: Comparison of estimates of exercise performance in respiratory disease, *Br. Med. J.,* **2**:241–243 (1978).
12. Bruce, R. A., F. Kusumi, and D. Hosmer. Maximal oxygen intake and nomographic assessment of functional aortic impairment in cardiovascular disease, *Am. Heart J.,* **85**:546–562 (1973).
13. Matell, G., Time courses of changes in ventilation and arterial gas tensions in man induced by moderate exercise, *Acta Physiol. Scand.* (Suppl.), **58**: 206 (1963).
14. Diamond, L. B., R. Casaburi, K. Wasserman, and B. J. Whipp, Kinetics of gas exchange and ventilation in transition from rest or prior exercise, *J. Appl. Physiol.,* **43**:704–708 (1977).

15. Owles, W. H., Alteration in lactic acid content of the blood as a result of light exercise, and associated changes in the CO_2 combining power of the blood and in the alveolar CO_2 pressure, *J. Physiol. (Lond.)*, **69**:214–237 (1930).
16. Kay, J. D. S., E. S. Petersen, and H. Vejby-Christensen, Mean and breath-by-breath pattern of breathing in man during steady-state exercise, *J. Physiol. (Lond.)*, **251**:657–669 (1975).
17. Borg, G., Relative response and stimulus scales. Reports from the Institute of Applied Psychology, University of Stockholm, No. 1 (1970).
18. Aitken, R. C. B., Measurement of feelings using visual analog scales, *Proc. R. Soc. Med.*, **62**:989–993 (1969).
19. Cotes, J. E., Assessment of disablement due to impaired respiratory function, *Bull. Physiopathol. Respir.*, **11**:210P–217P (1975).
20. McKerrow, C. B., M. McDermott, and J. C. Gilson, A spirometer for measuring the forced expiratory volume with a simple calibrating device, *Lancet*, **1**:149–151 (1960).
21. Musk, A. W., C. Bevan, M. J. Campbell, and J. E. Cotes, Factors contributing to the clinical grade of breathlessness in coalworkers with pneumoconiosis, *Bull. Eur. Physiopathol. Respir.*, **15**:343–355 (1979).
22. Peress, L., P. McLean, C. R. Woolf, and N. Zamel, Ventilatory muscle training in obstructive lung disease, *Bull. Eur. Physiopathol. Respir.*, **15**:91–92 (1979).
23. De Coster, A., Évaluation du déficit respiratoire et du handicap, *Bull. Physiopathol. Respir.*, **14**:59–64P (1978).
24. Widdicombe, J. G., Reflexes from the lungs in the control of breathing. In *Recent Advances in Physiology*, 9th Ed. Edited by R. J. Linden, Churchill, Edinburgh, Livingstone, 1974, pp. 239–278.
25. Cole, T. J., J. E. Cotes, G. R. Johnson, H. de V. Martin, J. W. Reed, and M. J. Saunders, Ventilation, cardiac frequency and pattern of breathing during exercise in men exposed to O-chlorobenzylidene malononitrile (CS) and ammonia gas in low concentrations, *Q. J. Exp. Physiol.*, **62**: 341–351 (1977).
26. Cotes, J. E., G. R. Johnson, and A. McDonald, Breathing frequency and tidal volume: Relationship to breathlessness. In *Breathing: Hering-Breuer Centenary Symposium. A Ciba Foundation Symposium.* Edited by R. Porter. London, Churchill, 1970, pp. 297–314.
27. Cotes, J. E., G. Berry, L. Burkinshaw, C. T. M. Davies, A. M. Hall, P. R. M. Jones, and A. V. Knibbs, Cardiac frequency during submaximal exercise in young adults; relation to lean body mass, total body potassium and amount of leg muscle, *Q. J. Exp. Physiol.*, **58**:239–250 (1973).
28. Cotes, J. E., A. M. Hall, G. R. Johnson, P. R. M. Jones, and A. V. Knibbs, Decline with age of cardiac frequency during submaximal exercise in healthy women, *J. Physiol. (Lond.)*, **238**:24P–25P (1974).
29. Cotes, J. E., C. Dicken, D. L. Evans, G. R. Johnson, E. B. Kalinowska, I. M. MacIntyre, and M. J. Saunders, Prediction of Harvard pack index from the result of an 11 min progressive exercise test and anthropometric measurements in coal miners, *Ergonomics*, **22**:1353–1361 (1979).
30. Andersen, K. L., R. J. Shephard, H. Denolin, E. Varnauskas, R. Masironi, F. H. Bonjer, J. Rutenfranz, and Z. Fejfar, *Fundamentals of Exercise Testing*. Geneva, World Health Organisation, 1971.

7

Contribution of Immunologic Techniques to Current Understanding of Occupational Lung Disease

MERLIN R. WILSON, REYNOLD M. KARR, and JOHN E. SALVAGGIO

Tulane University School of Medicine
New Orleans, Louisiana

I. Introduction

Recent advancements in immunological technology have allowed occupational lung diseases to be studied from a new and different aspect. The application of immunological testing to workers with occupational asthma, hypersensitivity pneumonitis, and fibrotic pulmonary disease secondary to silica and asbestos exposure have allowed immunological mechanisms to be suggested in the pathogenesis of these diseases. Modern techniques have identified several types of allergic tissue injury [1] which are important in the pathogenesis of occupational lung disease. For example, in many types of occupational asthma, immediate-type hypersensitivity responses (type I) mediated by IgE antibodies which produce the release of mediators from tissue basophils and mast cells may be the immunological event that is important. However, the mechanisms operative in other types of occupational asthma such as that secondary to toluene diisocyanate (TDI) vapor inhalation are still not clear and may involve altered β-adrenergic activity in the absence of an underlying primary immunological aberration. It has been suggested that immune complex (type III) and cell-mediated (type IV) responses may be the most important types of allergic tissue injury in patients with hypersensitivity pneumonitis due to inhalation of biological dust such as that observed in farmer's lung and pigeon-breeder's disease. Finally, the pulmonary fibrosis seen in patients with silicosis and asbestosis may be in part the end of a smoldering inflammatory response caused by activation of certain serum proteins such as the complement system to produce tissue injury or by mediators released from macrophages through immunological means which ultimately affect the function of fibroblast and produce collagen deposition. It is possible that the inflammatory response could be the result of the direct effects of the particles on various alveolar cell types. Therefore, the data of most studies of patients with occupational lung disease indicate there are several types of immune mechanisms which ultimately result in tissue injury.

In this chapter, we will discuss some of the immunological techniques currently used to evaluate individuals with occupational lung disease and illustrate, when possible, how these techniques have been employed in the diagnosis and pathogenesis of these lung diseases.

II. Skin Testing

The immediate-type (type I) sensitivity skin reaction is mediated by reagin or skin-sensitizing antibody, IgE [2]. Immediate-type skin reactivity depends on exposure of sensitized individuals to small amounts of antigen. There are basically two techniques for this type of skin testing, the prick and the intradermal test. In prick testing, a drop of antigen in solution (1:10 weight/volume) is placed on the subject's back or the volar surface of the forearm. The skin is gently pricked through the solution with a needle, and observed approximately 20 min for the development of a wheal and erythema reaction. The advantages of this assay are that it can be performed rapidly with crude antigen and with little risk to the patient. Since minute amounts of antigen are employed and can be wiped from the skin, the possibility of an untoward reaction is small. The method is easily performed and large study populations can be rapidly screened. A disadvantage of prick testing is that its sensitivity is less than that of intradermal testing.

In the intradermal test, the antigen solution is injected by needle into the superficial layers of the skin. Since there is a risk of a systemic reaction with this technique, a very dilute solution of antigen is employed (usually 100- to 1000-fold less concentrated than that of the prick test. In practice, for purposes of safety, the prick test is performed first and an intradermal test is performed only if the prick test is negative.

In selecting the proper dilution of a suspected occupational antigen to be employed, the antigen should first be evaluated by prick and intradermal testing in a nonatopic control group to determine the irritant threshold. If the prick test is negative using a 1:10 weight/volume solution of antigen, 1 million fold dilutions can be injected intradermally, and progressive increase in dosage at logarithmic increments being administered every 20 min until a positive reaction occurs or the threshold irritant level reached.

Immediate pricked intradermal reactions can be graded by many methods. Among these are a semiquantitative method employing a negative to 4-plus gradation. In this scheme a 4-plus reaction is generally characterized by greater than 40 mm of erythema and a weal greater than 15 mm with pseudopod formation. A 3-plus reaction consists of 31–40 mm of erythema and weal of 10-15 mm without pseudopod formation. In a 2-plus reaction, the erythema is 21-30 mm and 5-10 weal, and 1-plus reactions are characterized by 11-20 mm and a 2-10 mm weal. Other methods of grading, perhaps more accurate in nature, stress only weal size and discount erythema, considering the importance of the axon reflex in developing erythema and the evanescence of this component. Epinephrine, aminophylline, and antihistamine may interfere with the expression of positive weal and erythema reactions. However, corticosteroids have no effect on these reactions.

Immediate-type skin tests have been beneficial in studying workers with occupational asthma associated with exposure to certain antigens. Of most importance is the use of these tests in preemployment screening of prospective workers both for atopic status and if an appropriate antigen is available, for evidence of preexisting or work-associated sensitization.

Immediate skin tests are also of great importance in studying the pathogenesis of certain types of occupational airway diseases as well as in performing large epidemiological surveys designed to detect susceptible populations or diagnose overt occupational airway disease. There are, however, limitations to the usefulness of immediate skin tests. For example, in studies of individuals sensitized to previously encountered antigens via the respiratory tract route, positive weal-and-flare skin tests develop initially, followed in weeks or months by symptoms, and finally by demonstrable circulating IgE antibody. After cessation of exposure the level of circulating IgE antibody decreases rapidly, but skin reactivity persists. Thus, a positive weal-and-flare skin reaction may be noted in (1) the presence of past allergic disease, (2) the presence of current allergic disease, or (3) the absence of overt disease but with potential to develop clinically manifest disease at some future time.

Table 1 outlines the industrial material and the industry in which skin testing has been valuable in determining the relevant antigen. Pepys and coworkers have reported positive skin testing to enzymes to *Bacillus subtilis* in factory workers employed in the detergent industry [3]. These investigators have also used skin testing to show the reactivity of workers in the metal refining industry to complex salts of platinum [4]. Karr and associates have also utilized skin testing to identify important antigens in coffee worker's asthma [5]. Therefore,

Table 1 Types of Occupational Asthma in which Skin Tests Have Been Used to Determine the Probable Etiology

Industry	Industrial material	Reference
Veterinarians, animal and poultry breeders, laboratory workers, fishing	Animal, bird, fish, and insect serum, dander and secretions	6,7
Castor bean	Oil and food industry	8
Enzymes of *B. subtilis*	Detergent industry	3
Green coffee bean	Coffee	5
Hog trypsin	Plastics, rubber, and resin industry	9
Complex salts of platinum	Metal refining	4
Flour	Bakers, farmers	10
Grain	Grain elevator operators	11
Wood dusts	Wood mills, carpenters	12
Vegetable gums (*Acacia karaya*)	Printers	13

immediate skin testing has been useful in determining relevant antigens in asthma associated with several occupations. If possible, positive weal and erythema responses to an antigen should be confirmed by Prausnitz-Küstner's passive serum transfer test for serum reaginic activity. This has been done in several reported studies to confirm the presence of reagin [4,9,13]. Also, the radioallergosorbent test (RAST, see below) has been used by certain investigators to demonstrate specific IgE in the serum of exposed workers [5,8].

The delayed hypersensitivity skin reaction is important in the evaluation of the cellular immune response of an individual. Tuberculin reactivity is considered to be the classic example of a delayed-type reaction. This assay is generally performed by injecting 0.1 ml of antigen solution intracutaneously. The results are recorded at 24, 48, and 72 hr in terms of millimeters of induration and erythema. Greater than 5 mm or more of induration at the test site 48 hr after injection of the test antigen is considered a positive reaction.

Most investigators use a panel of five or six antigens to evaluate the cellular immune competence of a subject. The most common antigens used are candida, coccidiodin, streptokinase-streptodornase (SK/SD), trichophyton, and purified protein derivative of tuberculin (PPD). The panel of antigens, and concentrations employed in our clinical immunology laboratory are listed on the next page.

More than 90% of the normal population will show a positive response to two or more antigens if a panel of antigens is employed. Thus, delayed-skin testing is useful in evaluating a study population for an intact cellular immune system.

Antigen	Trade Name	Strength: Inter-mediate	Strength: Secondary	Source
Candida	Dermatophytin 0	1:100	1:10	Hollister-Stier Laboratories, Spokane, Washington
Cocci	Coccidioidin	1:100	1:10	Cutter Laboratories, Berkeley, California
PPD	PPD (stabilized	2 μg/ml	50 μg/ml	Connaught Medical Research Laboratories, Toronto, California
SK-SD	Varidase	40 U/10 U	400 U/100 U	Lederle Laboratories, American Cyanamid Company, Pearl River, New York
Tricho-	Dermatophytin	1:30	–	Hollister-Stier Laboratories, Spokane, Washington

In certain types of occupational lung disease, skin testing may be useful if a relevant antigen could be determined. For example, in asthma induced by toluene diisocyanate fumes, the skin testing of individuals exposed to TDI with a protein-hapten conjugate of this antigen has not been reliable in determining which individuals may be sensitive to TDI [14]. Although it is possible that this type of asthma may not be immunologically mediated, it is also possible that investigators have been unable to conjugate TDI to the proper protein to reveal the important antigenic determinants.

III. Radioallergosorbent Test (RAST)

The radioallergosorbent test (RAST) is a solid-phase radioimmunoassay employed for the serological determination of specific IgE antibody. In the RAST, the antigen is usually coupled to a cyanogen bromide-activated insoluble carbohydrate matrices, paper disks, or the walls of polystyrene tubes. The basic principle of the RAST is simple. The antigen-coated particles are incubated with the patient's serum. All classes of antibody, including IgE, will bind to the antigen during this phase of the reaction. The antigen-antibody-coated particles are washed, and a second incubation step is performed with highly purified radiolabeled anti-IgE antibody. The amount of radioactivity bound to the particle is directly related to the amount of IgE in the patient's serum which is specific for the test antigen.

The results of RAST compare favorably to clinical information obtained by immediate-type weal and erythema skin test response. False positive RAST may result when complex allergens are employed which may nonspecifically bind IgE. Therefore, it is important to include appropriate controls in each assay to determine the amount of IgE which nonspecifically binds. Perhaps the main disadvantage of the RAST, when compared to skin test, is that RAST are more expensive because of the need to have specialized equipment to measure radioactivity. Also, most investigators agree that the RAST is less sensitive than skin testing since an individual may have a positive skin test to an antigen, but no detectable specific IgE in the serum by RAST.

Among the major advantages of the RAST are its usefulness in studying the specific IgE immune response of workers to certain antigens. A standard RAST, in this setting, has the advantages of being more easily quantitated and reproducible than skin testing. It is frequently difficult and expensive to gather workers at a convenient time to perform skin testing. However, a serum sample can be obtained, mailed, stored, and tested under controlled conditions. Thus, RAST allows the sera of various study populations to be evaluated by use of serum banks.

The RAST has been useful in the study of occupational asthma associated with various occupational materials. Specific IgE antibodies to enzymes from *B. subtilis* have been detected in the sera of workers in the detergent industry [3]. Zeiss and associates have demonstrated specific IgE antibody to trimellitc anhydride (TMA) conjugate in the sera of workers in the plastics industry [15]. These investigators attached the antigen to polystyrene tubes rather than paper disks. In a study of coffee worker's asthma, Karr and co-workers [5] demonstrated positive RAST using crude extract of green coffee bean and castor bean as antigens. Therefore, by using RAST, these investigators have demonstrated a specific IgE response to antigens present in the worker's environment.

The standard RAST can be modified to give additional information about antigens present in a worker's environment. The RAST may be inhibited by absorbing the specific IgE from a standard reference serum with free antigen. If performed at antigen-antibody equivalence, this will render the serum devoid of detectable specific IgE using the solid-phase antigen. This is the basis for the RAST inhibition assay which is currently used clinically to standardize certain allergenic extracts. Lehrer and associates have adapted this assay to study dust samples from coffee bean sacks to which workers were exposed. They demonstrated that certain sacks were contaminated with castor bean antigen which probably contributed to the asthma described in these workers [5].

IV. Immunodiffusion and Immunoelectrophoresis

The double immunodiffusion method of Ouchterlony is an assay which allows for direct identification of antigen in unknown samples by comparison with known antigens. Also, it permits comparison of unknown antibody with known antibody [16]. Usually, in this assay, a Petri dish is coated with 1% agar in a buffered solution. The buffer solution will vary according to the antigen-antibody system that this assay is used to detect. Frequently, several buffer systems must be tried to achieve optimal precipitin lines. A center well and six circumferential wells are cut in the agar equal distances apart. In most instances, when this assay is used to detect antibodies in a patient's sera, the antigen is placed in the center well and the sera to be tested are placed in the circumferential wells. Also, reference sera are placed in the outer wells. The antigen and sera are allowed to diffuse toward each other. If precipitating antibody is present in a subject's serum, a precipitin line will form between the center and outer wells. If the patient's sera is compared to control reference sera in an adjacent well, one of three types of precipitin lines may form; lines of complete identity, partial identity, or nonidentity. If the precipitin line of the unknown serum fuses with the precipitin line of the reference serum in the adjacent well, this is a line of complete identity and indicates antibodies from both reference and unknown sera recognize the same antigenic determinants. If the precipitin line of the unknown serum forms a spur with the reference precipitin line, this is a line of partial identity, and demonstrates that some antibodies from the unknown and the reference sera have common specificities, but other antibodies in these sera recognized different antigenic determinants. If the precipitin lines of the unknown and reference sera cross, these are lines of nonidentity and indicate different antigenic determinants are recognized by antibodies from these sera.

The double immunodiffusion assay has been used by several investigators to demonstrate antibody in the sera of subjects exposed to various antigens which are important in occupational pulmonary disease. A good example of the usefulness of this assay is in the determination of precipitins in the sera of patients with hypersensitivity pneumonitis. In this assay, the thermophilic actinomycetes antigen is placed in the center well of the Ouchterlony plate. The patient's serum and a reference serum are placed in the outer well. The plates are allowed to develop in a moist chamber. Precipitin line(s) will form between the antigen and sera wells if the patient's serum contains precipitins to the thermophilic actinomycetes antigen. Most subjects with hypersensitivity pneumonitis demonstrate serum antibodies which specifically precipitate with the offending organic dust or animal protein antigen. For example, approximately 90% of patients with farmer's lung have precipitating antibodies in their serum to thermophilic actinomycetes, 87% are to *Micropolyspora faeni* and 3% to other species [17]. Poorly standardized crude extracts of actinomycetes species, certain true fungi, organic dust, and avian protein are commercially available for patient screening. Unfortunately, the diagnostic usefulness of this test is somewhat in doubt because serum precipitin may be found in normal subjects who have been exposed to moldy hay. Of normal farmers who have been exposed to moldy hay, 18% demonstrated serum precipitins to hay antigen [17]. Also, 40% of subjects exposed to pigeon droppings have serum precipitin to pigeon protein but no evidence of disease. A false negative test may occur if a certain batch of antigen extract is not sufficiently potent to give precipitin lines. Other limitations to the gel immunodiffusion test include improper antigen-antibody combining ratios. If antigen concentration is too high or too low, the precipitin line may not occur between the wells. Therefore, it is important to test sera with various antigen concentrations until optimal precipitin lines are obtained.

Since commercial antigen preparations are poorly standardized, it is important in any case of hypersensitivity pneumonitis to check the suspected organic dust for antigenic activity by double immunodiffusion using the patient's serum, a positive reference serum, and a negative control from an unexposed subject. If the patient's serum demonstrates precipitins, the crude dust extract can be presumed to contain the offending antigen and further precipitin tests can be performed with purified antigenic components of the dust. Occasionally, it may be useful to prepare cultures from suspected antigen sources in order to identify possible etiologic microorganisms and to develop a source for preparation of diagnostic antigens for immunodiffusions. Overall, it should be stressed that precipitins against organic dusts are found in many exposed individuals without overt disease and that a positive precipitin test must be interpreted in the light of clinical symptoms in establishing a diagnosis.

Another useful technique commonly employed in the evaluation of patients with occupational pulmonary disease is immunoelectrophoresis. The basic principle of this assay is to separate proteins by their electrophoretic mobility. A uniform electric field is used to segregate each protein by its net electric charge. At the given pH, the net charge of a protein molecule, and, therefore, the electrophoretic mobility, depends on the content of amino acid with ionizable side chains. At its isoelectric point, the molecule has no electrophoretic mobility and will remain at the point of origin. In routine electrophoresis of serum, the pH of the buffer is chosen so that all molecules will be negatively charged (alkaline buffer pH 8.0–9.0) and will all move to the positive pole. The protein having the highest mobility will be prealbumin and albumin and the lowest will be gammaglobulin.

Immunoelectrophoresis is a method that combines the principles of zone electrophoresis with antigen-antibody reactions in gel in a two-step procedure. In the first step, the protein is separated by zone electrophoresis in a supporting medium such as agar, agarose, or cellulose acetate. In the second step, groups of proteins separated by their electrophoretic mobility are analyzed with specific antisera to allow development of arcs of precipitation. For this purpose, a long narrow trough is cut parallel to the direction of electrophoretic separation. The trough is filled with antibody solution. The antigens and antibody diffuse toward each other, and precipitin lines appear as ellipsoid arcs.

One of the basic uses of immunoelectrophoresis by investigators has been to separate and identify antigens in a complex mixture. An excellent example of this is the use of immunoelectrophoresis in the separation of the antigenic components of *M. faeni.* The eight major antigenic components of *M. faeni,* the most important source of actinomycetes antigen in moldy hay, have been studied by immunoelectrophoreses and labeled according to their electrophoretic mobility [18]. Purification and immunochemical analysis has lead to partial characterization. Antigen 1, the major precipitin line in the "C" region, is a heat-stable (100°C) glycopeptide with an average Mw of 85,000 and is associated with the mycelial cell wall. Antigen 2, the major precipitin line in the "A" region, is a heat-labile protein with a Mw of 44,000 demonstrating chymotrypsin-like activity. Antigen 3, the major precipitin line in the "B" region, is a heat labile protein with a Mw of 77,000 with demonstrable enzymatic activity. Antigen 4, a fast anodally migrating line, is a heat-labile protein with high sugar content and a Mw of 101,000.

Another application of the immunoelectrophoretic assay has been to study and characterize proteins derived from feathers, serum, and excrement of several avian species that have been shown to produce hypersensitivity pneumonitis in patient's exposed to these proteins. Antigens contained in pigeon serum and droppings are known to cause disease in sensitized subjects [19] and have been extensively studied [20]. These analyses were performed on a soluble, non-dialyzable pigeon extract (PDE). After immunoelectrophoresis of this material, four dominant precipitin arcs were observed and labeled serially PDE 1 through 4, with increasing mobility. Thus, immunoelectrophoresis has been used to separate and characterize antigens important in hypersensitivity pneumonitis by their electrophoretic mobility.

V. Cellular Assays

Cell-mediated immunity (CMI) can currently be evaluated by several methods. An in vivo method, the delayed-hypersensitivity skin test, has previously been discussed in this chapter. A variety of in vitro assays of CMI have been developed since it was discovered that phytohemagglutinin (PHA) transformed small lymphocytes into proliferating lymphoblasts in tissue culture [21]. Since then, mitogen-induced lymphocyte transformation has become a useful experimental tool and currently is used to define immune defects in clinical diseases.

Briefly, this assay is performed usually be separation of lymphocytes from whole blood on Ficoll-Hypaque gradients [22]. There are, however, several other methods for lymphocyte separation such as cell separators or filtration on sterile glass bead or nylon colums. The lymphocytes are placed in a tissue culture medium where the cells can be stimulated by mitogens such as phytohemagglutinin, conconavalin A, or pokeweed mitogen. Also, they can be stimulated by antigens such as candida, or other suspected antigens which may be of interest. The amount of DNA synthesis is measured by the incorporation of radioactively labeled thymidine, a precursor of DNA synthesis, into the cells during stimulation. Two to four days of incubation is necessary to detect optimal DNA synthesis in response to mitogens, and 4.5 to 7 days of incubation is for optimal lymphocyte reactions to antigens. This assay is quantitative and a very sensitive indicator of antigen or mitogen stimulation of lymphocytes.

In addition to lymphocyte transformation, in vitro assays of mediator production are also important in assessing CMI. Sensitized lymphocytes, when activated by mitogen, produce soluble factors which are known as lymphokines. Numerous lymphokines have been described and are listed below. One lymphokine, macrophage migration inhibitory factor (MIF), has been extensively studied in certain types of occupational lung disease. This factor is produced by activated lymphocytes and retards the migration of macrophages from capillary tubes.

Cellular assays have been very useful in determining immunological mechanism which may be important in occupational lung diseases. One disease studied most thoroughly by cellular methods is the hypersensitivity pneumonitis seen in patients with farmer's lung or pigeon-breeder's disease. Since the histopathology of hypersensitivity pneumonitis resembles cell-mediated type IV hypersensitivity, recent efforts have been focused on defining a possible contribution of CMI in the pathogenesis of this disease. For example, in studies of patients with pigeon-breeder's disease, in vitro avian antigen stimulation of peripheral blood lymphocytes derived from symptomatic subjects but not from

Lymphokines
Macrophage migration inhibitory factor (MIF)
Macrophage activating factor (MAF)
Macrophage aggregation factor
Chemotactic factors for macrophages, leukocytes, eosinophils, and basophils
Leukocyte inhibitory factor (LIF)
Mitogenic factors for lymphocytes
Factors enhancing antibody formation
Factors suppressing antibody formation (SIRS)
Cytotoxic factors–lymphotoxin (LT)
Osteoclastic factor (OAF)
Colony-stimulating factor

asymptomatic exposed individuals supported a role of type IV hypersensitivity reaction [23]. This finding has been shown to correlate with disease activity but has also been noted in some exposed subjects without overt disease [24]. Other human studies have demonstrated that peripheral blood lymphocytes stimulated by avian protein produce MIF. This phenomenon occurs in most symptomatic patients, but not in asymptomatic exposed subjects [25]. These data suggest that CMI is an important mechanism in the pathogenesis of this disease.

In addition to studies of peripheral blood lymphocytes, currently investigators are studying the possibility that a local organ-restricted immune mechanism may be important in the lung. Several techniques have been described to study bronchoalveolar wash cells from patients with occupational lung diseases. For example, it has been reported that bronchoalveolar cells from a patient with pigeon-breeder's disease transformed and produced MIF in response to pigeon antigen, while peripheral blood lymphoid cells taken concurrently from the same subject demonstrated no reactivity to the same antigen [26]. In another study of bronchoalveolar washings in hypersensitivity pneumonitis, Reynolds and co-workers [27] found a higher proportion of lymphocytes, higher IgE and IgM levels, and higher T/B cell ratios than in washings from controls. Thus, studies of cells obtained from bronchoalveolar washing of patients with hypersensitivity pneumonitis have revealed different cellular ratios and different reactivity to antigens than peripheral blood lymphocytes taken from the same patients. This type of approach may be rewarding in determining if local immunological reactivity of the lung is important in the pathogenesis of certain types of occupational lung disease.

The importance of the bronchopulmonary macrophage in the etiology of hypersensitivity pneumonitis is strongly suggested by the pulmonary histopathology after exposure of humans and experimental animals to actinomycetes antigen. The pulmonary infiltrates are predominently mononuclear and characteristically granulomatous with a number of alveolar wash cells increasing to approximately three times normal. Macrophage migration inhibition production by *M. faeni*-sensitized bronchopulmonary lymphocytes provide the only direct evidence supporting a role of delayed hypersensitivity and macrophage involvement in disease pathology. On the other hand, more conclusive evidence for such a role was obtained by monitoring directly the physiological function of actinomycetes-exposed bronchopulmonary macrophages in correlating their immunological activity with the pathogenesis of disease. It is known that macrophage activation or the enhanced ability to phagocytize nonspecifically and kill microorganisms reflects increased hydrolytic enzyme formation and represents a sensitive in vitro measure of cellular physiological activity that often occurs in association with antigen-specific cell-mediated immunity. Studies of alveolar macrophage activation in animals inoculated with actinomycetes antigen has indeed demonstrated marked activation up to several weeks after initiation of immunization. Of great importance is the fact that this bronchopulmonary macrophage activation is capable of specific recall in actinomycetes-sensitized animals receiving a booster injection of antigen that did not activate normal wash cells. This recall of bronchopulmonary macrophage activation is also accompanied by a marked migration of mononuclear cells into the lung and a return of positive delayed skin reaction upon intradermal injection of actinomycetes antigen. These observations are important in that they confirm the occurrence of immunologically activated bronchopulmonary macrophages in animals inoculated via the respiratory tract route with actinomycetes antigen and they suggest a correlation between macrophage activation and histopathology.

Although several hypotheses have been proposed to define the etiology of hypersensitivity pneumonitis, these findings would argue against a nonspecific induction of disease and would favor the importance of cellular immunological involvement. For example, it is known that there is an initial polymorphonuclear cell migration into the lung after respiratory tract inoculation with actinomycetes antigen. Although it is conceivable that acute inflammation could nonspecifically lead to activation of mononuclear phagocytes, the abovementioned recall data favor an alternative immunological mechanism of action. The recall in previously immunized animals of macrophage activation, mononuclear infiltration, and pulmonary pathology with doses of actinomycetes antigen that do not produce any of these alterations in unimmunized animals clearly suggest an immune mechanism in disease pathogenesis. Briefly, it might be hypothesized that T-cell sensitization to actinomycetes antigen occurs after exposure via the respiratory tract route. This would result in the release of chemical mediators that activate the bronchopulmonary macrophage. It is further possible that enzyme activation and release would cleave the third and fifth components of the complement system generating split products that have chemotactic activity for macrophages. Thus, a continuing chemotactic stimulus and an accumulation of mononuclear phagocytes would ultimately produce a granuloma. Throughout this proposed model of disease pathogenesis the activated macrophage would play an interoral role and therefore would represent an important factor in disease management. This all-inclusive hypothesis would involve the activation of macrophages by such diverse agents as lymphokines, perhaps antigen antibody complexes, and perhaps nonspecific events including the presence of endotoxins and related material in organic dust.

The cellular immunity of patients with silicosis has been assessed with various in vitro and in vivo cellular assays [28]. Skin tests for delayed hypersensitivity, peripheral blood T- and B-cell quantitation, and lymphocyte transformation with pokeweed mitogen and phytohemagglutinin were all comparable to control group values; however, lymphocyte transformation with low-dose concanavalin A was diminished from control group values. These investigators have also demonstrated impaired lymphocyte MIF production following stimulation with specific antigens such as SK/SD. A cellular influence is also suggested by the finding of increased numbers of type II alveolar cells in bronchial lavage fluid from affected subjects. Continued search for a defect in cellular, specifically in T-cell regulatory function, may provide further clues to the complex interrelationship between silica, autoantibodies, immune complexes, and interstitial pulmonary fibrosis in patients with silicosis.

VI. Complement

The complement system is a multiprotein sequence which when activated is a major mediator of tissue injury. The sequence can be activated via proteins of the classic or alternative pathways. The activation of the classical pathway, C1, C4, and C2, can be initiated by antigen-antibody complexes. The classic pathway C3 convertase, $\overline{C42}$, cleaves C3 to C3a and C3b which activates C5. This results in the generation of the C5b through C9 complex. However, C3b may enter a feedback amplification loop and interact with factor B which has been cleaved by factor D to form $\overline{C3bBb}$, the alternative pathway C3 convertase. The $\overline{C3bBb}$ complex is stabilized by properdin. The alternative or properdin pathway can be activated indirectly by the feedback mechanism via the classic pathway or directly by certain substances such as zymosan, endotoxin, or C3 nephritic factor. Activation of the complement protein sequence results in the formation of biologically active proteins such as chemotactic factors, opsonins, and cytolytic factors which mediated an inflammatory response.

It has been demonstrated that the alternative complement pathway can be activated independently of the classic pathway by endotoxin. This may explain why most organic dust which contain endotoxin are efficient activators of the alternative pathway. A hypothesis for the development of hypersensitivity pneumonitis has been formulated requiring the initial activation of complement by inhaled antigen with the subsequent generation of chemotactic factors and C3b [29]. B lymphocytes sensitized by the antigen mature into plasma cells and secrete antibody to the inhaled antigen. Introduction of more inhaled antigen results in formation of immune complexes which activate complement and are opsonized. They are ingested by macrophages leading to their activation, and an inflammatory response results. Persistent inflammation may result in fibrosis possibly through a macrophage-mediated influence on fibroblasts. The pathogenetic focal point, according to this hypothesis, is the activated alveolar macrophage which serves as a functional link between an inhaled offending antigen and the consequent production of pulmonary lesions. Thus, pathogenesis of hypersensitivity pneumonitis may involve both local and systemic immune and nonimmune mechanisms linking the inhaled offending agent with the unique host response to result in disease.

Thus far, the results of most studies of complement in occupational lung disease have not been rewarding. Although complement levels drop in immune-complex diseases such as systemic lupus erythematosus, in acute phases of pigeon-breeder's disease serum complement remains in the normal range or increases following natural exposure or bronchoprovication challenge [30–32]. A possible explanation for the lack of positive findings is that the techniques to measure serum complement, hemolytic and radial immunodiffusion assays, may not be sensitive enough to detect different prechallenge and postchallenge serum complement levels. Studies of complement protein metabolism to determine turnover and half-life of radioactively labeled complement proteins are more sensitive methods to demonstrate complement utilization. It may be necessary to use these methods to demonstrate the importance of complement in these diseases.

VII. Antinuclear Antibody Assays

Antibody to nuclear antigens are detected commonly in the sera of patients with connective tissue diseases such as systemic lupus erythematosus. The assay commonly employed to detect antibodies is an indirect immunofluorescent technique which uses mouse or rat kidney or liver as a tissue substrate. Briefly, the tissue is snap frozen and cut into sections 4 μm thick and placed on glass microscope slides. The patient's serum is serially diluted. A drop of diluted serum is placed on the tissue section and incubated for 30 min at room temperature. The slide is washed. Next, the tissue is overlaid with a drop of antiserum to human immunoglobulin conjugated with fluorescein isothiocynate (FITC), and incubated for another 30 min. After a second wash, a coverslip is mounted and the slide is ready for viewing with a fluorescence microscope. Approximately 4% of normal individuals and up to 30% of normal elderly individuals may have a positive low-titer anti-nuclear antibody.

It has been reported that 44% of the sera of a group of 39 patients with silicosis were positive for anti-nuclear antibody [33]. Also, 28% of the sera of patients with asbestosis were reported to be positive [34]. It was noted that the patients with silicosis who were positive for ANA had more confluent lesions on chest x-ray than those with negative ANA. It is not clear why autoimmunity develops in these fibrotic lung diseases. It is possible that during tissue injury produced by asbestos or silica, these particles may interact with certain nuclear proteins and render them antigenic by revealing neoantigens, thus the patient produces an antibody response to them. Another explanation is that these particles may in some way interfere with the T-suppressor cell regulation of antibody produced by B cells. This deregulation of the B cell would allow abnormal antibodies to be produced to nuclear antigens by the matured plasma cell.

VIII. Assays for the Detection of Immune Complexes in Serum

Currently, there is increasing interest in the detection of immune complexes in biological fluids. Several techniques are available which are sensitive enough to measure minimal amounts of circulating immune complexes in sera of patients. The Clq binding assay utilizes the Clq molecule, a subunit of the first complement component, which binds monomeric IgG and IgM, but its binding is greatly enhanced by aggragation of these immunoglobulins. The Clq is labeled with radioactive iodine. It is reacted with patient serum, then the immune complexes which are bound to Clq labeled with ^{125}I are precipitated by polyethylene glycol [35]. The amount of radioactivity in the precipitate is directly proportional to the amount of immune complexes in the serum. This assay can measure immune complexes to a level of 50 μg of aggregated human gammaglobulin (AHG) equivalent per milliliter of serum, and is, therefore, very sensitive.

The Raji cell assay which detects immune complexes by complement receptors on the surface of a lymphoblastoid cell has produced interesting results. In this assay, a human lymphoblastoid cell, the Raji cell, which is devoid of membrane-bound immunoglobulin and has Fc receptors for IgG of low avidity, is used because it has a large number of receptors for C3-C3b, C3d, and Clq [36]. Consequently, these receptors can be used to detect complement-fixing immune complexes in animal and human sera. The assay can detect levels of circulating immune complexes at levels of 6 μg AGH equivalent per ml of serum. This assay was used by Dreisin and associates to demonstrate circulating immune complexes in the sera of patients with idiopathic interstitial pneumonia occurring during the cellular phase of the disease [36]. Thus far, no one has reported the use of this assay to study patients with occupational pulmonary disease such as silicosis or asbestosis.

When the Clq binding and Raji cell assays have been used to measure immune complexes in sera from patients with disease such as SLE, vasculitis, and rheumatoid arthritis, different values for circulating immune complexes have been obtained. These data may be explained by the fact that each assay detects immune complexes in a different way, and may, therefore, measure different properties of the complex. Thus, the assays currently available must be compared in each suspected immune-complex pulmonary disease to determine which technique may be most useful in demonstrating the immune complexes that are pathogenic.

References

1. Gell, P. G. H., and R. R. A. Coombs, *Clinical Aspects of Immunology*. Philadelphia, F. A. Davis Company, 1969.

2. Ishizaka, K., and T. Ishizaka, Human reaginic antibodies and immunoglobulin E., *J. Allergy,* **42**:330–363 (1968).
3. Pepys, J., I. D. Wells, M. F. D'Souza, and M. Greenberg, Clinical and immunological responses to enzymes of *Bacillus subtilis* in factory workers and consumers, *Clin. Allergy,* **3**:143–160 (1973).
4. Pepys, J., C. A. C. Pickering, and E. C. Hughes, Asthma due to inhaled chemical agents—complex salts of platinum, *Clin. Allergy,* **2**:391–396 (1972).
5. Karr, R. M., S. B. Lehrer, B. T. Butcher, and J. E. Salvaggio, Coffee worker's asthma: A clinical appraisal using RAST, *J. Allergy Clin. Immunol.,* **62**:143–148 (1978).
6. Lincoln, T. A., N. E. Bolton, and A. S. Garrett, Occupational allergy to animal dander and sera, *J. Occup. Med.,* **16**:465–469 (1974).
7. Frankland, A. E., Rat asthma in laboratory workers. In *Allergology.* Edited by Y. Yamamura, O. L. Frick, Amsterdam, Excerpta Medical Foundation, 1974, p. 123.
8. Pepys, J., and R. J. Davies, Occupational asthma. In *Allergy: Principles and Practice.* Edited by E. Middleton, E. Ellis, and C. E. Reed. C. V. Mosby, Co., St. Louis, 1978, pp. 812–842.
9. Colton, H. R., P. L. Polakoff, S. F. Weinstein, and D. Strieder, Immediate hypersensitivity in hog trypsin from industrial exposure, *J. Allergy Clin. Immunol.,* **55**:130 (1975).
10. Hendrick, D. J., R. J. Davies, and J. Pepys, Baker's asthma, *Clin. Allergy,* **6**:241–250 (1976).
11. Davies, R. J., M. Green, and N. McC. Schofield, Recurrent nocturnal asthma after exposure to grain dust, *Am. Rev. Respir. Dis.,* **114**:1011–1019 (1976).
12. Chan-Yeung, M., G. M. Barton, L. MacLean, and S. Gazybowski, Occupational asthma and rhinitis due to western red cedar (*Thuja plicate*), *Am. Rev. Respir. Dis.,* **108**:1094–1102 (1973).
13. Bohner, C. B., J. M. Sheldon, and J. W. Trevis, Sensitivity to gum acacia, with a report of ten cases of asthma in printers, *J. Allergy,* **12**:290–314 (1940).
14. Butcher, B. T., J. E. Salvaggio, H. Weill, and M. Ziskind, Toluene diisocyanate (TDI) pulmonary disease: Immunologic and inhalation challenge studies, *J. Allergy Clin. Immunol.,* **58**:89–100 (1976).
15. Zeiss, C. R., R. Patterson, J. J. Pruzansky, M. M. Miller, M. Rosenberg, I. Suszko, and D. Levitz, Immunologic and clinical aspects of trimellitic anhydride respiratory disease, *J. Allergy Clin. Immunol.,* **60**:96–103 (1977).
16. Ouchterlony, O., Diffusion in gel methods for immunological analyses II, *Prog. Allergy,* **6**:30–54 (1962).
17. Pepys, J., and P. A. Jenkins, Precipitin (FLH) test in farmer's lung, *Thorax,* **20**:21–35 (1965).
18. Edwards, J. H., The isolation of antigens associated with farmer's lung, *Clin. Exp. Immunol.,* **11**:341–355 (1972).
19. Fink, J. N., V. L. Moore, and J. J. Barboriak, Cell-mediated hypersensitivity

in pigeon breeder's, *Int. Arch. Allergy Appl. Immunol.*, **49**:831–836 (1975).

20. Fredericks, W., Antigens in pigeon dropping extracts. In *The NIAID Workshop on Antigens in Hypersensitivity pneumonitis.* Edited by Jordon Fink and John Salvaggio. *J. Allergy Clin. Immunol.*, **61**:221–223 (1978).
21. Nowell, P. C., Phytohemagglutinin: An initiator of mitosis in cultures of normal human leucocytes, *Cancer Res.*, **20**:462–466 (1960).
22. Boyum, A., Ficoll Hyapaque method for separating mononuclear cells and granulocytes from human blood, *Scand. J. Clin. Lab. Invest. (Suppl.)*, 77 (1977).
23. Hanson, P. J., and R. Penny, Pigeon breeder's disease: Study of the cell mediated immune response to pigeons by the lymphocyte culture technique, *Int. Arch. Allergy Appl. Immunol.*, **47**:498–507 (1974).
24. Schatz, M., R. Patterson, J. Fink, and V. Moore, Pigeon breeder's disease. II. Pigeon antigen induced proliferation of lymphocytes from symptomatic subjects, *Clin. Allergy*, **6**:7–17 (1976).
25. Caldwell, J. R., C. E. Pearce, C. Spencer, T. Leder, and R. H. Weadman, Immunologic mechanisms in hypersensitivity pneumonitis, *J. Allergy Clin. Immunol.*, **52**:225–230 (1973).
26. Schuyler, M. R., T. P. Thigpen, and J. E. Salvaggio, Local pulmonary immunity in pigeon breeder's disease, *Ann. Intern. Med.*, **88**:355–358 (1978).
27. Reynolds, H. T., J. D. Fulmer, J. A. Kazierowski, W. C. Roberts, M. M. Frank, and R. G. Crystal, Analysis of cellular and protein content of bronchoalveolar lavage fluid from patients with idiopathic pulmonary fibrosis and chronic hypersensitivity pneumonitis, *J. Clin. Invest.*, **59**: 165–175 (1977).
28. Schuyler, M., M. Ziskind, and J. Salvaggio, Cell-mediated immunity in silicosis, *Am. Rev. Respir. Dis.*, **116**:147–151 (1977).
29. Schorlemmer, H. V., J. H. Edwards, P. Davies, and A. C. Allison, Macrophage responses to mouldy hay dust, *Micropolyspora faeni* and zymosan, activators of complement by the alternative pathway, *Clin. Exp. Immunol.*, **27**:198–207 (1977).
30. Stiehm, E. R., C. E. Reed, and W. H. Tooley, Pigeon breeder's lung in children, *Pediatrics*, **39**:904–915 (1967).
31. Moore, V. L., J. N. Fink, J. J. Barboriak, L. L. Ruff, and D. P. Schleuter, Immunologic events in pigeon breeder's disease, *J. Allergy Clin. Immunol.*, **53**:319–328 (1974).
32. Moore, V. L., G. T. Hensley, and J. N. Fink, An animal model of hypersensitivity pneumonitis in the rabbit, *J. Clin. Invest.*, **56**:937–944 (1975).
33. Jones, R. N., M. Turner-Warwick, M. Ziskind, and H. Weill, High prevalence of antinuclear antibodies in sandblaster's silicosis, *Am. Rev. Respir. Dis.*, **113**:393–395 (1976).
34. Turner-Warwick, M., and W. R. Parkes, Circulating rheumatoid and antinuclear factors in asbestos workers, *Br. Med. J.*, **3**:492–495 (1970).

35. Nydegger, V. E., P. H. Lambert, H. Gerber, and P. A. Miescher, Circulating immune complexes in the serum in systemic lupus erythematosis and in carriers of hepatitis B antigen. Quantitation by binding to radiolabeled Clq, *J. Clin. Invest.*, **54**:297–309 (1974).
36. Dreisin, R., M. Schwarz, A. Theofilopoulos, and R. Stanford, Circulating immune complexes in idiopathic interstitial pneumonias, *N. Engl. J. Med.*, **298**:353–357 (1978).

8

Inhalation Challenge Testing

A. J. NEWMAN TAYLOR

Cardiothoracic Institute
Brompton Hospital
London, England

ROBERT J. DAVIES

St. Bartholomew's Hospital
London, England

I. Introduction

Charles Harrison Blackley [1] was almost certainly the first person to perform bronchial provocation tests with allergens. His study, which included nasal and conjunctival tests, convinced him of the importance of grass pollen in the etiology of these diseases. This use of inhalation challenge techniques in diagnosis was continued into the twentieth century, but in 1934 Stevens [2] suggested the routine diagnostic use of such tests should be abandoned because attacks of asthma lasting several days were occasionally provoked. In 1947, Lowell and Schiller [3] showed that inhalation of aerosols of pollen extract provoked a fall in the vital capacity of the lungs in asthmatic patients. Since that time, bronchial challenge techniques, in which the reaction has been monitored with lung function tests, have been extensively used in the investigation of patients with asthma and hypersensitivity pneumonitis due to an identifiable extrinsic agent. Bronchial challenge testing using soluble antigens which also elicit an immediate skin test reaction is recognized to be a safe procedure provided appropriate precautions are taken. In over 9000 bronchial provocation tests with a wide variety of allergens in 1035 children no anaphylactic or other severe reactions were noted [4].

Bronchial provocation testing, however, does remain a potentially hazardous method of investigation, particularly where testing is being conducted with agents met in the working environment such as vapors, fumes, or dusts, whose test exposure is less easily controlled than the soluble antigens, and where the degree of reactivity of the patient to the particular material can be difficult to assess. Such testing is inappropriate where the extrinsic cause of the patients respiratory reaction can be identified on clinical grounds and where support for the diagnosis from specific skin test reactions or serological tests is available, as is frequently the case in hypersensitivity pneumonitis. The method is now used primarily to identify those causes of allergic lung disease where such supporting evidence is not available. In a large proportion of such cases now met in clinical practice, exposure to the causal agent has occurred in the working environment. Bronchial provocation testing is generally unnecessary in an individual with a clear history of work-related respiratory symptoms exposed at work to a well-recognized cause of occupational asthma or hypersensitivity pneumonitis, particularly where a relationship can be demonstrated between occupational exposure and changes in lung function. However, it must be recognized that the diagnosis of a work-related allergic respiratory reaction usually implies the need for the affected individual to minimize, or avoid completely, further exposure to the causal agent. This often requires a change of job, a recommendation no physician would wish to make without as great a degree of confidence as is reasonably practicable in the diagnosis.

Bronchial provocation testing is a method used to obtain specific information on which to base decisions about the future management of an individual patient. Physicians will vary in the extent to which in any individual case they will require such information to reach a decision. However, although such differences in emphasis exist, it is possible to describe circumstances in which there is a wide agreement that such tests should be carried out.

1. Where the pattern of respiratory disease has not previously been recognized or has unusual features. "Humidifier fever," which has been described in recent years, was an example of this situation. Although the symptoms and functional abnormalities observed were very similar to those found in hypersensitivity pneumonitis, some features of this disease differed from hypersensitivity pneumonitis. Symptoms and functional changes which occurred within a few hours of returning to work after an absence, such as a weekend or holiday, resolved with continuing daily exposure, but recurred on returning to work after an absence over a weekend or on holiday. Chest radiographs had been normal in other reported cases, and no evidence of progression to pulmonary fibrosis had been observed [5].

2. Where an individual is suspected of reacting to an agent as yet unrecognized or poorly documented as a cause of occupationally related allergic respiratory disease. Although occupational asthma due to naphthylene diisocyanate (NDI) has been reported, this had not been validated at the time of investigation of three patients who were exposed to this agent at work. Bronchial provocation testing with NDI provoked an asthmatic reaction in all three [6].
3. Where an individual with work-related respiratory symptoms is exposed to several different agents, each recognized as causes of the particular disease.
4. Where genuine doubt about the diagnosis of work-related asthma or hypersensitivity pneumonitis still remains after all other appropriate investigations (including skin tests, serology, and work records of lung function) have been completed.
5. Where the respiratory symptoms experienced at work are of such severity that it is thought unjustifiable for the affected individual to be further exposed in the working environment. Obtaining work records of lung function is not justified by the risk.

Bronchial provocation whose sole purpose is in support of a legal claim is, we believe, unjustifiable.

In this chapter, the techniques of bronchial provocation testing will be considered with particular reference to testing with industrial agents. The limited information in relation to mechanism of reaction will be discussed as well as interpretation of the physiological changes observed during the reactions.

II. Techniques of Bronchial Provocation Testing

The techniques of bronchial provocation testing have been increasingly used not only to diagnose occupational asthma, hypersensitivity pneumonitis, and related diseases but also to study their physiology, immunopharmacology, and treatment. For these reasons many investigators have questioned the adequacy of much of the previous methodology used for bronchial provocation testing and attention has been increasingly focused on a number of factors which influence the respiratory reaction. These include the method of delivery of the provoking agent and the most appropriate method for measuring the respiratory reaction.

The traditional method for performing bronchial provocation tests is to use a nebulized extract of allergen or pharmacological agent. This method of administration bears little resemblance to natural exposure, particularly to those agents which normally occur in particulate form. Further, there is little similarity in terms of dose, rate of administration, presentation of allergen, or site of deposition within the respiratory tract.

Studies of occupational asthma particularly have led to the development of a different type of bronchial provocation test. Pepys and co-workers have developed simple and safe techniques for simulating work exposure within the hospital environment [7]. The patient is exposed to the industrial dust, gas, vapor, or fume in the form in which it is encountered in the factory. Since it is now frequently possible to assess factory exposure accurately, the "occupational type" of bronchial provocation test can be refined to allow the subject to be tested with the particular industrial material in the same form and in the same concentration (for a shorter duration) as that encountered at work.

Studies using this type of bronchial provocation testing have provided much information about the patterns of bronchopulmonary reactions and their response to therapeutic agents. Further, on-site observations in industry have allowed correlation between the types of respiratory reaction seen at work and those that can be reproduced in the hospital laboratory.

III. Delivery Systems

There is no method currently available which will allow the dose of material reaching the respiratory tract during a bronchial provocation test to be determined or predicted accurately. The majority of material inhaled is deposited in the nose, mouth, and oropharynx. The proportion reaching the respiratory tract and its site of deposition within the respiratory tract will depend upon a number of variables, which include the particle size of the aerosol or dust, the rate and depth of breathing, and, where aerosols are being generated by a nebulizer, by the output of the nebulizer. Nebulizers vary greatly, both in the size of the particles which they generate and in the flow rates they produce, which determine their output. Variation in the depth and rate of breathing produces changes in the site of deposition of the inhaled material. Uniform central and peripheral deposition occurs with slow tidal breathing. With increased speed and depth of ventilation, deposition becomes increasingly central. Hargreave [8] has reported that in challenge tests with histamine, variation in nebulizer output and in speed and depth of ventilation each produce changes in histamine dose-response curves. Similar studies in challenge testing with specific agents have not been reported.

Where the aim of a bronchial provocation test is simply to induce an identifiable reaction, standardization of the conditions of bronchial provocation testing is less important. However, where repeated tests need to be compared, as in the assessment of pretest drugs on the reaction, the accuracy and reproducibility with which particular doses of the pharmacological or occupational agent are administered becomes critical. At the present time there is no standardized or universally accepted technique for bronchial provocation testing, and each has its own problems. It is of considerable importance to test individual methods for uniformity of delivery, and the same equipment should be used for each patient throughout the investigation.

IV. Extracts and Solutions

The traditional method for bronchial provocation testing is to use a nebulizer to produce an aerosol which can be inhaled. Many techniques have been employed involving a number of different nebulizers including the Wright's, de Vilbiss, and Bird nebulizers. One method is illustrated in Figure 1. This shows a bronchial provocation test with an allergen solution. The Wright's nebulizer driven by

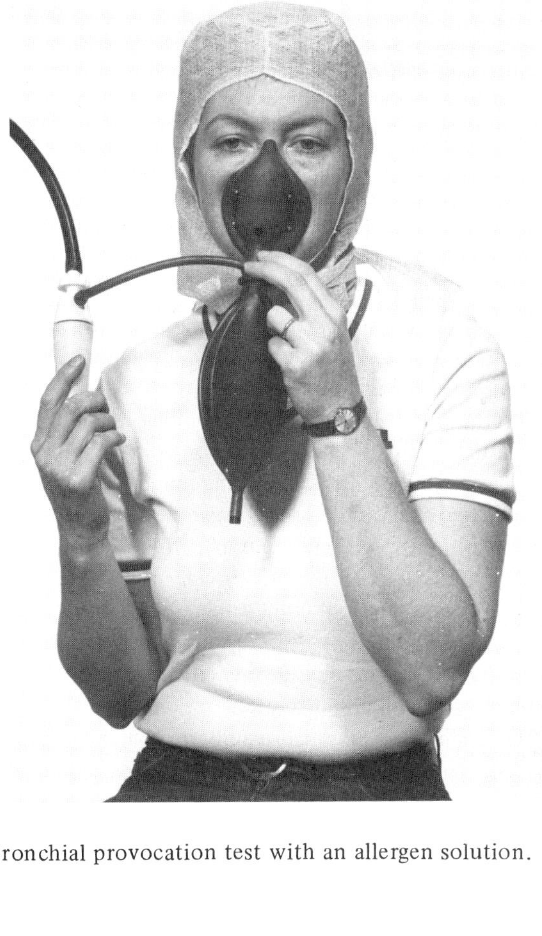

Figure 1 Bronchial provocation test with an allergen solution.

oxygen at 8 liters/min is connected to a face mask and rebreathing bag. The patient is instructed to breathe naturally around his or her functional residual capacity (FRC) during the inhalation test which may be continued for up to 2 min [9]. While some investigators favor the inhalation of aerosols throughout tidal breathing, Chai and co-workers [10] suggest the use of a Johnn Hopkins dosimeter which injects a timed bolus (usually 0.6 per sec) into the inspirate. This modification has some advantages, but the amount of aerosol reaching the lung will depend on the depth of inspiration. Improvements in technique of aerosol delivery should aim for more accurate measurement of the inhaled dose. Orehek and co-workers [11] used a nebulizer to fill a spirometer bell with a known concentration of fresh aerosol and the subject was instructed to inspire a fixed volume from FRC and to breath-hold for 4 sec to ensure maximal particle retention. The inhalation of fresh aerosol could be repeated, and with knowledge of the concentration and the volume of the aerosol inhaled, the dose reaching the patients mouth, if not the respiratory tract, could be calculated.

V. Occupational Materials

Pepys and co-workers at the Brompton Hospital in London developed a series of simple tests for assessing the effects of occupational dusts, gases, vapors, and fumes in bronchial provocation tests in the hospital laboratory. The principle of the system is to simulate the patient's work environment in the hospital laboratory. This occupational type of bronchial provocation testing should be carried out in an isolated chamber with adequate extraction procedures. It is very important to prevent the escape of any test materials into the atmosphere of the laboratory. This is desirable not only for the protection of the staff but also because of the exquisitely high degree of sensitivity of some patients which may result in continuing provocation after the patient is removed from the challenge chamber. Such occupational materials as grain or wood dust [12] can be tested directly by getting the patient to tip the material from one receptacle to another in the challenge chamber (Fig. 2). Agents such as antibiotics [13], the complex salts of platinum [14], and piperazine hydrochloride [15], which are highly allergenic and which exist in a fine powder form, are best mixed with a vehicle such as dried lactose before being tested. The lactose should be dried overnight at 105°C. A small quantity of the occupational material is mixed with 250 g of lactose and the patient instructed to create dust in the atmosphere of the challenge chamber by tipping the mixture from one tray to another. The vapors that arise from soldering fluxes can readily be tested by asking the subject to repeat the soldering maneuver in the challenge chamber (Fig. 3) [16]. One of

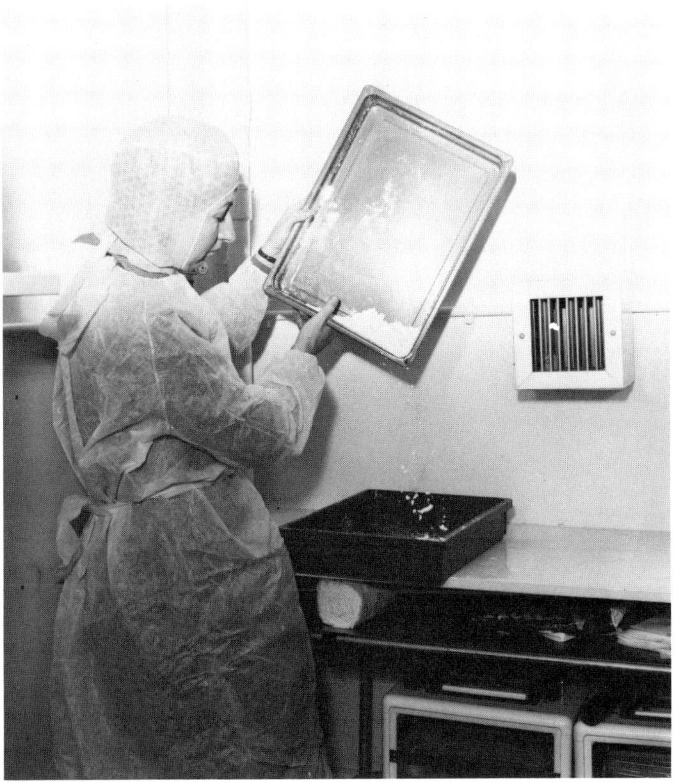

Figure 2 Bronchial provocation test. Occupational-type exposure to dust.

the problems with these techniques has been the lack of knowledge of the dose of material inhaled by the patient. Measurements, at least of the atmospheric concentration of the occupational material produced in the challenge chamber, should be made whenever possible and compared with those found at work. This has proved possible when conducting bronchial provocation tests with toluene 2,4-diisocyanate (TDI). Two main methods have been described. In one the subject varnishes on a board (Fig. 4) with varnish resin to which increasing concentrations of TDI are added on separate test days to produce a known maximum exposure concentration [17]. In the second method atmospheric concentrations of TDI are produced by passing air at a known flow rate over TDI in a gas washing bottle. The flow of air through the gas washing bottle can be adjusted until a steady-state concentration of TDI is reached at the required

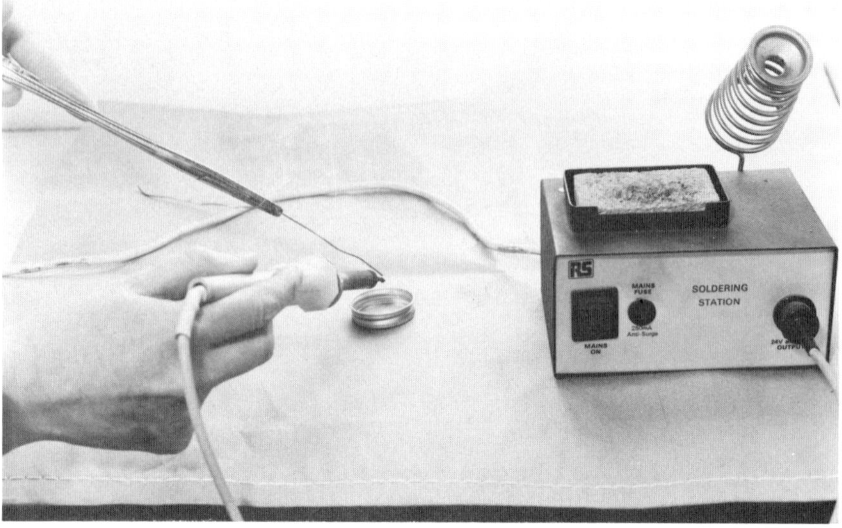

Figure 3 Bronchial provocation test. Occupational-type exposure to solder flux vapor.

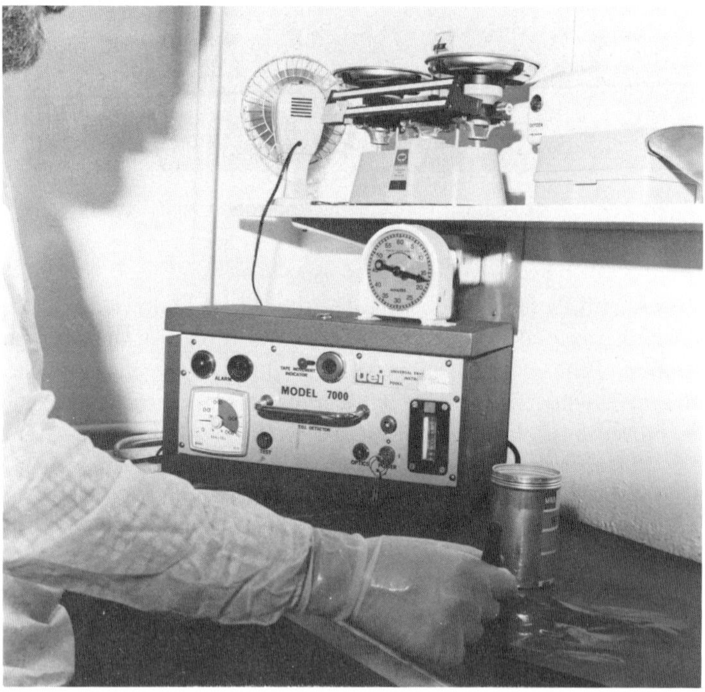

Figure 4 Bronchial provocation test. Occupational-type exposure to TDI vapor. Atmospheric TDI concentration monitored with EU1 monitor (model 7000) in challenge chamber.

level [18]. With both methods air in the challenge chamber is circulated by fans, and the atmospheric concentration of TDI is measured using a Universal Instruments Model 7000 TDI monitor.

VI. Dose and Exposure Time

The concentration at which to start challenge testing with a nebulized extract of allergen can be gauged with allergens such as rat and mouse urine protein, which elicit immediate skin test reactions, from the size of the weal provoked by different concentrations of allergen [19]. The initial bronchial provocation test reaction should be made with the allergen concentration which has provoked a reaction with weal diameter of less than 3 mm [9]. Exposure should initially be for 1 min, followed by a further 2 min exposure if no reaction has occurred after 15 min, followed by a final 2 min exposure (giving a total 5 min exposure) if again no reaction has occurred after the first 2 min exposure. If no reaction is provoked by a 5 min exposure to the concentration of extract on one day, a 10-fold increase in concentration of extract may be used for testing in the same way on a separate day.

Unfortunately, skin test reactions cannot be used to test many of the agents causing both occupational asthma and hypersensitivity pneumonitis, either because type I allergic mechanisms may not be involved in the pathogenesis or because it has not been possible to prepare suitable extracts for skin testing. In these circumstances it is necessary to gauge the test dose from careful knowledge of the patient's history and work conditions. In general, it is essential to start with extremely low exposures in order to avoid any untoward reactions. For example, with the complex salts of platinum, skin test reactions can be elicited at concentrations as low as 10^{-9} M, and marked asthmatic reactions can result from exposure to as little as 10 mg of the complex salts mixed with 250 g of lactose [14]. The amount of the occupational material used in the bronchial provocation test should be increased in two- to fivefold stages when the previous test was negative.

Precise measurement of personal levels of exposure to occupational materials at work can provide the necessary information about initial dosage and enable accurate reproduction in the hospital laboratory. At the present time, experience suggests that the occupational type of bronchial provocation test should be continued for between 15 and 30 min. This length of time will obviously vary according to the concentration of material being tested. With some occupational agents single breaths may be sufficient; for example, a single inhalation of epoxy resin fume [20] provoked marked changes in respiratory function. For this reason, extreme caution must be exercised when new materials are tested for the first time and very careful note must be taken of the history of the patients reactions at work as a guide to "level of sensitivity."

Whenever possible, patients for bronchial provocation testing should be taken off all forms of medication for at least 48 hr before the test. This includes antihistamines, the β-adrenoceptor stimulants, phosphodiesterase inhibitors, and corticosteroid drugs. Patients who are unable to stop treatment even when no longer exposed to the occupational material or who have persistent airway narrowing producing an FEV_1 of less than 2 liters are unlikely to be suitable candidates for bronchial provocation testing. In some patients with asthma, however, it is possible to obtain sufficient improvement in lung function with regular (usually every 4 hr) administration of a β-adrenoreceptor stimulant, such as salbutamol, on control and test days, to allow a bronchial provocation test to be undertaken. In general, these drugs, although inhibiting immediate asthmatic reactions, will not prevent the development of a nonimmediate asthmatic reaction.

VII. Measurement of Respiratory Reactions Provoked by Bronchial Provocation Testing

The respiratory reactions provoked by bronchial provocation testing with specific occupational agents can be measured by a number of different tests of lung function. The choice of test depends primarily on the expected outcome of the bronchial provocation test. An asthmatic reaction is usually quite adequately followed by observing changes in spirometry—forced expiratory volume in one second (FEV_1) and forced vital capacity (FVC)—or in peak expiratory flow rate (PEF). The development of an obstructive ventilatory defect, with a fall in FEV_1 of 15% or more following the bronchial provocation test when compared with the control day values, is conventionally accepted as evidence of a provoked asthmatic reaction. More sensitive tests of airway narrowing elicited by bronchial provocation testing can be obtained from measurements of specific airway conductance and from measurements of points on the maximum expiratory flow-volume curve at low lung volumes. Generally, these tests have been found to have little advantage over spirometric measurements in identifying asthmatic reactions to provocation tests, although they have been found to show greater proportional changes from the pretest values than spirometric tests [21]. They may, however, be useful in identifying small changes provoked in airway caliber which do not produce changes in FEV_1. In a study of a group of patients with occupational asthma due to Western red cedar, Chan-Yeung [22] observed immediate falls in flow rates at low lung volumes in some patients, which were not accompanied by changes in FEV_1. Measurement of specific airway conductance in the whole body plethysmograph can be of value in identifying asthmatic reactions in those individuals in whom forced expiratory maneuvers induce airway obstruction.

Where it is anticipated that the respiratory reaction provoked by a challenge test will involve the peripheral gas-exchanging parts of the lung, as in cases of hypersensitivity pneumonitis, in addition to measurement of FEV_1 and FVC, carbon monoxide gas transfer should be measured and expressed both as transfer factor (DL_{CO}) and transfer coefficient (K_{CO}). Lung volumes, total lung capacity (TLC) and residual volume (RV) should ideally also be measured to allow a confident identification of the site of reaction.

Measurement of FEV_1 and FVC and of PEF should be made on two separate occasions, half an hour and immediately before the bronchial provocation test. Identification of an asthmatic reaction during the bronchial provocation test is best done by the patient using a peak flow meter; this allows measurement of lung function without interruption of the test, which should, however, be stopped immediately if a definite asthmatic reaction occurs during the test. Measurements of FEV_1 and FVC or of PEF should be made every 5 min after the test for an hour and hourly thereafter for the rest of the day. Because of the need to identify nonimmediate reactions it is essential that bronchial provocation tests be conducted first thing in the morning. FEV_1 and FVC or PEF should also be measured during the night after a challenge test if the patient is awakened by respiratory symptoms.

Where carbon monoxide gas transfer and lung volumes are being measured, these should be done immediately before the test, at intervals of 4 hr for 12 hr after the test and then, if possible, at 12 hr intervals until the values have returned to pretest levels.

In addition to measurement of lung function, where bronchial provocation tests are expected to provoke a reaction affecting the peripheral gas-exchanging parts of the lung, oral temperature should be measured before the test and hourly thereafter for the rest of the day and on the following day until its value is consistently normal. A sample of venous blood should also be taken before the test and at 6, 12, and 24 hr after to look for the development of a polymorphonuclear leukocytosis.

Exposure to agents causing occupational asthma both in the working environment and in bronchial challenge testing have been shown to provoke reactions which can persist for prolonged periods. Serial peak flow measurements in those with occupational asthma due to colophony [23] and to diisocyanates [24] have shown that recovery from occupational exposure frequently takes several days and, particularly with diisocyanates, may take several weeks. Short exposures to occupational agents in bronchial challenge tests have also been found to provoke prolonged reactions. Asthmatic reactions occurring on several successive nights, with partial or complete recovery of lung function in the intervening daytime, have been provoked by a single bronchial challenge test exposure to a variety of materials (Fig. 5) which include ampicillin [13], penicillin [25], Western red cedar [26], grain dust [27], toluene diisocyanate [28], and formaldehyde [29].

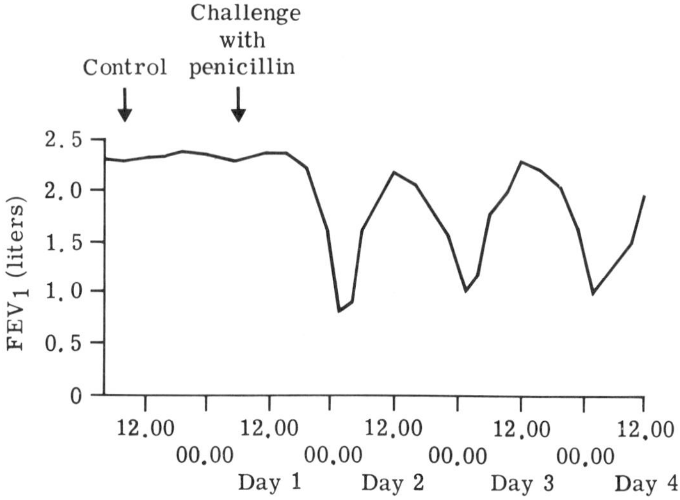

Figure 5 Bronchial provocation test. Recurrent nocturnal asthmatic reaction provoked by single exposure to penicillin dust (10 mg in 250 g lactose).

It is essential if reactions are to be correctly attributed to the appropriate agent, that the interval between occupational exposure and bronchial provocation test, and between bronchial provocation tests, particularly where exposure to different agents is undertaken, is adequate to allow complete recovery from any previous reaction. Regular estimations of lung function during the daytime and evenings, and if necessary during the night, must be undertaken before and between bronchial provocation tests to ensure that no previous reaction is persisting.

VIII. Patterns of Bronchial Provocation Test Reactions and Their Interpretation

Bronchial challenge tests may provoke transient reactions which develop either within minutes of exposure, "immediate" reactions, or one or more hours after exposure, "nonimmediate" reactions.

Immediate reactions start within 10-15 min of exposure, are maximal by 15-30 min, and resolve spontaneously within 1 or 2 hr. The reactions affect the airways and cause transient airway narrowing (i.e., asthma; Fig. 6). They are not associated with either a systemic reaction (fever, malaise, etc.) or with the development of a polymorphonuclear leukocytosis. They may be accompanied by a blood eosinophilia which is maximal at about 24 hr after the test. Im-

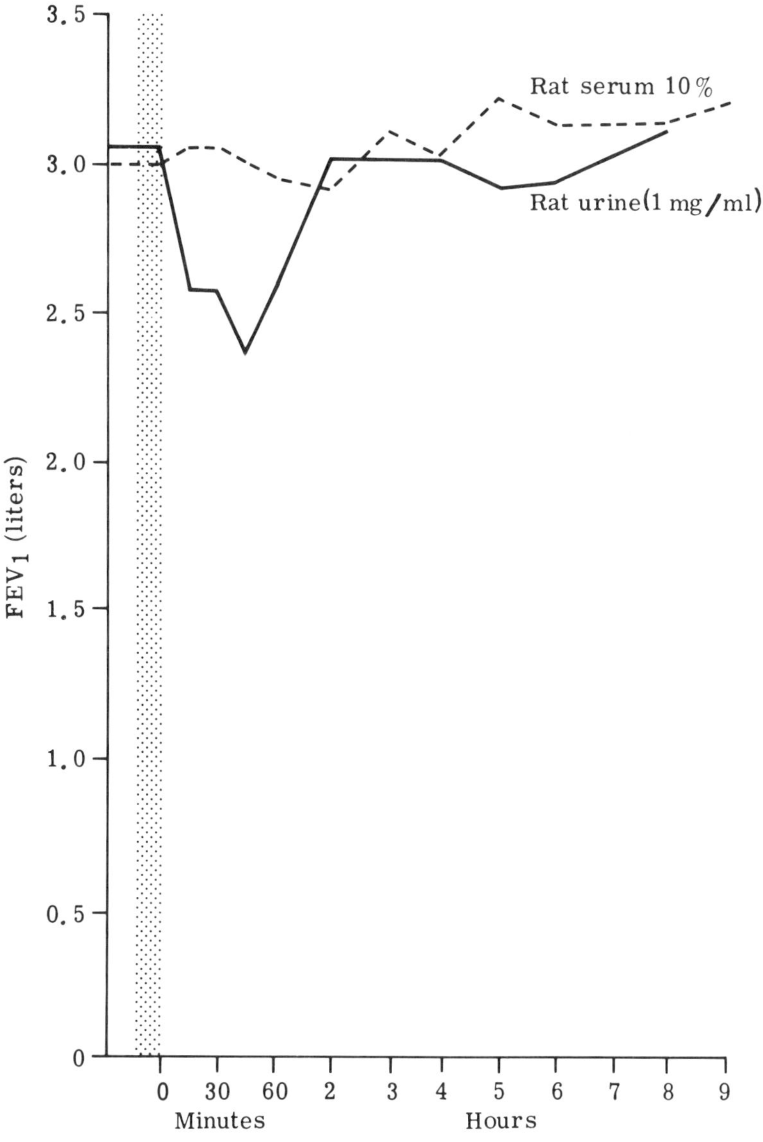

Figure 6 Bronchial provocation test reaction. Immediate asthmatic reaction provoked by exposure to rat urine (1 mg/ml). No reaction provoked by rat serum (10%).

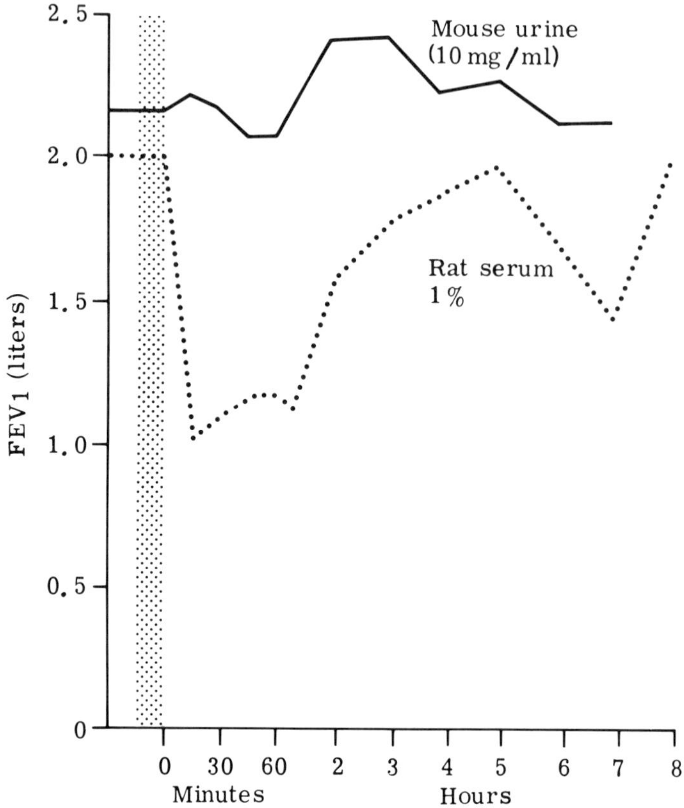

Figure 7 Bronchial provocation test reaction. Dual asthmatic reaction provoked by exposure to rat serum (1%). No reaction to mouse urine (10 mg/ml).

mediate asthmatic reactions may be inhibited by pretest β_2-adrenoreceptor stimulants, such as isoproterenol or albuterol, and by sodium cromoglycate. They are unaffected by pretest corticosteroids taken either by mouth or by inhalation. The reaction can be rapidly and completely reversed by the inhalation of a β_2-adrenoreceptor stimulant.

Nonimmediate reactions develop an hour or more after the challenge test, most commonly after 4–6 hr. They develop more slowly than immediate reactions and persist for between 24 and 48 hr, or longer in the case of recurrent nocturnal reactions. Three separate types of nonimmediate reaction may be distinguished: asthmatic reactions, peripheral respiratory reactions, and systemic reactions. A nonimmediate reaction preceded by an immediate reaction is described as a dual reaction (Fig. 7).

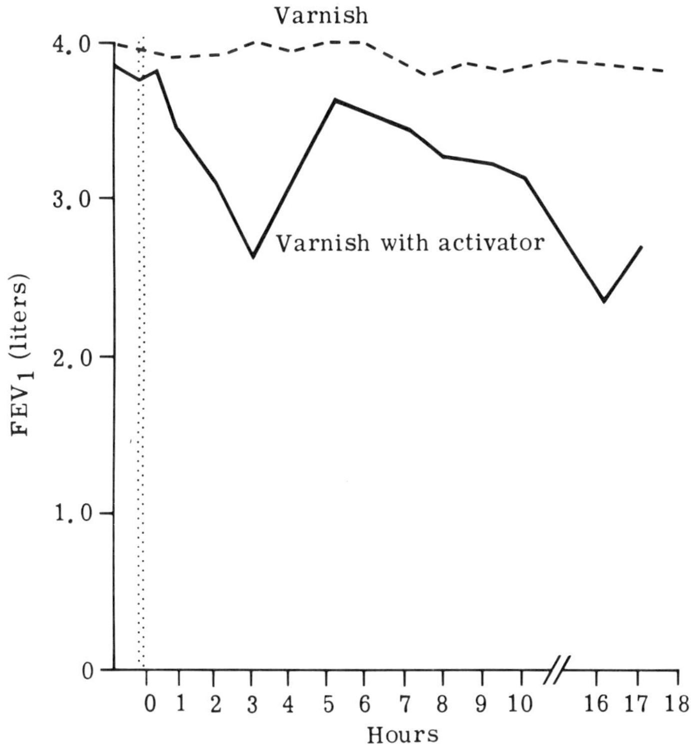

Figure 8 Bronchial provocation test reaction. Two distinguishable nonimmediate asthmatic reactions provoked by exposure to TDI. Onset of initial reaction 1 hr after exposure, and of second reaction 5 hr after exposure.

Pepys and Hutchcroft [30] have distinguished three different patterns of nonimmediate asthmatic reaction: those starting 1-2 hr after exposure which persist for up to 3 hr (Fig. 8), those starting within 4-8 hr of exposure persisting for 24 hr or more (Fig. 9), and those which develop in the early hours of the morning on the day after the challenge test and which tend to recur without further challenge test exposure on several subsequent nights, with a partial or complete return to normal lung function in the intervening daytime period (recurrent nocturnal reaction; Fig. 5).

The nonimmediate asthmatic reaction commencing at 4-8 hr is often completely inhibited by oral or inhaled corticosteroids taken pretest and during the day of the test. They may also be partially or completely inhibited by sodium cromoglycate taken pretest and during the day of the test. β_2-adrenoreceptor stimulants produce a partial and only temporary improvement in lung function.

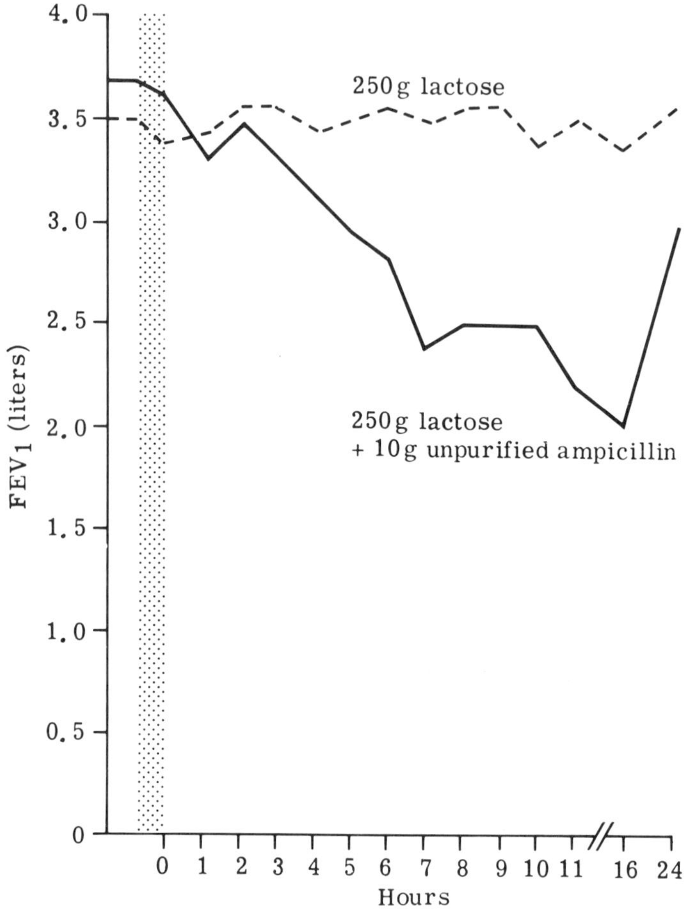

Figure 9 Bronchial provocation test reaction. Single nonimmediate asthmatic reaction provoked by exposure to ampicillin dust (10 g in 250 g lactose).

The two other patterns of nonimmediate asthmatic reaction are much less common and have not been sufficiently studied in relation to drug effects.

Whether these different patterns of nonimmediate reaction are due to real differences in underlying mechanisms is not known. It is of interest that Chan-Yeung in her study of a group of patients with nonimmediate reactions provoked by Western red cedar found that with repeated challenges on successive days, the interval between exposure and the onset of the reaction decreased, and the reactions became more severe [31]. In another study of patients with Western red cedar asthma, Lam et al. [32] found that in those in whom nonimmediate reactions were provoked, reactivity to methacholine had increased at

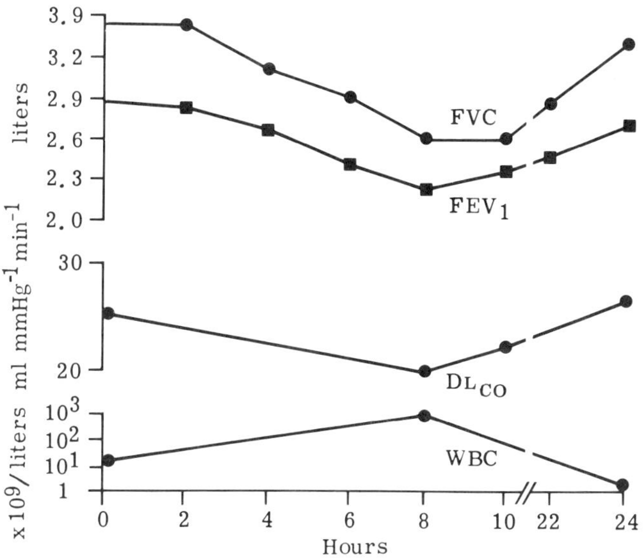

Figure 10 Bronchial provocation test reaction. Peripheral respiratory reaction with polymorphonuclear leukocytosis provoked by exposure to *M. faeni* at time 0. (By kind permission of Professor M. Turner-Warwick.)

24 hr after the challenge test as compared to pretest, on average 30.8-fold. Differences in the timing and severity of nonimmediate reactions may therefore in part reflect differences in airway reactivity at the time of the test.

Peripheral respiratory reactions are distinguished from asthmatic reactions by the provocation of transient changes in tests of ventilatory function, without evidence of airway narrowing, or a transient fall in gas transfer, or of both. They develop 4-6 hr after the challenge test, persist for 24-48 hr, and are frequently accompanied by a systemic reaction and polymorphonuclear leukocytosis (Fig. 10). They are partially or completely inhibited by pretest oral corticosteroids. In most studies reported, the measurements of lung function made have been of FEV_1, FVC, and DL_{CO}, and the reaction identified by a fall in FEV_1 proportionate to the fall in FVC, or a fall in DL_{CO}, or both. As peripheral respiratory reactions were provoked in patients with clinical, radiographic, and on occasions histologic evidence of hypersensitivity pneumonitis, they were attributed to a reaction occurring in alveolar walls, and have therefore been described as "alveolar" reactions.

A reaction occurring in the peripheral airways rather than within alveolar walls could produce a similar pattern of change in FEV_1 and FVC, together with a fall in DL_{CO} consequent upon the reduction in alveolar volume. Pathological changes in hypersensitivity pneumonitis have been reported to affect both alveoli and bronchioles, and some studies of patients with hypersensitivity pneumonitis in whom more detailed measurements of lung function have been made have demonstrated changes involving both alveoli and peripheral airways. Schleuter et al. [33] studied 13 patients with pigeon-breeder's lung, of whom 8 with acute reactions following pigeon exposure were studied 24 hr after exposure to their birds. FEV_1 and FVC were normal in all at this time, and DL_{CO} was normal in all but one. Total lung capacity (TLC) was increased in two and residual volume (RV) in five of the eight. Unfortunately, the distinction between those patients with asthma and those with hypersensitivity pneumonitis is not clearly made; five of the eight patients had normal chest radiographs. Serial measurements of lung function were made in two of the eight patients, both of whom had normal chest radiographs after exposure to the pigeons. Proportionate falls in FEV_1 and FVC were observed, maximal between 6 and 7 hr, with the development of basal inspiratory crackles in the lungs. In one patient TLC and RV were decreased and static compliance increased, suggesting a reaction in alveolar walls. In the other, TLC remained unchanged; RV increased and was associated with a fall in static compliance and increased frequency dependance of compliance, suggesting a reaction predominantly affecting peripheral airways. Allen et al. [34] studied nine patients with hypersensitivity pneumonitis due to pigeon-breeder's lung. Eight had abnormal chest radiographs, and all were nonsmokers. Evidence of airway disease was found in all nine. In five, FEV_{25-75} was decreased. Two showed increased frequency dependance of compliance and in two maximal expiratory flow rates were decreased when related to elastic recoil at different lung volumes. Warren et al. [35] studied a group of 14 nonsmoking patients with hypersensitivity pneumonitis 1 week and 4–6 weeks after exposure to the causal agent. TLC, RV, and FVC and steady-state CO extraction were reduced in all 14 when compared to controls, but the FEV_1/FVC ratio was normal. However, maximum midexpiratory flow rates were reduced in all 14, and in 3 of the 14 maximum expiratory flow rates were decreased when related to elastic recoil at different lung volumes, suggesting an increase in upstream resistance. Schofield et al. [36], however, in a study which included six patients with hypersensitivity pneumonitis in whom TLC, RV, and FVC were reduced and FEV_1/FVC ratio normal at the time of investigation, found no evidence of peripheral airway narrowing. In none of their patients were maximum expiratory flow rates decreased when related to elastic recoil at different lung volumes.

Evidence from studies of lung function in patients with hypersensitivity pneumonitis therefore suggests that at least in some patients narrowing of peripheral airways as well as changes in alveolar walls contributes to the functional abnormalities which occur in the disease. As yet, sufficiently detailed studies of patients at the time of a peripheral respiratory reaction elicited by bronchial provocation testing have not been undertaken, and a confident identification of the site of the reaction cannot be made.

The systemic reaction provoked by bronchial challenge tests is characterized by fever often associated with malaise, shivers, myalgia, and headache, and the development of a polymorphonuclear leukocytosis. The fever and systemic symptoms usually develop within 4-10 hr of exposure and may persist for 24-48 hr. The polymorphonuclear leukocytosis develops usually between 6 and 12 hr after the test, but may take 24 hr to develop. Nonimmediate systemic reactions after bronchial provocation testing were initially described by Williams [37] in a group of patients with farmer's lung, and subsequently reported with many of the different causes of hypersensitivity pneumonitis, including pigeon-breeder's lung, bagassosis, and malt-worker's lung. In their study of allergic reactions in bird fanciers, Hargreaves and Pepys [38], reported that of 31 patients with nonimmediate reactions provoked by avian serum proteins a fever developed in 29, systemic symptoms in 25, and a polymorphonuclear leukocytosis in 22. The systemic reaction accompanied the nonimmediate peripheral respiratory reaction in each case in which it was provoked, and developed in some but not all of those with nonimmediate asthmatic reactions. In 16 patients the systemic reaction provoked was unaccompanied by changes in ventilatory function or gas transfer, and fever was the only objective evidence of reaction.

IX. Pathological Mechanisms Underlying Bronchial Provocation Test Reactions

Both occupational asthma and hypersensitivity pneumonitis are diseases characterized by pathological responses to a specific inhaled extrinsic agent. They also have in common clinical characteristics which have been used to distinguish hypersensitivity reactions from other types of reaction, such as a toxic reaction. The disease develops only after an initial symptom-free episode or period of exposure. It occurs only in a proportion of those exposed, and reactions are provoked by exposure to concentrations not affecting other exposed individuals, and which previously did not provoke a reaction in the affected individual. Based on such observations, an immunologic basis for the disease processes has been suggested, whose nature has been in part deduced from studying the patterns of respiratory reaction provoked by bronchial provocation testing.

The immediate asthmatic reaction is similar in speed of onset and duration to the immediate weal and flare skin test reaction. Pretreatment corticosteroids are without effect on either reaction, but antihistamines, which have little effect on the immediate asthmatic reaction, can inhibit the immediate skin test reaction. By analogy it has been considered that the immediate asthmatic reaction may be the consequence of IgE or IgG-STS dependent mast cell degranulation in the airways, similar to the reaction identified as causing such immediate reactions in the skin. In support of this, specific IgE antibody directed against several of the agents causing occupational asthma has been demonstrated in the sera of those affected, as well as in some of those exposed but not affected. Specific IgE antibody has been identified to several of the biological agents which cause occupational asthma, including the *Bacillus subtilis* enzyme, Alcalase [39], rat and mouse urinary proteins [19], castor bean and green coffee bean [40], and wheat and rye flour [41]. Recently, specific IgE antibody to some of the chemical agents causing occupational asthma has also been reported, including the complex platinum salt, ammonium hexachlorplatinate [42], toluene moniisocyanate in workers with asthma due to a reaction to toluene diisocyanate [43], and the epoxy resin curing agents, phthalic acid anhydride [44] and trimellitic acid anhydride [45]. Evidence for the presence of specific IgE antibody, however, is still lacking for several of the agents which cause occupational asthma, and which can provoke immediate reactions on bronchial challenge testing. This may be a reflection of the difficulty of working with highly reactive chemicals in test systems in vitro, or possibly due to the involvement of specific IgG-STS rather than IgE antibody, which has been found in the sera of some platinum refinery workers directed against ammonium hexachlorplatinate. Alternatively, nonimmunologic mechanisms may be involved in these reactions. Davies et al. [46] showed that toluene diisocyanate inhibits the isoproterenol- and prostaglandin E-induced increase in lymphocyte intracellular cyclic AMP in a dose-related fashion, suggesting that TDI may be exerting its effect partly or wholly through a pharmacologic, rather than immunologic effect, causing asthma in those with preexisting bronchial hyperreactivity. Butcher et al. [18] found that 7 of 10 patients who reacted on bronchial provocation testing to TDI had a greater than 20% fall in FEV_1 elicited by methacholine, whereas in only 1 of 10 TDI nonreactors was a greater than 20% fall in FEV_1 provoked; whether the hyperreactivity preceded or followed the development of occupational asthma can only satisfactorily be determined by serial measurements of bronchial reactivity in an exposed cohort, with the initial measurements made before their first exposure to TDI. Some evidence suggesting that the increase in bronchial reactivity is a consequence rather than a predisposing factor in occupational asthma comes from a study of Lam et al. [32]. They found that methacholine reactivity was increased in a group of patients with occupational asthma due to Western red cedar when compared to controls. In those patients in whom serial methacholine studies from the time of diagnosis had been made, methacholine reactivity decreased significantly in those who had subsequently avoided exposure, but remained unchanged in those who had continued to be exposed.

The similarity in speed of onset and duration of both the nonimmediate asthmatic reactions which commence at 4–8 hr and of the peripheral respiratory reactions, to the late cutaneous (Arthus-type) skin test reaction, as well as the finding of specific precipitating antibody in the sera of affected individuals, particularly in those with hypersensitivity pneumonitis, has led to the suggestion that these nonimmediate reactions are a consequence of local immune complex formation in the airways or peripheral lung. In their study of allergic respiratory reactions in bird fanciers, Hargreave and Pepys [38] found that 26 of 31 patients with nonimmediate reactions had precipitins to avian serum proteins, whereas these were found in 1 of the 5 with a lone immediate reaction, and in 5 of the 45 in whom bronchial challenge testing did not provoke a reaction. Of the 30 patients with nonimmediate reactions in whom intracutaneous skin tests with avian serum protein were done, 26 had a late cutaneous reaction; this reaction was elicited in 1 of the 3 tested who had a lone immediate reaction, and in 2 of the 22 not reacting on bronchial provocation testing. Immunofluorescence studies of biopsies taken from some of the patients with late skin test reactions provoked by avian serum proteins demonstrated the presence of perivascular immunoglobulin and complement [47]. In a study of two patients with farmer's lung, Ghose et al. [48] found IgG and IgM antibody and C3 component of complement within blood vessel walls and in surrounding tissue in lung biopsies taken in one patient 36 hr after a natural exposure, and in the other following a bronchial provocation test.

In a study of enzyme detergent workers with occupational asthma, Dolovich et al. [49] found that although the immediate skin test reaction to intracutaneous Alcalase correlated well with the presence of specific IgE antibody in the serum, there was no correlation between the presence of specific serum IgG antibody and the development of a late skin test reaction. Immunofluorescence studies of biopsies of the late skin test reaction revealed neither immunoglobulin or complement. Furthermore, they were able to provoke not only an immediate, but also a late, skin test reaction at passively sensitized sites in the skin of nonsensitive recipients (Prausnitz-Kustner reaction) both with Alcalase and with the $F(ab)_2$ portion of anti-IgE. In a similar study using different antigens, Solley et al. [50] obtained similar results. These studies together suggest that specific IgG or IgM precipitating antibodies are not an obligatory requirement for the development of the late skin test reaction, which can be solely dependant upon an IgE-mediated reaction. Evidence for the involvement of specifically sensitized lymphocytes in the pathogenesis of hypersensitivity pneumonitis has been obtained, both in experimental animals and in humans. This may help to explain why precipitins to *M. faeni* have been found in 18% of farmers without disease [51], and in 40% of healthy pigeon breeders [52], and also the characteristic granulomatous reaction found in the lungs of patients with this disease. Delayed-type hypersensitivity reactions, however, have not been reported as being elicited in patients with hypersensitivity pneumonitis by the specific causal agent, and the timing of the respiratory reactions is at variance with the time course of delayed-type hypersensitivity reactions.

It seems most probable that hypersensitivity pneumonitis is the end result of several interrelated reactions, both immunologic and nonimmunologic, such as activation of the alternate pathway of complement, which Edwards has demonstrated can be activated by *M. faeni* [53]. Which of these mechanisms underlies the peripheral respiratory reaction provoked by bronchial provocation testing is unclear, but this provoked reaction, although not the whole disease process, is probably still best explained by a local immune-complex-mediated reaction.

X. Conclusion

Although concern is sometimes expressed about the use of such tests in clinical investigation, if used only where appropriate indications exist by those with experience of the methods, they constitute a safe and important means of patient investigation.

Understanding of both occupational asthma and hypersensitivity pneumonitis has been helped by analyses of bronchial provocation test reactions. However, the site of the peripheral respiratory reaction in the lung, and the pathological mechanisms underlying nonimmediate reactions, both asthmatic and peripheral, remains unclear. Further investigation of these problems is required.

References

1. Taylor, G., and J. Walker, Charles Harrison Blackley—Review article, *Clin. Allergy,* **3**:103 (1973).
2. Stevens, F. A., A comparison of pulmonary and dermal sensitivity to inhaled substances, *J. Allergy,* **5**:285 (1934).
3. Lowell, F. C., and I. W. Schiller, Reduction in the vital capacity of asthmatic subjects following exposure to aerosolised pollen extracts, *Science,* **105**:317 (1947).
4. Aas, K., Bronchial provocation tests in asthma, *Arch. Dis. Child.,* **45**:221 (1970).
5. Newman Taylor, A. J., C. A. C. Pickering, M. Turner-Warwick, and J. Pepys, Respiratory allergy to a factory humidifier contaminant presenting as a pyrexia of undetermined origin, *Br. Med. J.,* **2**:94 (1978).
6. Harries, M. G., P. S. Burge, M. Samson, A. J. Newman Taylor, and J. Pepys, Isocyanate asthma: Respiratory symptoms to 1, 5 naphthylene di-isocyanate, *Thorax,* **34**:762 (1979).
7 Burge, P. S., and J. Pepys, Berufsbezogenes bronchaler Provokationstest, *Allergologie,* **2**:7 (1979).

8. Hargreave, F. E., Paper presented at symposium on The Reactive Airway. Leicester, England, 1979.
9. Davies, R. J., Bronchial provocation tests with common allergens and chemical vapours and fumes, 197
10. Chai, H., R. S. Farr, L. A. Frochlick, D. A. Matthison, J. A. McLean, R. R. Rosenthal, A. L. Schaffer, S. L. Spector, and R. G. Townley, Standardization of bronchial inhalation procedures, *J. Allergy Clin. Immunol.*, **56**:333 (1975).
11. Orehek, J., P. Gayrard, A. P. Smith, C. Grimaud, and J. Charpin, Airway response to Carbachol in normal and asthmatic subjects: Distinction between bronchial sensitivity and reactivity, *Am. Rev. Respir. Dis.*, **115**:937 (1977).
12. Pickering, C. A. C., J. C. Batten, and J. Pepys, Asthma due to inhaled wood dusts: Western Red Cedar and Iroko, *Clin. Allergy*, **2**:213–218 (1900).
13. Davies, R. J., D. S. Hendrick, and J. Pepys, Asthma due to inhaled chemical agents: Ampicillin, benzyl penicillin, 6-aminopenicillanic acid and related substances, *Clin. Allergy*, **4**:227 (1974).
14. Pickering, C. A. C., Inhalation tests with chemical allergens: Complex salts of platinum, *Proc. R. Soc. Med.*, **65**:272 (1972).
15. Pepys, J., C. A. C. Pickering, and H. W. G. Loudon, Asthma due to inhaled chemical agents–piperazine hydrochloride, *Clin. Allergy*, **2**:189 (1972).
16. Fawcett, I. W., A. J. Newman Taylor, and J. Pepys, Asthma due to inhaled chemical agents, fumes from "Multicore" soldering flux and colophony resin, *Clin. Allergy*, **6**:577 (1976).
17. O'Brien, I. M., A. J. Newman Taylor, P. S. Burge, M. G. Harries, I. W. Fawcett, and J. Pepys, TDI induced asthma. II. Inhalation challenge tests and bronchial reactivity studies, *Clin. Allergy*, **9**:1 (1979).
18. Karr, R. M., R. J. Davies, B. T. Butcher, S. B. Lehrer, M. R. Wilson, V. Dhamarajhan, and J. E. Salvaggio, Occupational asthma, *J. Allergy Clin. Immunol.*, **61**:54 (1978).
19. Newman Taylor, A. J., J. L. Longbottom, and J. Pepys, Respiratory allergy to urine proteins of rats and mice, *Lancet*, **2**:847 (1977).
20. Fawcett, I. W., A. J. Newman Taylor, and J. Pepys, Asthma due to inhaled chemical agents–epoxy resin systems containing phthalic anhydride, trimellitic anhydride and triethylene tetramine, *Clin. Allergy*, **7**:1 (1977).
21. Haydu, S. P., D. W. Empey, and D. T. D. Hughes, Inhalation challenge tests in asthma: An assessment of spirometry, maximum expiratory flow rates and plethysmography in measuring responses, *Clin. Allergy*, **4**:371 (1974).
22. Chan-Yeung, M., Maximal expiratory flow and airway resistance during induced bronchoconstriction in patients with asthma due to Western Red Cedar (*Thuja plicata*), *Am. Rev. Respir. Dis.*, **108**:1103 (1973).
23. Burge, P. S., I. M. O'Brien, and M. G. Harries, Peak flow rate records in the diagnosis of occupational asthma due to colophony, *Thorax*, **34**:303 (1979).

24. Burge, P. S., I. M. O'Brien, and M. G. Harries, Peak flow rate records in the diagnosis of occupational asthma due to isocyanates, *Thorax,* **34**:317 (1979).
25. Newman Taylor, A. J., R. J. Davies, D. J. Hendrick, and J. Pepys, Recurrent nocturnal asthmatic reactions to bronchial provocation tests, *Clin. Allergy,* **9**:213 (1979).
26. Gande via, J., and J. Milne, Occupational asthma and rhinitis due to Western Red Cedar (*Thuja plicata*) with special reference to bronchial reactivity, *Br. J. Ind. Med.,* **27**:235 (1970).
27. Davies, R. J., M. Green, and N. McC. Schofield, Recurrent nocturnal asthma after exposure to grain dust, *Am. Rev. Respir. Dis.,* **114**:1011 (1976).
28. Siracusa, A., F. Curradi, and G. Abbrilli, Recurrent nocturnal asthma due to toluene di-isocyanate: A case report, *Clin. Allergy,* **8**:195 (1978).
29. Hendrick, D. J., and D. J. Lane, Occupational formalin asthma, *Br. J. Ind. Med.,* **34**:11 (1977).
30. Pepys, J., and B. J. Hutchcroft, Bronchial provocation tests in aetiological diagnosis and analysis of asthma, *Am. Rev. Respir. Dis.,* **112**:829 (1975).
31. Chan-Yeung, M., G. M. Barton, L. MacLean, and S. Grzybowski, Occupational asthma and rhinitis due to Western Red Cedar (*Thuja plicata*), *Am. Rev. Respir. Dis.,* **108**:1094 (1973).
32. Lam, L., R. Wong, and M. Chan-Yeung, Non-specific bronchial reactivity in occupational asthma, *J. Allergy Clin. Immunol.,* **63**:28 (1979).
33. Schleuter, D. P., J. N. Fink, and A. J. Sosman, Pulmonary function in pigeon breeders' disease. A hypersensitivity pneumonitis, *Ann. Intern. Med.,* **70**:457 (1969).
34. Allen, D. H., G. V. Williams, and A. J. Woolcock, Bird breeders' hypersensitivity pneumonitis: Progress studies of lung function after cessation of exposure to provoking antigen, *Am. Rev. Respir. Dis.,* **114**:555 (1976).
35. Warren, C. P. W., K. S. Tse, and R. M. Cherniack, Mechanical properties of the lung in extrinsic allergic alveolitis, *Thorax,* **33**:315 (1978).
36. Schofield, N. McC., R. J. Davies, I. R. Cameron, and M. Green, Small airways in fibrosing alveolitis, *Am. Rev. Respir. Dis.,* **113**:729 (1976).
37. Williams, J. V., Inhalation and skin tests with extracts of hay and fungi in patients with farmer's lung, *Thorax,* **18**:182 (1963).
38. Hargreave, F. E., and J. Pepys, Allergic respiratory reactions in bird fanciers' provoked by allergen inhalation provocation tests, *J. Allergy Clin. Immunol.,* **50**:157 (1972).
39. Pepys, J., I. D. Wells, M. F. D'Souza, and M. Greenberg, Clinical and immunological responses to enzymes of *Bacillus subtilis* in factory workers and consumers, *Clin. Allergy,* **3**:143 (1973).
40. Karr, R. M., S. B. Lehrer, B. T. Butcher, and J. E. Salvaggio, Coffee workers asthma: A clinical appraisal using the RAST test, *J. Allergy Clin. Immunol.,* **62**:143 (1978).
41. Bjorksten, F., A. Backman, A. J. Jarvinen, H. Lehti, E. Savilahti, P. Syvanen, and T. Karkkainen, Immunoglobulin E specific to wheat and rye flour, *Clin. Allergy,* **7**:473 (1977).

42. Cromwell, O., J. Pepys, W. E. Parish, and E. G. Hughes, Specific IgE antibodies to platinum salts in sensitized workers, *Clin. Allergy,* **9**:109 (1979).
43. Karol, M., H. H. Ioset, and Y. C. Alarie, Tolyl specific IgE antibodies in workers with hypersensitivity to toluene di-isocyanate, Paper presented to American Industrial Hygiene Conference, May 1978.
44. Maccia, C. A., I. L. Bernstein, E. A. Emmett, and S. M. Brooks, In vitro demonstration of specific IgE in phthalic anhydride hypersensitivity, *Am. Rev. Respir. Dis.,* **113**:701 (1976).
45. Zeiss, C. R., R. Patterson, J. J. Pruzansky, M. M. Muller, M. Rosenberg, I. Suszko, and D. Levitz, Immunological and clinical aspects of trimellitic anhydride respiratory disease, *J. Allergy Clin. Immunol.,* **60**:96 (1977).
46. Davies, R. J., B. T. Butcher, C. E. O'Neill, and J. E. Salvaggio, The in vitro effect of toluene di-isocyanate on lymphocyte cyclic adenosine monophosphate production by isoproterenol prostaglandin and histamine, *J. Allergy Clin. Immunol.,* **60**:223 (1977).
47. Pepys, J. M. Turner-Warwick, P. L. Dawson, and K. F. W. Hinson, Arthus (type III) skin test reactions in man. Clinical and immunopathological features. Edited by B. Rose, M. Richer, A. Schon, and S. W. Frankland. In *Allergology*. Amsterdam, Excerpta Medica, 1968, p. 221.
48. Ghose, T., P. Landrigan, R. Killeen, and J. Dill, Immunopathological studies in patients with farmers' lung, *Clin. Allergy,* **4**:119 (1974).
49. Dolovich, J., F. E. Hargreave, R. Chalmers, K. J. Shier, J. Gauldie, and J. Bienenstock, Late cutaneous allergic responses in isolated IgE dependant reactions, *J. Allergy Clin. Immunol.,* **52**:38 (1973).
50. Solley, G. O., G. J. Gleich, R. E. Jordan, and A. L. Schroeter, The late phase of the immediate weal and flare skin reaction. Its dependence upon IgE antibodies, *J. Clin. Invest.,* **58**:408 (1976).
51. Pepys, J., and P. A. Jenkins, Precipitin (FLH) test in farmer's lung, *Thorax,* **20**:21 (1965).
52. Fink, J. N., A. J. Sosman, J. J. Barboriak, D. P. Schleuter, and R. A. Holmes, Pigeon breeder's disease, *Ann. Intern. Med.,* **68**:1205 (1968).
53. Edwards, J. H., A quantitative study on the activation of the alternate pathway of complement by mouldy hay dust and thermophilic actinomycetes, *Clin. Allergy,* **6**:19 (1976).

9

Lung Morphometry

COOLEY BUTLER

University of New Mexico School of Medicine
Albuquerque, New Mexico

JEROME KLEINERMAN

Mount Sinai School of Medicine
New York, New York

I. Introduction

In general, there are two broad types of morphologic problems amenable to quantitative study in occupational disorders affecting the lung. While the maximum extent and severity of many of these classic pneumoconioses are well defined [1], little if any quantitation of the morphologic lesions in the population at risk has been accomplished, and the relationship of the morphometric evaluation to epidemiological data and radiographic information has barely been initiated. Several limitations are inherent in performing adequate morphometric correlations on autopsy material. (1) The findings at autopsy often represent the advanced and terminal anatomic picture. At this time changes may be present which result from complicating or associated disease states, not necessarily related to the primary pneumoconiosis. Separation of the pertinent anatomic features of the pneumoconiosis and correlation with the relevant historical exposure information may be extremely difficult. (2) Nonoccupational lesions may mimic those associated with occupational exposures; for example, healed disseminated histoplasmosis may simulate nodular silicosis, and nonindustrial soot deposits may mimic the uncomplicated macule of the coal worker. (3) Terminal complicating diseases or lesions such as pneumonia or non-specific interstitial fibrosis may mask the occupationally initiated lesions and make quantitative study of the lung difficult. (4) The quantitative morphometric observations cannot be directly correlated with the specific function tests performed in life, and only to a limited extent with the finding in antero-posterior and lateral chest radiographs. This problem is made even more difficult by nonoccupational factors such as cigarette smoking and environmental pollution which may contribute to the functional compromise observed.

One source of anatomic material, which could provide early lesions of pneumoconiosis, is from individuals who die suddenly from natural causes such as coronary occlusions or from accident, foul play, or suicide. This case material has not been systematically collected or studied, but could provide important information not now available. These efforts would be greatly augmented if autopsies were mandatory in all such cases where compensation is requested, assuming the lungs are prepared and studied by appropriate methods. This anatomic and morphometric information would still require correlation with exposure histories including dust concentrations to which the victims were exposed, cigarette smoking history, and associated medical (respiratory disease) information. It is the only available means by which relatively early lesions of the pneumoconioses in humans can be evaluated morphometrically.

Despite these drawbacks, systematic quantitation of pulmonary abnormalities in persons with known or suspected occupational exposures is worthwhile. The correlation of the quantitative anatomic data with antemortem lung function tests, chest radiographs, and exposure histories remains an area of important study. Moreover, in certain disorders (e.g., silicosis, asbestosis) the intrapulmonary concentrations and chemical nature of the noxious dust or agent can be measured at autopsy [2]. Although the lung content reflects the combined effects of exposure and lung clearance, and only indirectly mirrors either total or maximum exposure, this correlative information is of great value in comparing morphometric data with total dust burden, and to evaluate individual differences in the response to similar dust exposures, particularly the extent of the lung reaction and residual dust in the lung.

Some current problems in occupational lung diseases which are amenable to investigation by morphometric techniques are listed.

1. What is the relationship between functional deficit and destruction of lung substance in occupational lung diseases characterized by fibrosis, such as progressive massive fibrosis (PMF) in coal workers and conglomerate silicosis (CS)? Does the emphysema usually present in association with these zones of fibrosis result in substantial loss of diffusing surface and/or capillary bed? What proportion of the complement of small arterial vessels are narrowed or obliterated by the

fibrosis? To what extent does the loss of capillary bed and the degree of luminal narrowing of the small arteries and arterioles correlate with the presence of pulmonary hypertension? Is the anatomic basis of the limitation to air flow observed in PMF and/or CS related to significant reduction in the total cross-sectional area of small airways?

2. Does exposure to coal dust and/or free crystalline silica (FCS) produce lung fibrosis in a predictable dose-response relationship? How does cigarette smoking influence the morphometric alterations produced by coal dust or FCS exposure? Is there a predictable response of the bronchial mucus glands and/or bronchial or bronchiolar goblet cells to dust concentrations and duration of exposure?

3. Do individuals engaged in working with radioactive dusts (e.g., uranium miners) have morphometrically defined nonneoplastic structural lung findings which can be used as indices of cumulative exposure? How are the findings influenced by concurrent cigarette smoking, or by the type of other minerals (e.g., siliceous rock) present in the ore?

4. In the disorders characterized initially by reversible airway obstruction, such as byssinosis, are there morphometrically definable structural changes in the airways? If so, what level of exposure is necessary to induce them? Is there a dose-response relationship associated with the exposure? What size airway is involved? Are the changes similar in nonsmokers and smokers with similar exposures? Do changes exist in nonsymptomatic, similarly exposed workers?

II. Techniques in Quantitative Pulmonary Pathology

A. Background

Tissue morphometry is a discipline employing techniques designed to quantify the proportion of one or more components in an organ or tissue. Because most tissue is opaque, direct measurement of this kind is not possible without preliminary destruction of architectural relations and physical separation of the components. Morphometric techniques, although largely optical, allow retention of at least some of the architectural relations within a tissue or organ. Therefore, they are almost all indirect forms of measurement which depend on a variety of statistical and geometric assumptions.

The basic concepts of tissue morphometry are actually derived from similar geologic techniques for the visual study of the composition of rocks and other compound minerals. The interested reader can find a valuable resume of these geologic studies, which were begun in the last century, in the work of Chalkley [3]. However, the landmark tissue morphometric study of the lung was the now-classic 1963 monograph by Weibel [4]. This publication was the first comprehensive quantitative anatomic study of any human organ system except for the brain and the blood, and has become a cornerstone for a very large body of information about quantitative normal and abnormal lung structure. This in turn has been immensely helpful in the understanding of the anatomic basis of ventilatory mechanics, the structural and functional correlation of various chronic obstructive lung diseases, and the intricacies of lung growth and development. As a result, the technical refinements and the number of publications in which the morphometric approach is utilized are greatest in studies of the lung. It is, therefore, somewhat paradoxical that so little use has been made of this readily available technology in the important area of occupational lung disease.

For example, our recent literature search by computerized techniques revealed only one English title [5] in the last 6 years for which the terms *morphometry* or *quantitative pathology*, on the one hand, and *pneumoconiosis, occupational lung disease*, or *hypersensitivity pneumonitis*, on the other hand, were indexed as keys. Further, in recent extensive "state-of-the-art" reviews of silicosis [6], lung disease in coal workers [7], and asbestos-induced lung injury [8], only two references were targeted toward a quantitative assessment of tissue injury. This deficit stands very much in contrast to the extensive literature on quantification of radiographic changes and indices of exposure in occupational lung disease, as well as the large body of information about quantitative aspects of normal lung structure and the techniques useful for measuring disease-related alterations in lung structure occurring in many non-occupational disorders such as emphysema.

B. Basic Morphometric Principles

There are several methods for the measurement of area proportions, but the simplest, least subject to various biases, and most widely applicable is point-counting. This method utilizes random placement of a grid system on the cut surface, most commonly a uniform grid composed of complete or incomplete equilateral triangular or rectangular lattices, and differential counting of the tissue components falling directly beneath the grid intersections. It is useful for measurements on gross material, microscopic slides, or photographs, and is unaffected by the shape of the components or the complexity of their spatial interrelationships. Compared to several other available techniques, it is less time consuming, and has the added advantage that it is conceptually compatible with automated video image analysis processes.

This method and most others involved in morphometric studies depend upon unbiased sampling of the organ to be studied. Because inferences about the whole-organ structure are to be made from very small portions of the parenchyma, it is essential that each part of the organ have the same probability as any other part of being included in the samples. Acceptable methods for obviating sample bias are stratified sampling and random sampling; most commonly they are employed in combination in pulmonary morphometry. Stratified sampling is exemplified by the creation of multiple, parallel, equidistant slices through an entire organ: once the plane of the first slice is chosen, either randomly or in respect to the organ geometry, the plane of all other slices is predetermined. In this example, the several cut surfaces constitute the primary samples. Random sampling is exemplified by the placement of the point-counting grid on the cut surface, which must be accomplished blindly, without regard for the relation of the grid to the slice, the shape of the slice, or the internal distribution of the components to be point-counted. A combination of stratified and random sampling is used to obtain blocks for tissue sections from the slice surface. Most commonly, consecutively numbered rectangles of the exact block size to be used are marked on an overlay transparency in a checkerboard fashion and dropped in random position on the slice surface. The rectangles beneath which blocks are taken are chosen sequentially with a table of random numbers. The overlay must be somewhat larger than the largest slice, so that the difference in area between slices can be taken into account by using the same number of random "tries" per slice: a greater number of tries will fall beyond the edges of the smaller slices, so that fewer tissue blocks are chosen from them. Although much of this procedure is randomized, the long axes of the various blocks from a given slice are oriented in a stratified fashion, and of course only the slice surfaces are sampled, not the interiors. Microscopic sampling is done by similar techniques: normally one slide per block is used, and if possible the desired measurement is made on the whole of that particular side. If only a part of the slide is sampled, a convenient technique is to choose microscopic fields with longitudinal and transverse coordinates on a stage vernier designated by random numbers; in this situation it is important to avoid partial remeasurement of previously chosen fields. Entirely analogous methods permit unbiased measurements from photographs, photomicrographs, projected microscopic fields, and electron micrographs.

It is implicit in the type of sampling procedures described above that the component to be measured is distributed randomly throughout the specimen, or at least that its distribution does not form some spurious correlation with the sampling procedures. An example of the latter situation might arise in the morphometric evaluation of the larger sizes of blood vessels in many organs, for these often are not uniformly distributed. Serious underestimation of the number of such vessels might arise because the organ slices were sufficiently thick and oriented in a plane which "buried" most vessels of the desired size inside the slices, with little exposure on the cut surface. There is no hard and fast rule available in these circumstances: proper slice thickness and orientation vary to some extent from problem to problem, and will obviously be quite different in dealing with the hypophysis as compared to the liver. However, there are some statistical considerations in planning the size and the intricacy of any morphometric study, which are useful to the investigator for assuring the desired level of precision. First, if the sampling procedure has multiple steps, such as the slicing of a gross organ, followed by the selection of microscopic slides from the slices, in turn followed by the selection of fields from each slide, the overall variance (S^2) of the procedure is related to the variance of the results from the individual steps in the following way:

$$S^2_{\text{overall}} = \frac{S^2\ \text{slices}}{a} + \frac{S^2\ \text{slides}}{ab} + \frac{S^2\ \text{fields}}{abc}$$

Where a = number of slices sampled, b = number of slides used, and c = number of fields used. The important point from the relationship is that variance is reduced most efficiently by increasing the number of primary samples (i.e., slices). It provides much greater accuracy to examine twice as many tissue slices (by making the slices half as thick) and retain the same number of slides per slice and fields per slide, than it does simply to double the number of fields examined per slide, even though the total number of fields examined is the same in each case.

The second statistical consideration in relation to sample size has to do with the prevalence of the component being measured within the whole organ or tissue. If p = the fraction of the organ occupied by the measured component, so that $0 < p < 1$, then the relative error of the morphometric measurement is proportional to the expression

$$\sqrt{\frac{1 - p}{pn}}$$

where n = sample size or number of observations. Relative error relates the standard error of the measurements of p to the size of the p itself, somewhat analogous to the coefficient of variation commonly applied to means. The important aspect of this relationship is that if p is small (the component is sparsely distributed), the sample size must be comparatively large to reach a given degree of statistical accuracy. It is much less time consuming to measure plentiful tissue components.

Finally, the processing of tissue influences the measurements made with these techniques. Fixation induces tissue shrinkage of varying degrees, depending on the fixation and the temperature, and the magnitude may be irregular if fixation is initially incomplete. Dehydrating and embedding chemicals produce further shrinkage, particularly alcohols, and section cutting may compress the tissue perpendicular to the cutting edge, thereby inducing differential shrinkage. The most reliable way to allow for these effects is to make direct linear measurements on the gross organ before and after fixation (or to take blocks prior to organ fixation) and to measure the size of the tissue block, before embedding, and compare it to the size of the fully processed section mounted on the slide. These latter comparisons should be made in two dimensions, to account for cutting compression. The resulting ratios are simply used as coefficients for correction of the raw morphometric data to yield measurements representative of the tissue elements without fixation and dehydration.

C. Special Morphometric Considerations in the Lung

One of the most important ways in which lung differs from other organs is its great elasticity, making it deformable and compressible. Furthermore the lung undergoes rapid changes in size, 15-35 times a minute in normal situations. As a result, particular effort must be taken to standardize the size of the lung during morphometric investigation. Modern methods of evaluating lung function in vivo commonly include measurement of lung volumes, which may be used as a basis for evaluating the degree of postmortem lung inflation. Many morphometric studies standardize lung size by controlling lung volume, in particular the degree of inflation, during tissue fixation. A simple technique is to instill fixative into the airways at a constant pressure, conventionally 25 cmH_2O, which is roughly the maximum attainable transpulmonary inflation pressure in life. This pressure is maintained for several hours until fixation is complete and the tissue has lost much of its elasticity. Removal of major intraluminal obstructions, such as mucus, is a necessary prelude to the proper application of this technique. When mucus plugging is severe and the secretions extremely viscous, as in cystic fibrosis, complete fixation and inflation may take a longer time or may not be possible.

There are two problems with the use of a constant inflation pressure as the sole control of lung size. First, there are age-related changes in the elastic recoil properties of lung and chest wall [9]. With age the human lung loses elastic recoil, the chest wall becomes more rigidly fixed, and the maximal pressures generated by muscular contraction of the diaphragm and intercostals are compromised. Thus a given inflation pressure in excised lungs may result in a volume within the accepted normal ranges for younger age-sex groups, but can produce a volume greater than the normal in vivo range in the lungs from older individuals. A second problem is that the elastic recoil properties of lung are frequently altered by disease, particularly emphysema or diffuse fibrosis, so that the use of a constant inflation pressure may lead to morphometric measurements which include the effects produced by disease in addition to the variables under study [10]. These differences must be evaluated in comparison with controls of appropriate ages and by elimination of specimens with significant amounts of intercurrent disease. The interpretation of a "significant" degree must be left to the individual investigator, but as a general guide should not exceed *10%* of the lung cut surface. With these limited reservations, inflation-fixation at 25 cmH_2O transpulmonary pressure is a satisfactory technique for almost all purposes. A cumbersome alternative is the performance of a preliminary pressure-volume study using air on each lung, after which an inflation pressure which will result in "full" inflation is selected for each lung [11]. This is time-consuming and not completely satisfactory because it does not necessarily ensure that the appropriate volume attainable in life is used, and because the pressure-volume characteristics of a given lung during air inflation are different from those observed during inflation with fixative, because of the effect on airspace surface properties of the fixative. For some morphometric purposes, such as measurement of total internal surface area, it has been a common practice to correct the volume obtained with the lung inflated to 25 cmH_2O pressure to either a constant volume, the measured antemortem total lung capacity, or the value predicted for total lung capacity from the individual's height, age, and sex [12,13]. The correction factor used for area-related measurements, such as surface area, is the two-thirds power of that ratio; for linear measurements, the cube root of the ratio applies. This correction is based on the assumption that the lung expansion occurs equally in all tissue components and is proportionately the same in all directions under the conditions of inflation-fixation. This practice is problematic because it makes assumptions which cannot be verified for the individual case.

Although inflation-fixation with liquid fixative, most commonly buffered 10% aqueous formalin, is the simplest, least expensive, and most commonly used technique, other methods may be used: inflation with air [14], with formalin vapor [15], or with other liquid fixatives such as Zenker's solution [16] or glutaraldehyde [17] has some advantages, but these techniques may also compromise histologic quality, are more difficult technically, and more expensive.

The compressibility of pulmonary tissue, even after fixation, demands very careful handling to prevent artifactual compression of tissue blocks during their preparation. A useful safeguard is to select blocks and excise them from the noncompressed slice surface while the slice is immersed in water. In subsequent handling to produce microscopic slides, the tissues must be vacuum embedded, and free of air and not compressed during embedding. Furthermore, considerable care must be taken not to squeeze or tear the tissue, and to produce sections of uniform thickness without folding or compression at the edges.

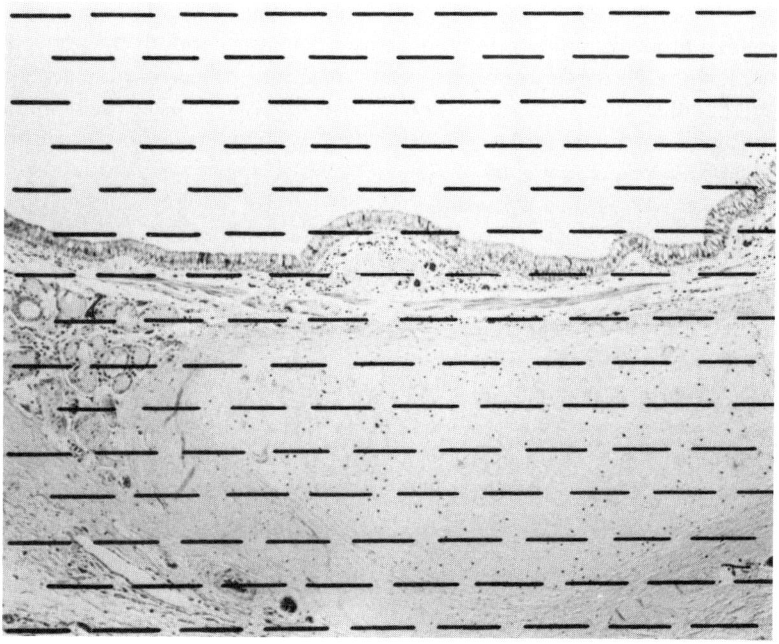

Figure 1 Bronchial wall component measurement. The microscopic image can be projected onto a grid such as that illustrated. Each end of each short line constitutes one point. The proportion of mucosal cells, cartilage, muscle, glands, other tissue, and lumen are easily measured. Data from different fields or slides can be pooled, as long as magnification is constant. (Magnification X48).

Our experience has taught us that tissue preparation for first-rate pulmonary morphometry requires specially trained and skilled histology personnel devoted to that activity and working in a separate and adequate area. Appropriate material can rarely be produced in a service-oriented laboratory.

III. Useful Specific Measurements in Lung

A. Bronchial Wall Component Measurement

A number of useful techniques have evolved for quantitative study of airway walls, particularly in the setting of chronic airflow obstructions. Smooth muscle mass [18], bronchial gland mass [19], and amount of cartilage [20] have all been measured, often concurrently. It is also possible to distinguish between longitudinal and circular muscle, and between basophilic (serous) and clear (mucous) cells in the glands by differential counting (Fig. 1). A number of closely related techniques can be used, but one of the simplest is to project the image of a bronchial cross section onto a point-counting grid. If the projection magnification and the separation of points are chosen properly, one can count several hundred points on a given section. Frequently, it is useful to stain the section with trichrome or Alcian Blue-PAS (pH 2.5) in order to sharpen the contrast between components.

The results yielded by this method are relative, so that some sort of normalization is necessary for comparison of different cases. A simple solution is to compare airways of the same branching generation, although this fails to take into account the large differences in central airway size among individuals of different size [21]. Direct measurement of airway diameter is accurate only if a true cross section at right angles to the long axis is selected, or if the smallest axis of an elliptical section is used. Measurement of lumen cross-sectional area during the point-counting procedure requires high-quality histologic sections without significant distortion. The validity of these measurements is dependent on adequate sampling techniques, the counting of significant numbers of airways, consistency in measurements, and comparison with normal populations studied by similar techniques.

The classic method of describing bronchial gland mass is the Reid index, which is the ratio of gland layer thickness to the thickness of bronchial mucous membrane, with the latter measured from the inner perichondrium to the basement membrane of the luminal epithelium [22]. This technique is much faster than point-counting, but less accurate because it doesn't measure the glands between cartilages, which may be extensive in chronic bronchitis, particularly in the distal bronchi [23]. Despite this objection, the Reid index has usefulness as a quick estimate of the comparative measure of bronchial gland mass for correlation with symptoms of mucus hyperproduction in life. Even with this simple method multiple measurements of the linear thickness of glands and mucous membranes should be done in any one bronchus section since these values may vary at different points in one bronchus by 100% or more.

B. Quantification of Gross Parenchymal Abnormalities

Techniques for estimating the severity of parenchymal involvement by disease have been applied most commonly in the study of emphysema; these methods can be applied to other diseases including pneumonic infiltrates, fibrosis, and metastatic neoplasm to name a few. In relation to occupational disease, quantification of the extent of emphysema and of fibrosis separately would yield important information (Fig. 2). Point-counting of gross slices cut at equal intervals will provide the relative proportions of uninvolved and involved parenchyma, as well as "nonparenchyma" (vessels and airways). For purposes of measuring emphysema, counting of two midsagittal slices (in order to provide

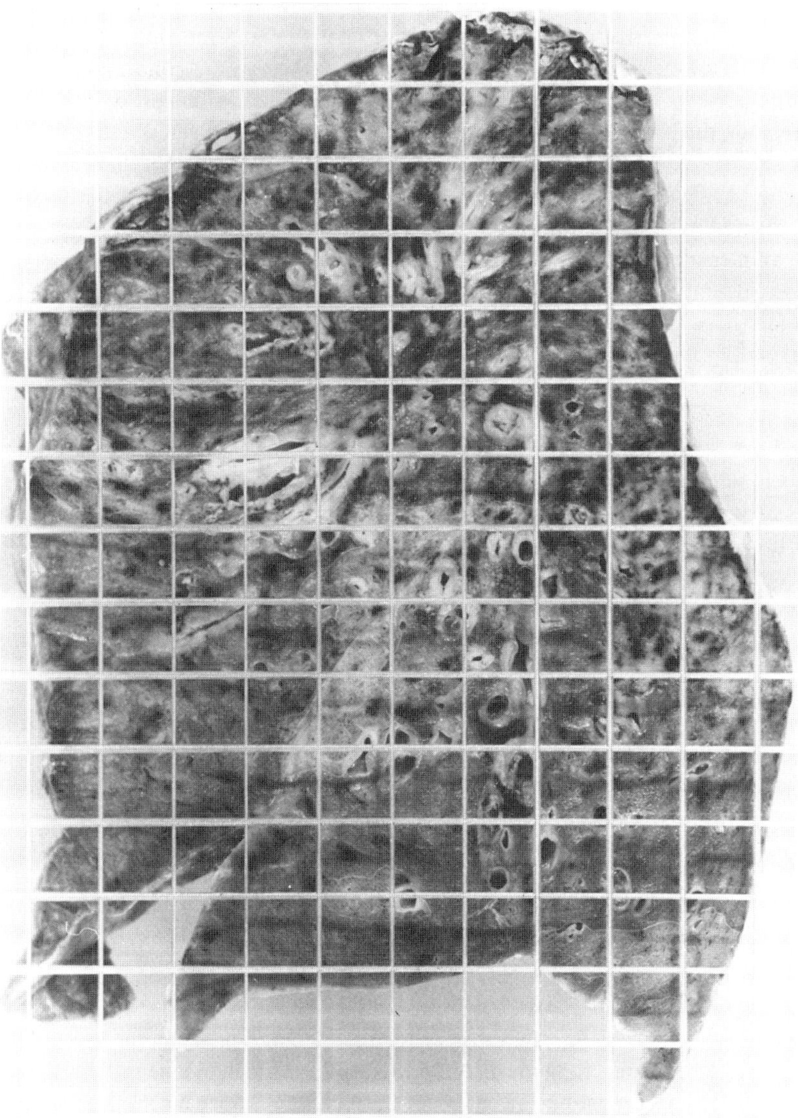

Figure 2 A sagittal slice of fibrotic, shrunken lung is covered by a plexiglass grid with engraved 1 cm squares. Using the corners as single points, the proportion of lung parenchyma which is grossly abnormal is readily obtained from one slice or from many.

counts of 200–250 points), is often adequate [24]; however, the less widespread the abnormality, the more important it becomes to count multiple slices sufficient to provide an adequate number of points falling on the abnormal areas, and to provide acceptable sampling. A major drawback to this procedure is that it records the presence or absence of the abnormality at a given point, but not the severity, so that, for example, similar point counts can be obtained from lung specimens with quite different degrees of emphysematous destruction. This problem may be less important in the estimate of focal fibrosis than of emphysema unless diffuse honeycombing is present. Alternative techniques for assessment of emphysema include comparison of specimens under study with standardized pictures of lesions of varying degrees of severity [25], measurement of light transmission through a section of specified thickness [26], and the semiquantitative estimation, by direct visual inspection, of regional severity [27]. One difficult problem inherent in all these techniques is that disease may change local tissue properties: for example, elastic recoil is lost in emphysema, resulting in comparative hyperinflation, whereas there is progressive volume loss in areas of fibrosis as the scars undergo remodeling with time [10]. As a result, the proportion of original parenchymal volume occupied by the abnormality can not be adequately assessed.

C. Microscopic Quantification of Structural Components of the Lung

Given adequate sampling as described previously, it is possible to measure the number of, and parenchymal proportion occupied by, the different kinds of bronchioles, alveolar ducts, and alveoli. The techniques for this kind of measurement presuppose that these structures are distributed and oriented in an essentially random way in regard to the plane of tissue section. This assumption is reasonable for small distal structures. Analogous methods may be used for small blood vessels, as described below. Two forms of quantification are possible: (1) the proportion of parenchyma occupied by each component, with the result expressed as a percentage and the data collected by point-counting; (2) the number of each kind of structure per unit area of the microscopic section [28,29]. The former figure is directly applicable as a volumetric proportion, whereas the latter must be corrected for both airway shape and the area-volume relationship to yield the number of structures per unit volume. One major problem with these techniques is the difficulty in distinguishing an alveolar duct from a respiratory bronchiole in the section: The distinction is based, respectively, on the absence or presence of discontinuous smooth muscle in the wall, and muscle may not be evident in a given plane of section. Further, these methods require the use of a rigid set of operational rules for the frequent circumstance where a point falls on the interface between two structures or where a structure is partially cut off by the edge of the section. Rules similar to those adopted in manual hematologic cell counting are usually employed. It is important to note that comparatively large structures are more likely to be influenced by the edge considerations than are small structures, because of the finite size of the section.

It is also possible to measure the diameter or cross-sectional area of the conducting airways, principally nonrespiratory bronchioles, and to develop mean values or frequency histograms from these data [30]. The principal difficulty has to do with any structure the long axis of which is sharply oblique to the plane of section; "true" or "greatest" diameter may not be in the section plane under these circumstances. The conventional solution is to measure only those structures more or less perpendicular to the section plane, which sharply reduces the number available from each section and requires extensive sampling for an adequate number of measurements. This method is very difficult to apply to more distal structures because the alveolation of gas-exchanging airways obscures precise delineation of the external limit of the structures.

A final comment about these methods is that, because of the mixed dichotomous and nondichotomous branching of the airways, more peripheral airway generations are more heavily represented in normal lungs. In fact, about half of all structures of a given class (e.g., nonrespiratory bronchioles) are of the most distal generation of that class. This fact must be taken into account in comparing normal lungs with lungs in which there is pathological alteration of these structures.

D. Internal Surface Area

A useful stereologic principle is that if a given length of line (L) is randomly cast on a tissue section, the ratio (S/V) of the surface area of complex randomly distributed structures, such as gas-exchanging surfaces, to the volume of the tissue, is inversely proportional to the mean linear intercept (L_M), or the average distance between intersections of that line with outlines of the structures (Fig. 3). In practice, surface/volume ratios in lung are measured by randomly placing a line of known length L on multiple tissue sections and counting the total number of intersections (n) of airspace wall and the line. If the line is placed S number of times to arrive at the total n, then:

$$l_m = \frac{n}{LS} \quad \text{and} \quad S/V = \frac{4}{l_m}$$

If the lung volume is known, and appropriate corrections are made for shrinkage of processing and for the percentage of the lung which is nonparenchyma, then total gas-exchanging internal surface area can be calculated directly. This is a

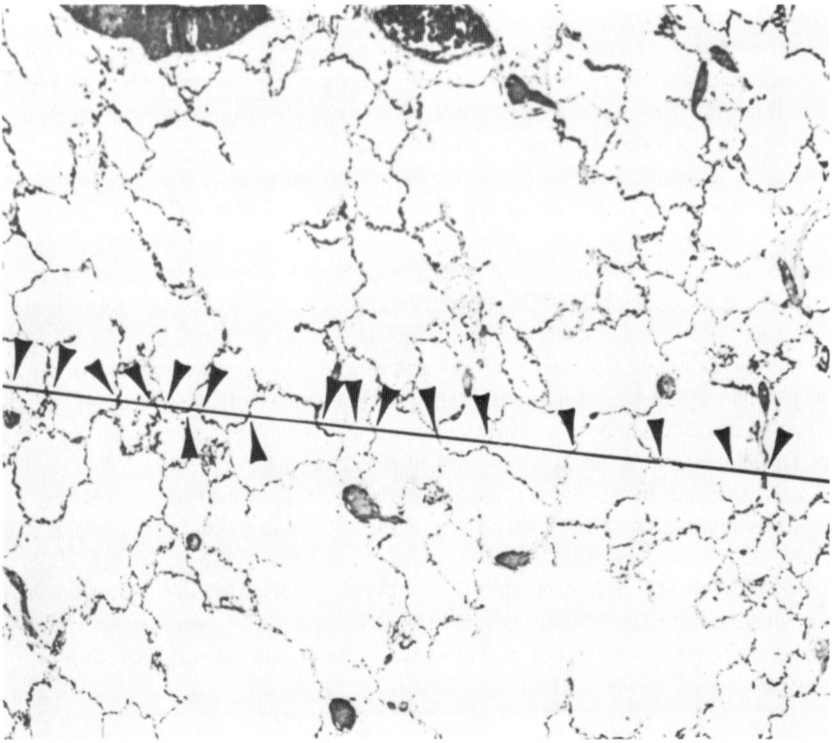

Figure 3 Mean linear intercept measurement: The central line may be in an eyepiece or on a projection screen. The field must be chosen in a random fashion (see text). The arrowheads represent intersections of the line with alveolar walls. LM is the average distance between intersections and is inversely proportional to internal surface area. (Magnification X 48).

most useful measurement in detecting subtle loss of lung tissue, as in emphysema, in which the total area and S/V ratio are diminished [31]. The utility of knowing lung volume in part is related to the decrease of S/V which may occur in hyperinflation without destruction: only by comparing actual lung volume with expected norms can hyperinflation be recognized and allowed for as described above.

On the other hand, comparatively little work has been done to assess the effect of interstitial lung diseases, particularly those resulting in restrictive ventilatory abnormalities and parenchymal fibrosis, on lung surface area. A technical difficulty is that in these disorders the airspaces are frequently enlarged and the walls are thickened so that intersections with the measuring line are not points, as is usually true in emphysematous or normal lung, but rather are broad zones. It is possible for the measuring line to be largely within, and parallel to the surface of, airspace walls, and difficulties in counting arise if the ends of the measuring line lie in such a position. Choice of a lower magnification for counting tends to reduce this difficulty.

E. Vascular Component Measurement

Previous efforts to study pulmonary vasculature quantitatively have largely been in relation to the pathogenesis of increased vascular resistance and, ultimately, cor pulmonale. Measurements most frequently employed have been medial thickness, lumen diameter, overall vessel size, and often the ratio between any two measurements of lumen and wall [32]. Generally, these measurements have been done on lung inflated in a controlled fashion, at times with the added control of vascular perfusion at constant pressure during fixation, but at least some measurements have been published in which the number or area of endothelial nuclei—presumed to be constant in a given vessel and unaffected by lung disease—has been used as a normalizing factor in uninflated lung [33]. Generally speaking, it is satisfactory to perform measurements of the smaller arteries and veins on sections of inflated lung, using elastic stain such as the Verhoff method counterstained with van Gieson stain. This stain enhances the distinction between arteries and veins, allows easy recognition of totally thrombosed vessels, and precisely delineates the media of small muscular arteries, the vessels most severely affected in hypertensive pulmonary disease. As with small airways, obliquity to the plane of section must be dealt with; it is simple to limit measurements to those vessels with an elliptical presentation on section not exceeding a 2:1 ratio for the long to short axes, a tactic which in our experience eliminates all tangential sections and makes avoidance of branch points much simpler. Because the vessel is assumed to be cylindrical, measurements along the short axis of the ellipse are the equivalent of "true" measurements perpendicular to the long axis of the vessel. A convenient way to gather relevant morphometric information about small vessels is to "size" them by measuring from external media to internal media along the short axis of the ellipse, and to point-count the respective medial and luminal areas, all on projected sections. The absolute cross section of the media can be calculated as:

$$\frac{\pi D^2}{4}\left(\frac{M}{L+M}\right)$$

where D is the short axis measurement, and M and L are the number of points on media and lumen, respectively. In analogous fashion.

$$\frac{\pi D^2}{4}\left(\frac{L}{L+M}\right)$$

yields absolute lumen cross section. These formulae presuppose that there is no significant subintimal thickening; however, a substantial subintimal zone, if present, is readily dealt with by point-counting it separately and including the count (I) in the denominator of the calculation above:

$$\frac{\pi D^2}{4}\left(\frac{L}{L+M+I}\right)$$

(for absolute lumen size).

The pulmonary capillary bed can be measured using electron microscopic sections if certain geometric assumptions are accepted. These techniques, similar to those above for measurements of internal surface area, yield data on the surface available in the vast plexus of vessels. However, for most purposes we recommend the measurement of capillary density (CD) [34]. CD is measured, on thick (50 μm) sections, as the frequency with which a random line parallel to the alveolar wall intercepts capillaries. These structures are easier to see when prefilled with an aqueous suspension of pigment* injected arterially under pressure. The thick sections are used to assure that many alveolar walls lie within and parallel to the plane of the section. CD is expressed in units of intercepts per millimeter of measuring line after correction for section shrinkage, and yields useful comparative (but not absolute) data about the number of capillaries in airspace wall.

IV. Conclusion

Consideration of the techniques and potential applications discussed in this chapter leads to the recognition of the important problems associated with this kind of investigation of occupational lung disease. For the most part, the methods are best applied at autopsy, but many of the disorders are compatible with longevity. Collection of material for study of early lesions is most difficult and can only reasonably be approached by studies of medical examiner populations. Many individuals with occupational lung diseases die in hospitals due to unrelated or nonrespiratory causes and often go unrecognized or unstudied. Pulmonary infections, which are frequent in hospital deaths, may produce changes which interfere with the application of methods for quantitative or morphometric study. Finally, the autopsy

*Monastral Pigments, Dupont Corporation, Wilmington, Delaware.

services of many hospitals are ill equipped and unprepared for these kinds of study, so that much of the available material is surely lost with regularity.

Although these problems are serious, there are two potential avenues for research scientists to gain this kind of material. The first is through cooperation with modern, thorough forensic pathologists in cases where occupational injury exists or is suspected. The problems occurring in hospital deaths are obviated in the frequent cases of sudden, traumatic, or otherwise unexpected death characteristic of the medical examiner's autopsy responsibility. Epidemiological support is necessary to verify the occupational history and exposure levels, as far as possible, in all cases studied. Participation in this sort of investigation is generally viewed favorably by forensic pathologists, who recognize that the resulting information is of considerable public interest, particularly in the areas of work safety and legislative regulation of industry.

The second available avenue, and one with considerable current precedent, is the establishment of federally sponsored centers for the study of occupational lung disease, with mandated authority to obtain autopsy material in all instances where industrial compensation is an issue. Such a project might be carried out on a regional basis and directed toward various occupations indigenous to the region, such as byssinosis in the Southeast, or hypersensitivity pneumonitis in the North Central states.

The results of the studies suggested in this brief review could add important information and provide significant benefits to the working population, as well as to industry and government, by making available objective data for use in adjudicating compensation claims and more detailed scientific information concerning the pathology and pathogenesis of the human diseases produced by inhalation of industrial dusts, gases, and aerosols.

References

1. Morgan, W. K. C., and A. Seaton, *Occupational Lung Diseases.* Philadelphia, W. B. Saunders, 1975.
2. Funahashi, A., K. Pintar, and K. A. Seigesmund, Identification of foreign material in lung by energy-dispersive x-ray analysis, *Arch. Environ. Health,* **30**:285–289 (1975).
3. Chalkley, H. W., Methods for the quantitative morphologic analysis of tissues, *J. Natl. Cancer Inst.,* **4**:47–53 (1943).
4. Weibel, E. R., *Morphometry of the Human Lung.* Berlin, Springer, 1963.
5. Divertie, M. B., S. M. Cassan, and A. L. Brown, Jr., Ultrastructural morphometry of the diffusion surface in a case of pulmonary asbestosis, *May Clin. Proc.,* **50**:193–197 (1975).

6. Ziskind, M., R. N. Jones, and H. Weill, State of the art: Silicosis, *Am. Rev. Respir. Dis.*, **113**:643–665 (1976).
7. Morgan, W. K. C., and N. L. Lapp, State of the art: Respiratory disease in coal miners, *Am. Rev. Respir. Dis.*, **113**:531–559 (1976).
8. Becklake, M. R., State of the art: Asbestos-related disease of the lung and other organs: Their epidemiology and implications for clinical practice, *Am. Rev. Respir. Dis.*, **114**:187–227 (1976).
9. Turner, J. M., J. Mead, and M. E. Wohl, Elasticity of human lungs in relation to age, *J. Appl. Physiol.*, **25**:664–671 (1968).
10. Macklem, P. T., and M. R. Becklake, The relationship between the mechanical and diffusing properties of the lung in health and disease, *Am. Rev. Respir. Dis.*, **87**:47–56 (1963).
11. Pratt, P. C., and G. A. Klugh, A technique for the study of ventilatory capacity, compliance and residual volume of excised lungs and for fixation, drying and serial sectioning in the infated state, *Am. Rev. Respir. Dis.*, **83**:690–696 (1961).
12. Thurlbeck, W. M., The internal surface area of non-emphysematous lungs, *Am. Rev. Respir. Dis.*, **95**:765–776 (1968).
13. Bignon, J., J. Andre-Bougaran, and G. Brouet, Parenchymal, bronchiolar, and bronchial measurements in centrilobular emphysema, *Thorax*, **25**: 556–567 (1970).
14. Blumenthal, B. J., and H. G. Boren, Lung structure in three dimensions after inflation and fume fixation, *Am. Rev. Tuberc.*, **79**:674–772 (1959).
15. Weibel, E. R., and R. A. Vidone, Fixation of the lung by formation steam in a controlled state of air inflation, *Am. Rev. Respir. Dis.*, **84**:856–861 (1961).
16. Wright, R. R., Elastic tissue of normal and emphysematous lungs: A tridimensional histologic study, *Am. J. Pathol.*, **39**:355–367 (1961).
17. Siegwart, B., P. Gehr, J. Gil, and E. R. Weibel, Morphometric estimation of pulmonary diffusion capacity. IV. The dog normal lung, *Respir. Physiol.*, **13**:141–148 (1971).
18. Hossain, S., and B. E. Heard, Hyperplasia of bronchial muscle in chronic bronchitis, *J. Pathol.*, **101**:171–184 (1970).
19. Bedrossian, C. W. M., S. D. Greenberg, and B. S. Duran, Bronchial gland measurements: A continuing search for a "yardstick," *Exp. Mol. Pathol.*, **18**:219–224 (1973).
20. Thurlbeck, W. M., R. Pun, J. Toth, and J. G. Frazer, Bronchial cartilage in chronic obstructive lung disease, *Am. Rev. Respir. Dis.*, **109**:73–80 (1974).
21. Jesseph, V. D., and K. A. Merendino, The dimensional interrelationships of the major components of the human tracheobronchial tree, *Surg. Gynecol. Obstet.*, **105**:210–214 (1957).
22. Reid, L., Measurement of the bronchial mucous gland layer: A diagnostic yardstick in chronic bronchities, *Thorax*, **15**:132–141 (1960).
23. Bedrossian, C. W. M., A. E. Anderson, Jr., and A. G. Foraker, Comparison of methods for quantitating bronchial morphology, *Thorax*, **26**:406–408 (1971).

24. Thurlbeck, W. M., The geographic pathology of emphysema and chronic bronchitis. II. Subjective assessment of emphysema, *Arch. Environ. Health,* **14**:21-28 (1967).
25. Ryder, R. C., W. M. Thurlbeck, and J. Gough, A study of interobserver variation in the assessment of the amount of pulmonary emphysema in paper-mounted whole lung sections, *Am. Rev. Respir. Dis.,* **99**:354-364 (1969).
26. Sherwin, R. P., Quantitation for the diagnosis and measurement of pulmonary emphysema. In *Pathology Annual 1968.* Edited by S. C. Sommers. New York, Appleton-Century-Crofts, 1968, 399-435.
27. Thurlbeck, W. M., M. S. Dunnill, W. Hartung, B. E. Heard, A. G. Heppleston, and R. C. Ryder, A comparison of three methods of measuring emphysema, *Hum. Pathol.,* **1**:215-226 (1970).
28. Anderson, A. E., Jr., and A. G. Foraker, Relative dimensions of bronchioles and parenchymal spaces in lungs from normal subjects and emphysematous patients, *Am. J. Med.,* **32**:218-228 (1962).
29. Matsuba, K., and W. M. Thurlbeck, The number and dimensions of small airways in non-emphysematous lungs, *Am. Rev. Respir. Dis.,* **104**:516-524 (1971).
30. Anderson, A. E., Jr., and A. G. Foraker, The non-respiratory bronchioles in pulmonary emphysema. In *Pathology Annual 1974.* Edited by S. C. Sommers. New York, Appleton-Century-Crofts, 1974, pp. 231-261.
31. Butler, C., Lung surface area in various morphologic forms of human emphysema, *Am. Rev. Respir. Dis.,* **114**:347-352 (1976).
32. Scott, K. W. M., Quantitation of thick-walled peripheral lung vessels in chronic airways obstruction, *Thorax,* **31**:315-319 (1976).
33. Naeye, R. L., and W. A. Laqueur, Chronic cor pulmonale: Its pathogenesis in Appalachian bituminous coal workers, *Arch. Pathol.,* **90**:487-493 (1970).
34. Butler, II, C., and J. Kleinerman, Capillary density: Alveolar diameter, a morphometric approach to ventilation and perfusion, *Am. Rev. Respir. Dis.,* **102**:886-894 (1970).

10

Tissue Mineral Identification

FREDERICK D. POOLEY

University College of Cardiff
Cardiff, Wales, United Kingdom

I. Introduction

The association of dust particles with production of disease has been recognized for many hundreds of years, and references from Hippocrates onward can be found concerned with mining operations and their related medical problems. It was only at the start of this century, however, that the first serious attempts were made to study airborne dusts and collect information concerning the particles being retained in the lungs.

The importance of the identification of material of nonbiological origin that may be found in lung tissue specimens obtained from diseased and control cases has in recent years received increasing attention because of the demonstratable association of cancer with the inhalation and retention of dust particles formed from certain mineral species [1]. It has become apparent that a more permanent and extended examination of the materials implicated in the incidence of lung fibrosis and cancer is required. No major effort in the research into diseases of the respiratory system and other related organs, which are presumed to be precipitated by the exposure to particulate materials, can therefore proceed without research which can provide adequate information concerning the quality and quantity of the particular dust materials involved.

Information of this type is often of vital importance in assessing the health hazard when exposure to dust clouds of particular compositions is taking place, and it also contributes significantly to the design and scientific interpretation of biological experimentation and epidemiological studies.

The establishment of the identity of the constituents of the foreign material to be found in tissue specimens presents many practical problems. These problems mainly arise from the fact that the deposits of material to be investigated are often only present in minute quantities and occur in a very finely divided form. The composition of dust deposited and retained in the lungs will vary tremendously, being related to an accumulation of particles from a variety of atmospheres over many years of occupational and nonoccupational exposure. Each tissue specimen examined must therefore be considered to be unique even though in many investigations the source of specimens consist of disease cases arising from a particular industry where individuals are assumed to have been exposed to airborne materials of an identical nature.

A survey of the literature covering investigations of the dust content of lung tissues shows that in most instances the identity of the materials observed have rarely been definitely established, the presence of a particular mineral being simply inferred from a physical or chemical observation of the dust. This situation still arises in present-day investigations where, for example, fibrous particles observed by optical microscopy are often identified as being asbestos minerals when they may just as easily be any one of several fibrous materials which may be found in our environment.

Naturally occurring minerals are defined by a combination of chemical and structural information which has been accumulated over the years for reference purposes. To identify a particular mineral in a dust requires therefore that structural and chemical information be collected and compared with the reference data. It is often very difficult to make such a satisfactory match, sometimes because of inadequate reference data, but usually because of the poor quality of the data collected from the dust specimen itself. In many cases an identification of a particular constituent may be impossible because of alterations in its chemical or physical properties or because of the lack of reference information. Many particles that are inhaled and retained are not produced from the size reduction of natural mineral grains but are the products of industrial activity. These particles may be amorphous, may vary considerably in their chemical composition and morphology, and may have no identity. The identification of such constituents of a dust is not therefore the prime objective of an analysis; rather, it must be accurately characterized both chemically and physically. If the information collected allows the identity of one particular fraction of the dust to be subsequently identified, then this may often be considered to be a bonus. It is rarely the case that only a single mineral is implicated in a disease response. The presence of other constituents in a dust must be considered as they may modify or enhance a pathological reaction. The effort in establishing the identity of only a portion of the dust material can produce data which may lead to biased conclusions.

The short history of research into the dust content of lung tissue is one closely linked to the development of analytical techniques. Optical microscopy and wet chemical analysis were initially the only methods available for characterization of dust samples; however, in recent years there has been a proliferation of techniques and instrumentation, some so sophisticated that they can provide chemical and physical data from only a single dust particle. With such an armory of analytical techniques available it is necessary to first consider the objectives required when designing an investigation into the dust content of diseased and control tissue samples. Many publications have appeared in recent years concerned only with the application of a particular technique or instrument, and few of these sophisticated methods have been used to generate practical information which can be usefully used for statistical purposes.

It is very important therefore, when designing an investigation into the dust content of tissue, to ensure that the tissue preparation techniques and instrumentation used are suitable to provide the necessary information required for correlation purposes.

II. Historical Review

At the start of this century the first serious attempts were made to study airborne dust and the particles being retained in the lungs. A large amount of this work was performed in South Africa, and it centered mainly around the use of the optical microscope which was employed to study the morphology and nature of the doubly refracting particles seen in sections of silicotic lungs [2]. The optical microscope until the 1950s was the only instrument available for the direct examination of dust specimens, and many publications were produced not all of which recognized the limitations of optical equipment in the examination of dust deposits in lung tissues. In 1963 [3] it was recorded that the petrological examination of dust could be made down to 5 μm and sometimes down to 3 μm but below this size, although particles could be seen, no information could be produced which could be used for identification. It was also noted [4] that many minerals had similar optical properties which made the discrimination between them in a mixture almost impossible, e.g., quartz and feldspar. Light microscopic examination of histologic sections of lung and dust residues extracted from lung did provide information on the size of dust particles but only on the optically visible size fraction. Unfortunately, the siliceous materials in tissue are in such a finely divided state that it led one author [5] to comment "the identification of dust particles chemically or petrographically leaves much to be desired." Optical examination did, however, reveal concentrations of dust in certain areas of the lung in diseased cases and indicated that the distribution and composition of dust material may have an important effect on its distribution and subsequent response in the lung [6]. This comment has also been made in more recent years [7], but dust composition could not be studied because of inadequacies of the analytical techniques available.

The use of optical microscopy for studying dust in tissue led to the implication of certain minerals such as sericite [8] as the main causative agents for certain of the pneumoconioses. This led to Haldane [9] to comment that "evidence was constantly accumulating that many scattered cases of fibrosis were occurring and that they seemed to arise from excess exposure to dusts of many kinds, not only silicates."

The fact that the majority of the disease cases from dust exposure were arising in situations where silicate dust clouds were being produced and inhaled meant that silica was considerably implicated in pneumoconiosis diseases. Therefore, the use of chemical methods to study the composition of dust extracts from lung tissue became of increasing importance. Many publications were produced which based their examination of dust samples extracted from tissue on chemical techniques, and the use of wet chemical methods was employed well into the early 1960s [4,10-12,13-25].

The wet chemical techniques were very varied but all were directed at obtaining a silicon dioxide (SiO_2) content of the dust extracted from tissue with one or two examples of iron and aluminium also being measured. The analytical procedures varied a great deal, with dust being extracted from tissues by digestion in strong alkalis and/or acids followed by ashing or sometimes direct ashing of the tissues. The SiO_2 content of the dust residues were then measured by colorimetric techniques after suitable digestion of the dust, or gravimetrically by treatment with hydrofluoric acid. The majority of the techniques were purely elemental measurements and did not reveal the minerals present. Some attempts were made to determine free silica or quartz chemically but they were not successful. The overall result thus obtained was that no correlation could be obtained of disease with an SiO_2 content of tissue material and that the various mineral fractions themselves would have to be determined.

In the late 1930s, the development of x-ray diffraction analysis using x-ray powder photograph methods provided a useful technique for the identification of mineral phases in extracted dust samples [26-28]. The x-ray photographic technique was found to be useful for identifying the presence of certain mineral phases but proved to be difficult to operate if more than two mineral phases were present. It was also not quantitative. Improvements in the design of x-ray equipment and the production of the x-ray diffractometer allowed quantitative techniques to be developed [29-32] for quartz and these were employed extensively in the 1950s [10,12,13,23,25,33] in the study of lung dust extracts, mainly from coal workers. The technique was not developed for the quantification of other mineral species, and it was shown to be difficult to obtain reproducible results, quantitative readings being dependent on particle size and the crystallinity of the mineral sample being examined.

Both wet chemical and x-ray diffraction techniques require fairly large quantities of dust for analysis, and whole lungs were often necessary to produce a suitable sample. The preparation and extraction of the dust was found to be critical, and extraction techniques were shown to influence results in a very major way. A typical procedure for the extraction of dust and its analysis is given below [12].

1. Lung material dried at 105°C and ground to minus 0.125 mm in particle size
2. Digestion in 25% sodium hydroxide
3. Residue after NaOH digestion weighed
4. Residue ashed at 380°C for 5-6 days until no black material remained, the weight loss being recorded as "coal" material
5. Ashed residues were washed in 2 N HCl for 24 hr then water-washed to remove iron, phosphorus, and carbonate material
6. Acid-washed ash residues then ignited in a crucible to determine weight of "siliceous" material
7. For SiO_2 determination 100 mg of ignited material fused with sodium carbonate and estimated chemically
8. Crystalline quartz determined from acid-washed ashed material by x-ray diffraction methods

The authors of the above procedure, which was used to study perhaps the largest collection of coal workers, tin miners, and granite quarry workers' lungs, commented themselves that the procedure destroyed certain mineral phases. They also produced results which showed that granite quarry workers and tin miners had 42% coal dust in their lungs. The only mineral identified in these various studies was quartz, all other minerals being grouped as kaolin and mica, which were not directly quantified.

The examination procedure just outlined represents the most comprehensive attempt at the quantification of lung dust residues. The combination of wet chemical, ashing, and x-ray diffraction techniques required large samples of dust, with the whole procedure being destructive. It must be stated that the results were the best that could be obtained with the techniques available. The inadequacy of the method is best illustrated by the results obtained for the examination of dust extracts from kaolin pneumoconiosis cases [23], where an average result of 50% kaolin, 10-20% mica, and 15-20% SiO_2 of an unknown source was reported.

III. Tissue Specimen Preparation

Before the dust contained in lung tissue specimens can be examined and analyzed some preparation of the biological material must be made. This may consist of preparing thin sections of the tissue for an in situ examination of the dust deposits or it may entail the extraction of the dust deposit from the tissue for an unhindered examination of the biologically foreign material. The choice of technique may often depend upon the availability of suitable pathological specimens, but both preparation procedures may be employed to obtain a complete picture of the composition and distribution of dust in a tissue sample.

A. Examination of Tissue Sections

The optical detection of dust particles in thin sections of lung tissue 6-10 μm thick is often a simple task, especially where an individual case is the result of an exposure to heavy airborne dust concentrations. Accumulation of dust in severe cases of pneumoconiosis can sometimes exceed 40 g of mineral in a whole lung, and the evidence of such heavy deposits can be seen with the naked eye in tissue sections. However, exposure levels vary significantly in industry, and often particles are extremely difficult to detect with an optical microscope in thin sections of tissue. Detection of dust particles may often be complicated by the fact that the tissue material may have similar optical properties to the mineral present so that the latter cannot be distinguished from the former. The tissues in some cases may have over a period of time reacted to the dust particles present, coating them with inorganic material, e.g., asbestos bodies, thus making it very difficult to distinguish dust particles from biological products. Particle resolution in thin sectiions of tissue can also be hampered by the presence of other materials which may have accumulated with the dust in the tissue, such as tar stains due to cigarette smoking and fine carbonaceous material derived from the inhalation of combustion products. In general pathological terminology, mineral deposits in tissue are referred to as dust foci or granuloma as the aggregated particles and other materials appear very simply as an optically different colored material, often opaque. The use of light microscopy in the localization of foreign material in the sections of tissue is extremely important in constructing a picture of particle deposition and progression of disease; however, very little information concerning the nature of the dust and its physical and chemical characteristics can be obtained from such an examination. Where the particles have a distinct morphology such as in the case of fibers some conclusions can be made that the material observed may be, for example, one of the asbestos minerals, and this may also be further supported by the detection of typical asbestos bodies. However, in the examination of most tissue specimens the pathologist may only record the presence of dust foci.

Dust particles in tissue sections often exhibit optical properties such as birefringence, but the observation of such phenomena is of little use in the analysis of such particles as many minerals exhibit birefringence while the fixation and preparation of the tissue itself can result in the production of birefringent material.

However, the examination of thin sections is still an important prelude to the further investigation of dust inclusions in tissue specimens, and it has been demonstrated [34] that with the use of selective staining compounds it is possible to indicate the presence of specific materials in tissue sections to which it is known that the individual had been exposed.

Histochemical textbooks contain many references to staining techniques for various compounds. However, these can be difficult to perform and produce nebulous results. The most used technique is perhaps that of the Prussian blue staining procedure to indicate iron; it does not differentiate, however, between iron of biological and nonbiological origins.

Microincineration of Tissue Sections

The optical examination of histologic sections still remains the most popular procedure for examining dust deposits in tissue specimens, even though the information obtained about the composition of the dust observed is negligible. It is very important as an aid in the further preparation of thin sections for examination by electron microscopy where only limited areas of tissue can be examined [35]. Thin sections of tissue with their wax embedding material removed by washing in xylene have been employed as specimens in studies of their dust content in scanning electron microscopes and electron and ion mass probe instruments [36-45]. The presence of the tissue complicates the detection of particles, and those particles that are deeply embedded in the tissues cannot be observed or analyzed satisfactorily. Tissue material can be destroyed by ashing or microincineration of sections either in a muffle furnace at 450°C or using plasma oxygen ashing equipment which will perform the ashing at approximately 100°C. Both techniques produce ashed tissue residue with the inorganic dust deposits spatially distributed as they were in the original tissue section. Organic dust particles are destroyed by this method of preparation, while inorganic material derived from the tissues themselves also remains to complicate the examination and analysis of the dust residues produced. Some alteration of the remaining dust particles may also have taken place; for example, many silicate particles such as kaolin undergo structural changes at temperatures above 350°C while other silicates will lose some water of crystallization at elevated temperatures. Carbon particles will also be altered by heat treatment with subsequent loss of CO_2, and iron oxide particles also may undergo phase changes. The effects of heating can, however, be minimized by ashing at low temperatures using an oxygen plasma ashing apparatus [46].

The dust materials revealed by ashing thin sections are still in such a finely divided state that their identification by optical means is still not possible. However, the residues can be prepared for examination by electron microscopy [47], enabling a more sophisticated analysis to be performed.

Figures 1a and 1b illustrate the type of preparations to be expected from the ashing of 6 μm histologic sections of lung tissue as prepared for examination [47] in a transmission electron microscope. Dust particles can be observed together with the inorganic remains of the tissue itself. Preparations of this type are extremely useful for studying the distribution and aggregation of mineral particles of different types and sizes in specimens. While the technique can be applied to tissue section as small as those produced from needle biopsies, this technique has been employed in several investigations of the inorganic mineral content of lung tissue [47-51].

Ultrathin Sectioning of Tissue

Ultrathin sections of tissue 100 nm thick prepared for electron microscope examination of cellular structure detail have been employed in many investigations [35,37,38,41,52-55] to study the close association of dust particles with tissue. The objective in the majority of these studies has not been to identify or quantify the dust particles present but rather to study cellular changes that occur because of the presence of dust. For the examination of dust particles such preparations are highly unsatisfactory as the preparation technique requires that the dust particles themselves have often to be sectioned. Sections containing dust can only be adequately prepared using diamond knives, and even so dust particles still have a tendency to shatter and very hard minerals such as quartz are often dislodged from the sections, leaving large holes and producing torn sections.

B. Bulk Extraction Procedures for the Release of Dust from Tissues

A more satisfactory preparation approach for the analysis of dust in tissue specimens has been to release the dust from large samples of biological material using a suitable extraction procedure. In this way a bulk dust extract can be

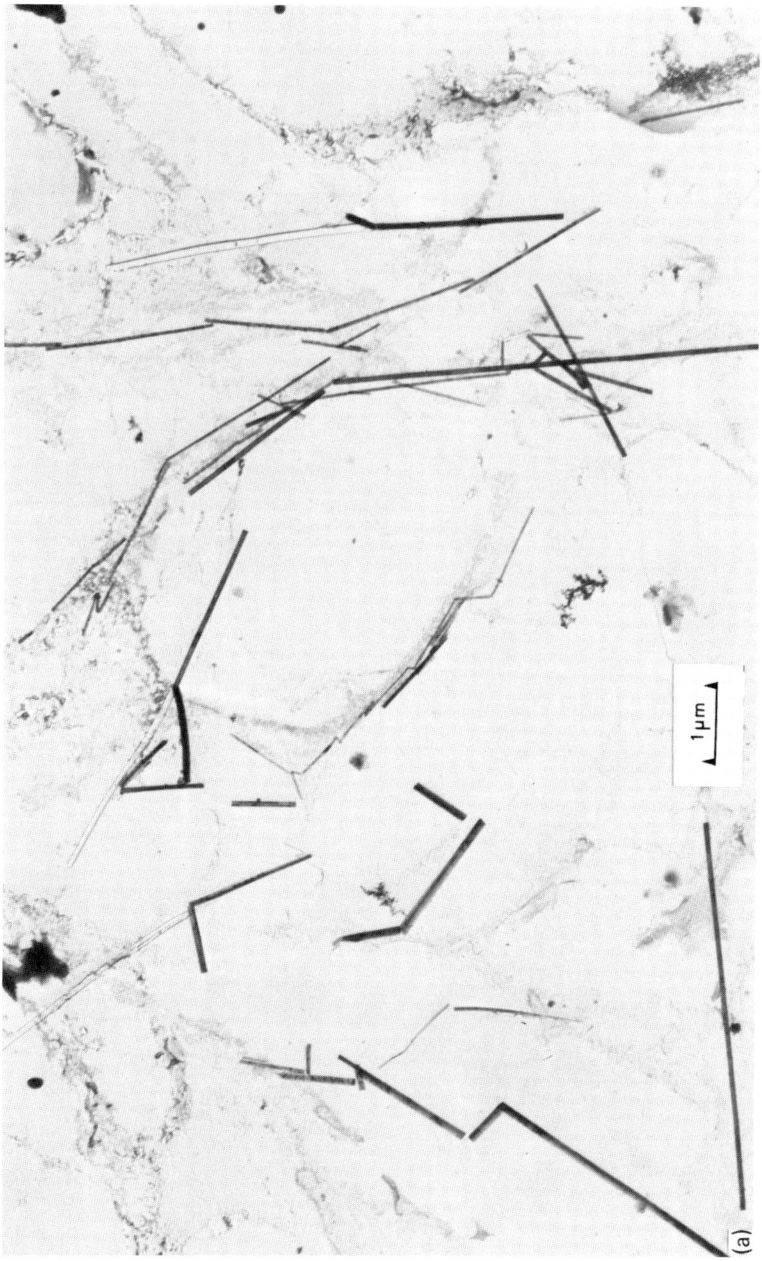

Figure 1a Electron micrograph of the residues obtained by the microincineration of 6 μm histological sections of lung tissue from a case of asbestosis (X7500).

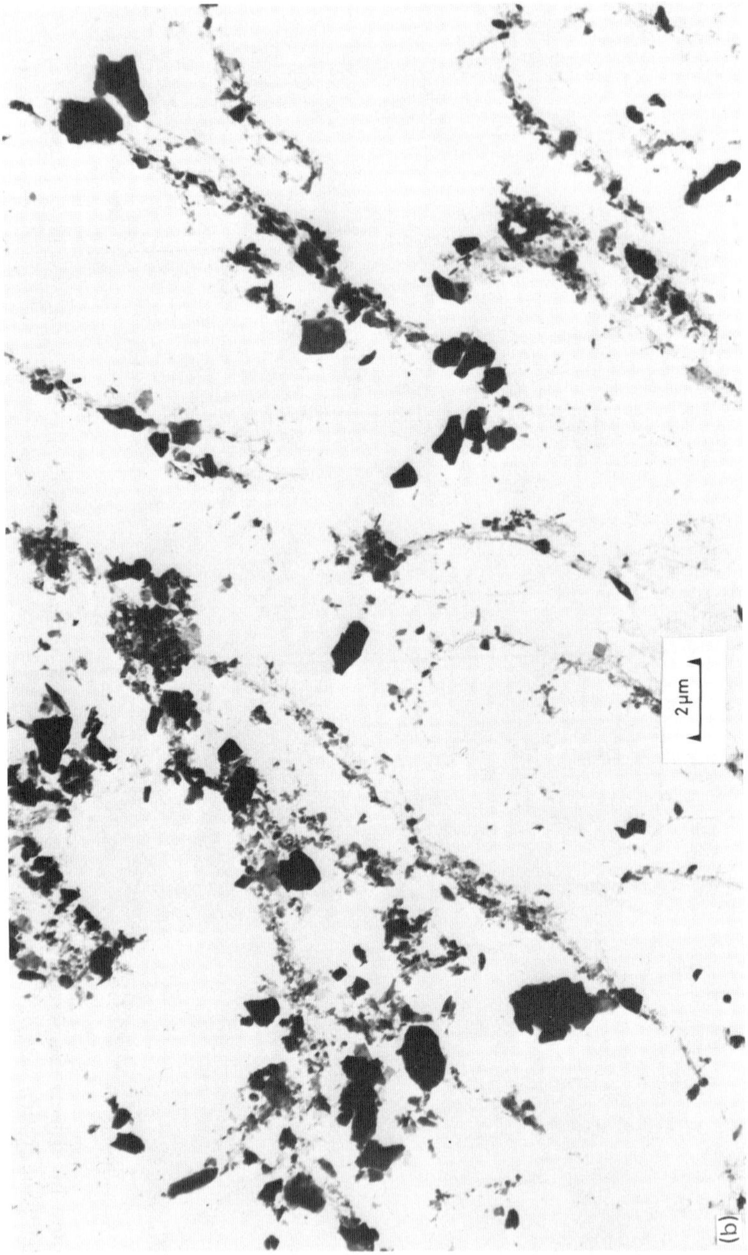

Figure 1b Electron micrograph of the residues obtained by the microincineration of 6 μm histologic sections of lung tissue from a case of silicosis in the slate quarrying industry (X5000).

produced which is more representative of the material contained in the tissue, while larger quantities of dust are also made available for examination by a variety of analytical techniques. Any results obtained from the dust analyses can be quantitatively related to the tissue sample (using known weights of dry or wet tissue). The methods for the bulk extraction of dust from tissue specimens fall into two categories: those employing chemical reagents for tissue digestion and those which rely upon ashing procedures for the tissue removal. In some cases combinations of digestive and ashing procedures have been adopted with the chemical digestion normally preceding any treatment of a specimen by ashing.

Digestive Techniques

Chemical digestive techniques have been by far the most popular preparation route that various investigators have applied, with the range of tissue solvents used and the experimental procedure employed varying with every publication of their respective results. An examination of the various techniques contained in the literature reveals that very few authors have ever taken the trouble to investigate whether the treatment they were giving to their tissue samples in any way affected the dust they were trying to extract. Many of the procedures were devised to examine only a single constituent of the dust being recovered, and many complicated washing stages were often added to separate or destroy unwanted constituents, especially organic particulates. The main emphasis in most of the techniques appears to have been the efficient removal of biological material sometimes at the expense of the dust material itself.

Acid Techniques

Hydrochloric acid solutions have been employed [56] in the investigation of coal workers' pneumoconiosis cases, especially where the emphasis was placed on recovery of coal material. Acid strengths ranging from 5 to 11 N have been used at temperatures ranging from 60°C to boiling, with the digestion taking place within 2 hr. No prior preparation of the specimens such as defatting was apparently required to produce a favorable result although it was noted that some loss of other minerals normally associated with coal occurred. Hot nitric acid solutions often in association with sulfuric acid and hydrochloric acid in a concentrated form were extensively employed [8,14] in the many early investigations into the siliceous mineral content of silicotic lung tissue. These acid combinations were normally followed by an ashing to a dull red heat to remove any remaining organic material prior to a total wet chemical determination of SiO_2 and an estimation of free SiO_2. This very severe acid treatment of specimens probably generated more free silica in the dust residues than originally existed in the tissue themselves, mainly by the leaching of cations from chemically unstable silicate minerals. Another procedure using glacial acid saturated with ammonium acetate at 130°C was devised [57] for the preparation of tissue from coal workers' pneumoconiosis cases. This digestion was then followed by a washing in concentrated formic acid at a temperature of 100°C. This technique was found to produce good extractions of coal dust and had a minimal effect upon other mineral particles contained in the tissue specimens.

The use of strong acids for digestion purposes would appear only to be justified where the aim of the investigation is to isolate only a particular component of the dust known to be stable under acid conditions. The use of strong acid solutions cannot be recommended for the routine extraction of dust from tissue where information regarding all the components of the dust are required.

Alkali Techniques

Solutions of both sodium and potassium hydroxide of varying strengths are well established as digestive reagents for the extraction of dust from lung tissue specimens, with digestions normally being performed using a water bath at a temperature of 100°C. A 25% solution of NaOH formed the basis of a well-established procedure [12] for the examination of tissue from coal workers' pneumoconiosis cases, the dust residues obtained from such cases being washed with alcoholic potassium hydroxide and dilute hydrochloric acid before determination of the coal content of the dust extracted. In recent years, KOH has been a more popular reagent, with 40% solutions usually being employed at 100°C. Many authors concerned with the extraction of asbestos fibers from tissue [58-61] have employed KOH as the basis of their extraction technique followed by repeated washings with distilled water. Both NaOH and KOH do not appear to be 100% efficient in the removal of biological material, and dust extracts prepared using either tissue solvent still contain some organic residues. The amount of this residue varies and appears to depend upon the manner in which tissues have been preserved, i.e., formalin fixed or frozen, and also upon the amount of fibrotic tissue present in the sample. Formalin-fixed fibrotic specimens would appear to be the most difficult to prepare by alkali digestions. This has led investigators [58,59] to ash (at 450°C) the residues they have obtained from alkali digestions in order to obtain a more readily examinable dust extract. Using NaOH and KOH solutions, digestions of tissue specimens can be performed in 20-60 min, but the effect of these strong alkali solutions upon the majority of mineral dusts is relatively unknown. They may be considered not to be as damaging to most dust components as are strong acid solutions, but as long as they are employed at low temperatures they can only again be recommended for those situations where only selective dust components which have been shown to be alkali resistant are to be studied.

Enzyme Techniques

The use of enzyme solutions to digest biological material is fairly well established in the biochemical literature, and their efficiency for use as lung tissue solvents has been investigated [62]. The enzymes ficin, bromelin, and pronase have been examined as suitable digestive reagents, with ficin having been shown to be comparable to NaOH for the preparation of lung tissue from coal workers' pneumoconiosis cases [62], with the time taken to produce a dust residue being in excess of 24 hr. The use of enzyme solutions would appear to require some degree of experimental skill in order to produce a satisfactory result as the efficiency of enzyme extraction is very dependent upon obtaining the correct temperature and environmental conditions for a digestion, the addition of other chemicals such as buffering agents being very important in obtaining an efficient digestion of tissue. Further investigations into the use of enzyme solutions and the application of new enzyme compounds would appear to be a very fruitful field of investigation in an effort to find a suitable tissue solvent which does not affect the physical and chemical properties of retained dust particles.

Formamide Techniques

Reagent-grade formamide employed at a temperature of 130°C has been used for digestion in the investigation of the asbestos fiber content of lung tissue specimens [63,64]. It is reported as having taken 4 days to complete the procedure, with repeated changes of formamide being employed followed by washing in water, methonal, chloroform, and n-hexane. Other residual organic material was removed from the dust residues produced by using perchloric acid at 180°C. The use of formamide is not a common technique; and from its description in the literature it would appear to be unsuitable for use as a quantitative procedure, as the loss of dust material, especially the finer particles, is likely to be very high with so many centrifugation, washing, and resuspension steps. An essential step prior to the use of formamide is the defatting of the tissue specimens with a suitable solvent such as acetone or benzene. Formamide has also been shown to readily attack carbonate minerals.

Sodium Hypochlorite Techniques

Sodium hypochlorite solutions in various forms have been most popular as digestive reagents in the preparation of lung tissue [65-69]. They have ranged from reagent grade 5% sodium hypochlorite solutions to commercial bleaches of unknown composition. Where they have been employed, digestion times ranging from 3 to 7 days are recorded, and prior to their use many research workers have found it necessary to defat their specimens with benzene or acetone. In many cases it is reported that considerable quantities of organic material of biological origin often remain undissolved, and to overcome this problem 65% sucrose solutions have been used to obtain a density separation of mineral matter and residual organic material. Other workers have employed chloroform and ethonal to produce a similar effect. Perchloric acid and ashing techniques have also been employed to obtain dust residues free of tissue material. Conventional sodium hypochlorite solutions appear to be very inefficient solvents for tissue with many changes of solution often being required to produce a satisfactory result. Some success with sodium hypochlorite has, however, been reported [70,71] where the procedure has involved the use of formulations of sodium hypochlorite in a dilute NaOH solution. Using such formulations, digestion of lung tissue has been completed in a matter of hours rather than days, while residual tissue material has been shown to be minimal in the dust extracts. Sodium hypochlorite solutions have not been shown to be destructive to any of the common minerals destroyed by strong acid or alkaline solutions [72]. If the digestion of tissue by sodium hypochlorite solutions is compared with published procedures using other solvents it would appear to be the most simple to operate and the least harmful to any dust material that may be recovered and as such is to be recommended.

Other Digestive Techniques

Hydrogen peroxide solutions are very rarely used for lung tissue digestion [72]. The major criticism of this reagent appears to be the excessive time required to complete a digestion coupled with necessary changes of the solvent and intermittent heating [72] up to 80°C in a water bath to accelerate the digestive process. Hydroxide of hyamine has been recommended as a suitable reagent for the recovery of inhaled dust from lung tissue, with solutions of this compound having very little effect upon a variety of minerals normally susceptible to damage [72]. For successful tissue digestion both hydrogen peroxide and hydroxide of hyamine required defatting of the tissue, while solutions of the latter compound reacted more rapidly in the presence of benzene and at a temperature of 60°C, the time taken for digestion being 24 hr. Another solvent used for tissue digestion and quoted in the literature is Solvene [73].

The digestive procedures that have been outlined vary considerably in their complexity of application and their efficiency of dust extraction. Many investigators using the same basic solvent often incorporate additional steps in their procedure to produce what they consider to be clean dust extracts. No single reagent appears to be capable of giving a completely tissue-free extract. Often very little thought has been given to the effect of the tissue solvent upon the inhaled dust particles themselves or the influence of repeated washing stages upon the loss of particles. Before the adoption of any digestive technique investigators should satisfy themselves that the procedure that they finally adopt does not introduce errors of such magnitude that they may mask the differences they are trying to detect.

Ashing Techniques Ashing of pathological specimens has been used in many research investigations as an alternative to the chemical digestion of lung tissue to release dust particles. It has also been adopted as a final treatment for residues obtained from initial chemical digestions [58,59]. The manner in which the ashing of specimens has been performed has varied considerably, with temperatures ranging from above 600°C to less than 100°C. So-called low-temperature ashing at 450°C in air was the most popular procedure, while a treatment at between 350°C and 400°C in the presence of oxygen has also been reported [74,75]. Very low temperature ashing of tissue at approximately 100°C can be performed using oxygen plasma equipment which over the past few years has been found to be of great value for removing organic material from dust samples. The one major drawback of all ashing techniques is that organic material, whether of inhaled dust or biological origin, is destroyed, and such techniques cannot therefore be employed to investigate organic particulates contained in tissue specimens. The inorganic material left after ashing lung tissue specimens not only contains inhaled particles but also very large quantities of inorganic residue derived from the tissue itself. This tissue ash is normally composed of the oxides of phosphorus, calcium, sodium, and iron, with the proportions of these elements in ashed residues varying between diseased and normal tissue specimens. Fibrotic lung specimens after ashing invariably contain very large quantities of calcium and phosphorus derived from calcified tissues. Attempts are sometimes made to remove tissue ash by washing with dilute acids; this can, however, affect certain mineral dust particles, altering both their chemistry and structure. Although ashing procedures may be normally performed at specific furnace temperatures it is most probable that, due to the exothermic reactions taking place during the ashing, the actual ashing temperature is well above that desired. The exception to this situation is tissue ashing performed in oxygen plasma devices. Elevated temperatures are known to alter the structure of minerals considerably, and temperatures in excess of 300°C can be detrimental [76]. The effect of elevated temperatures on dust particles is also magnified by the release of alkali oxides from the tissue itself which act as fluxing agents and can attack often refractory silicate particles, producing water-soluble silicate products. Detrimental effects of ashing at elevated temperatures can be reduced if the bulk of tissue material is first removed by chemical digestion. This especially alleviates the major problem of having dust extracts heavily contaminated with tissue ash, while the reduction in organic matter drastically reduces the excess heat generated from the ashing of large quantities of tissue. The most suitable ashing procedure available would appear to be the use of oxygen plasma devices where temperatures are very low; however, it is an extremely long technique, with several days being required to produce a satisfactory result from 0.5 g of dry tissue. The problem of tissue ash in the dust residue also remains with this technique. An examination of ashing procedures indicates that direct ashing, especially at temperatures in excess of

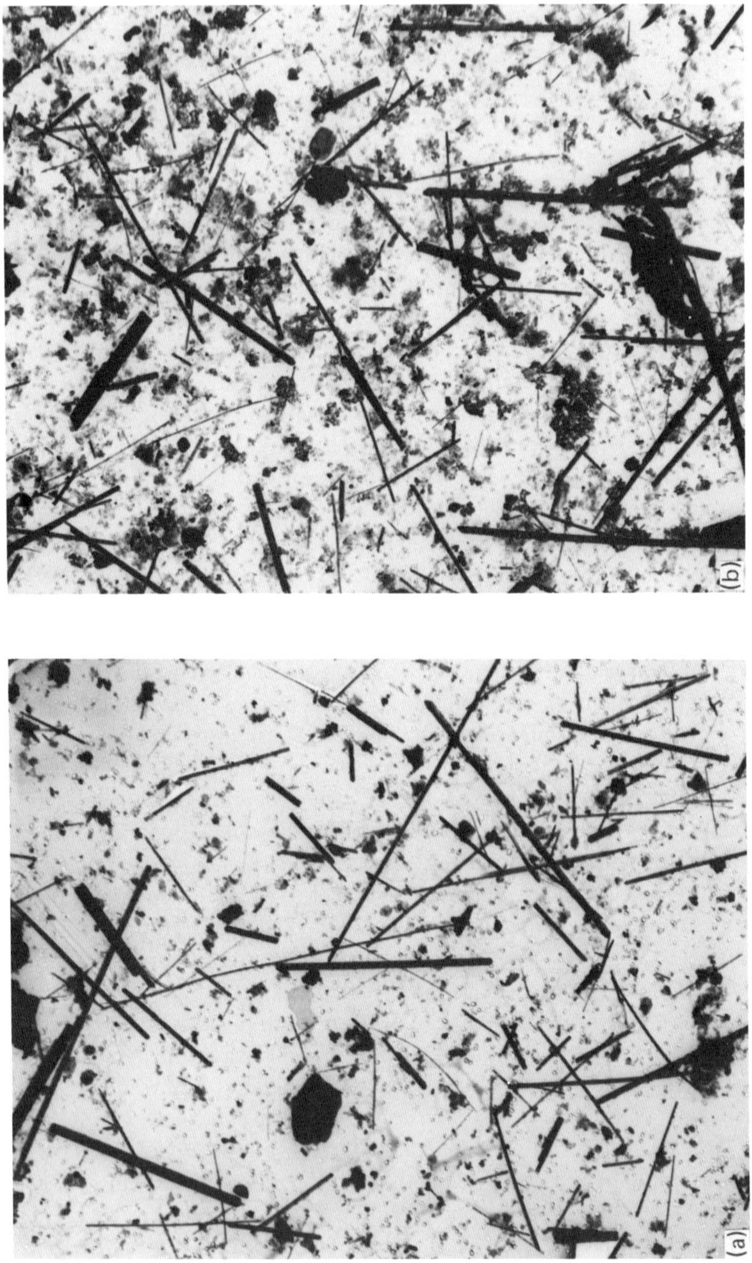
(b)
(a)

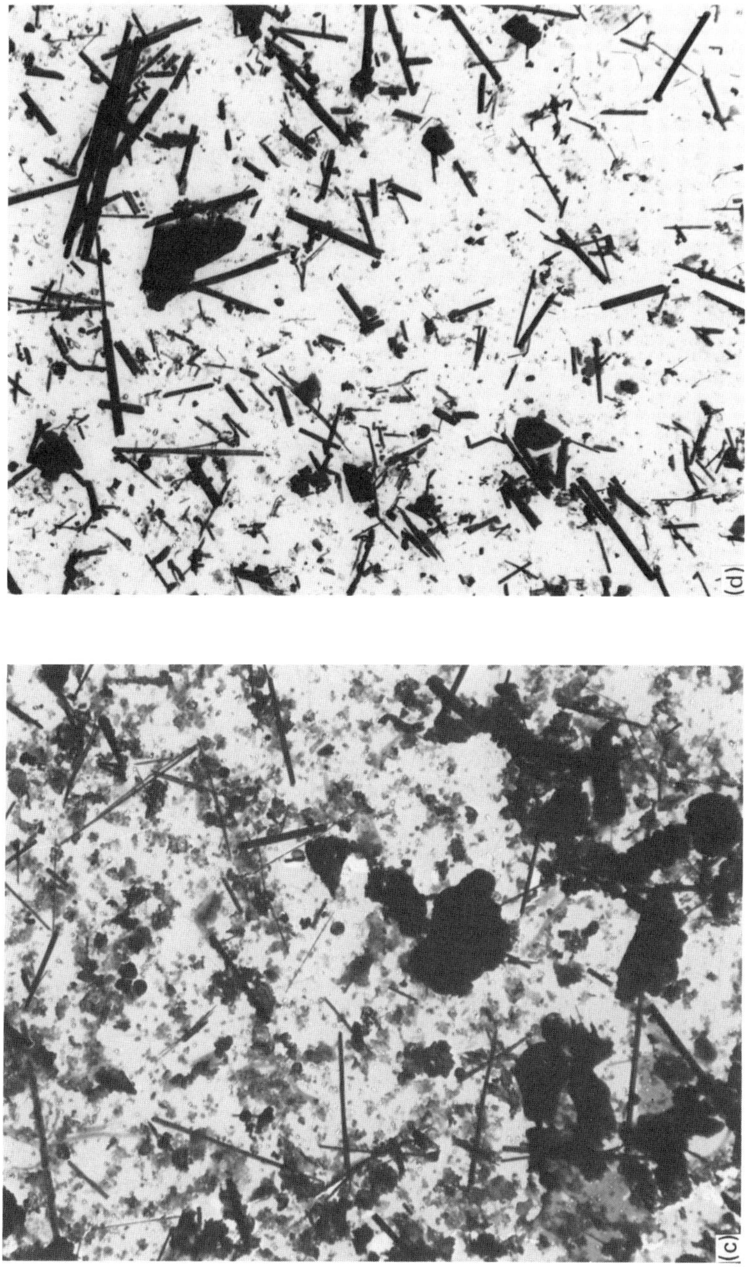

Figure 2 Electron micrographs of bulk extractions of dust from samples of lung tissue from a common source prepared in different ways. (a) Tissue digested in KOH at 90°C for 1 hr; residue ashed at 360°C and washed in dilute HCl at pH 1 for 10 min. (b) Tissue digested for 2–3 hr in sodium hypochlorite solution prepared in 0.1N NaOH. (c) Tissue ashed in an oxygen plasma ashing device. (d) Tissue ashed at 450–500°C, then washed with dilute HCl at pH 1 for 10 min.

100°C, is not a satisfactory method for the preparation of dust extracts from tissue samples [77]. Ashing at a low temperature with oxygen plasma equipment can, however, be useful for the final treatment of chemical digestion residues but only where investigation of inorganic dust materials are the sole objective of the extraction procedure [76].

Figure 2 is a group of electron micrographs of dust extracts which illustrate the physical differences that can be observed when samples of tissue from a common source are prepared in a number of different ways. It can be seen that the fibrous particles appear to be associated with varying amounts of other nonfibrous material, in the case of preparations illustrated by the micrographs in Figures 2b and c. This material for the greater part is tissue residue which is mainly organic in Figure 2b and inorganic in c. The preparation illustrated by Figure 2d shows the effect that ashing at high temperature has on the morphology of the fibrous particles: They are all considerably reduced in length. The most satisfactory preparation would appear to be that illustrated by Figure 2a.

IV. Analytical Techniques

It has been stated previously that the analysis of dust material contained in tissue specimens is complicated by the fact that it is always in a very finely divided state and often only small quantities are available for examination. It must also be recognized that unless the utmost care has been taken in the preparation of samples for examination that there are likely to be serious losses of certain components of the dust and perhaps alterations in the physical and chemical properties of others which may then negate the successful application of an analytical technique. Before attempting the examination of the dust content of a series of tissue specimens certain questions must be answered:

1. What physical and chemical parameters of the dust have to be measured?
2. Do the results have to be quantitative or qualitative?
3. Is it necessary to identify all the components of the dust contained in the specimens both organic and inorganic?
4. Have the results to be related to a known quantity of dry or wet tissue, or is the objective of the study to relate the dust composition to the anatomy of the tissue material?
5. Are the series of samples selected for examination representative of the cases of disease under investigation and are they matched with adequate control specimens?

The answers to these questions can only be obtained by the collaboration of individuals from the disciplines of medicine, materials science, and statistics, and they are necessary in order to select equipment and design procedures required to produce the information for statistical analysis and comparison with medical information.

After having selected a tissue preparation and analytical procedure, then both should be thoroughly tested and investigated to establish their suitability for obtaining the desired information. In many cases establishing a successful preparation and analytical procedure may take more time than the actual collection of the final experimental data as it may often involve the development of new procedures.

A. Optical Microscopic Techniques

As previously stated optical microscope techniques have been and are still the most inexpensive and practical methods employed to examine dust particles both in situ and extracted from lung tissue specimens. The optical examination of mineral specimens is a well-established mineralogical procedure [78] but it is normally confined to the study of particles which are very much larger than those encountered in dust samples. It is a technique mainly applicable to particles which are translucent. Very fine, opaque particles are extremely difficult to examine by normal optical techniques, with reflected light rather than transmitted light being used to examine polished specimens. To identify particles by optical means requires that certain optical properties of the unknown materials have to be established and compared with reference information.

The identification of mineral species by optical techniques involves a sequence of procedures which can be tabulated as shown on the following page. Identification on the basis of optical properties will then finally depend upon the possibilities suggested by each of the optical properties examined. Frequently many possibilities will remain, and materials with similar optical properties will be confused. It is also possible that if particles whose optical properties have not been recorded are encountered, identification by optical techniques is then impossible. It must be kept in mind that only larger particles can be fully characterized optically in a specimen. This task will be made even more difficult when several mineral phases are present, as each must be considered independently.

Optical properties do not therefore provide a unique characterization of particles, and supplementary results from other techniques such as x-ray diffraction or chemical analysis are required to produce a positive identification [79].

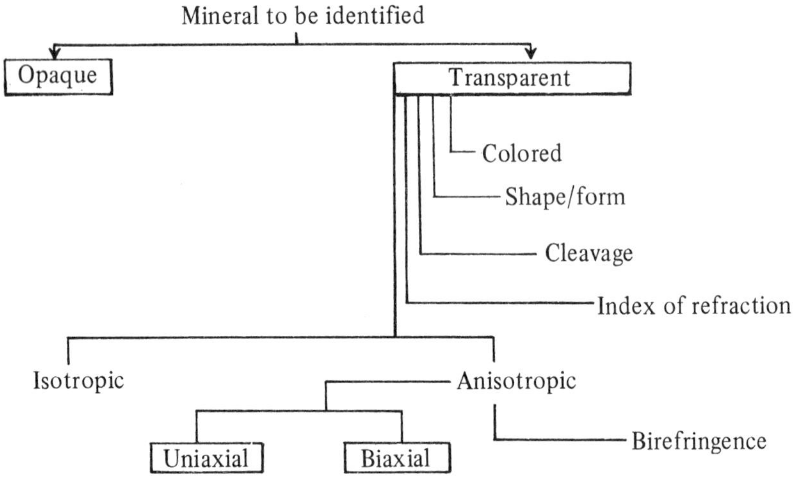

There are certain specific inadequencies in the use of optical microscopy for the examination of dust specimens. The first and most obvious is the resolution limitations of the optical microscope itself. It is claimed that particles as small as 0.2 μm can be observed by optical methods, but it is recognized that no measurement of optical properties can be made from particles which are so small [80]. Optical microscopy is most useful in studying the larger particles that occur in dust specimens and in this role can only be considered to be useful for obtaining morphological information. It can provide data concerning the number, concentration, size, and shape of particles present in tissue specimens, which may be of great value especially where the disease response is related to the mass of dust retained. In any dust sample the comparatively small percentage of large particles present may represent the major proportion of the mass of dust in a sample.

In the past the inexperienced use of optical microscopy has resulted in the production of some misleading results [8] with regard to the mineralogical composition of the dust contained in tissue specimens. Optical techniques must therefore be confined to the estimation of morphology and number and concentration of particles in tissue, except in those situations where independent measurement of the composition of the dust material allows the use of optical techniques to monitor changes in composition. Some attempts [80,81] have been made to extend the use of optical techniques such as dispersion staining for the determination of specific mineral species, but again they are only useful in those situations where the dust sample has been obtained from a known source or has been previously characterized. For unknown specimens it can be considered to be impractical. The technique is limited to particles larger than 1 μm.

Optical microscope techniques for the examination of dust in tissue specimens is therefore limited to the direct location of dust deposits in tissues and the morphological examination of optically visible particles in dust extracts.

B. X-ray Diffraction Techniques

X-ray diffraction techniques are very useful for the identification of the mineral constituents of bulk samples of powder or dust residues extracted from tissue samples. They can be used as a primary technique to establish the number and identity of various mineral phases in a sample, or they can be employed to estimate the quantity of a single mineral known to be present in an extract. These techniques are only useful, however, in the investigation of particulate materials which have crystalline structures, and they are not of any use for the examination of amorphous materials not detected by x-ray diffraction techniques.

The presence of large quantities of amorphous material in extracted dust samples can in fact seriously reduce the quality of information obtained by x-ray techniques concerning the crystalline phases present. Dust particles must therefore be released from tissue samples in order to apply x-ray diffraction techniques to their examination, and great care must be taken to ensure that the crystalline nature of the material is not interfered with by the extraction procedure itself as this may modify or introduce artifacts into the results obtained. The removal of all biological organic material should therefore be a major objective in the preparation of samples for x-ray diffraction examination, and where practical inorganic material of a biological origin should also be removed to produce as clear a diffraction result as possible from the crystalline dust material itself.

The theory and practice of x-ray diffraction techniques are extremely well documented in many good texts [82], and they are now considered as routine procedures to be used for analyzing crystalline materials. Although they may appear to be relatively simple to perform, the results obtained from samples may be very difficult to interpret and the limitations of precision and accuracy of these techniques when they are used must always be given very careful consideration. This is especially true when dust extracts from tissue specimens are being examined as these can be far from the ideal specimens for diffraction studies [83]. Samples may contain several crystalline phases and they are always present in a very finely divided state while the quantity of material available for study may also only just be sufficient to produce a suitable diffraction result.

There are two distinct x-ray methods which can be employed in the examination of dust samples: the x-ray powder photographic and x-ray diffractometer methods. X-ray powder photography is widely used to identify minerals as the powder photograph of a crystalline material is characteristic of the atomic arrangement of that material. It is similar to a fingerprint in that no two substances give identical powder patterns. There are many circumstances, however, when the differences are very small and other analytical results such as chemical composition and morphology of the particles producing the diffraction pattern are necessary to obtain a positive identification. X-ray powder photographs have two distinct characteristics: an accurate measurement of the position of lines on the photograph and an estimate of the relative blackness of lines are required to find what minerals are present in a sample. For identifying the minerals in a mixture, first the most probable major mineral phase is established and reflections in the sample data found to correspond with reference information for this phase are ignored while the remaining lines are compared against other standard data. In this procedure no account is taken of overlapping lines, and with mixtures containing four or more minerals ambiguous results can be obtained. This is particularly true when the minerals present produce similar powder diffraction photographs. Computer techniques can be used to help in the interpretation of complex powder photographs and they are extremely useful for locating standard x-ray information. Specialized powder cameras, suitable selection of x-ray wavelength, and sample orientation can also be employed to separate reflections that are very close together or to enhance reflections from certain minerals which have a particular morphology, e.g., fibrous or plate.

When interpreting powder photographs or any x-ray result obtained from a mixed mineral dust it is much better to have first obtained some chemical information regarding the sample and its various components so that the most probable standard data can be selected for comparison purposes. Of the powder photographic techniques, cameras employing the Debye-Scherrer procedure for recording the diffraction pattern are the most popular while the quantity of sample required to produce a result using photographic methods is only on the order of micrograms.

Although only microgram quantities of sample are required for powder photographic methods [83], milligram quantities of material are normally required for x-ray diffractometry; however, as the detection limit of approximately 1% by weight of any crystalline material in a sample can be obtained then microgram quantities can be detected by this technique [84-86]. Diffractometer results can be enhanced using "step scanning" techniques [87], where quantification of small percentages of specific minerals in a sample are required, but the technique is not useful for routine identification purposes.

Normally, x-ray powder photographic techniques are employed only for identification and other crystallographic purposes while x-ray diffractometry is used extensively for quantitative determination of the components of powder samples. Accurate quantitative results can be difficult to obtain by diffractometry as standard mineral specimens are required to produce calibration curves. These standards should be obtained preferably from the same geological or industrial source as the powder being investigated. They should also be prepared with the same physical characteristics, such as particle size distribution, as the material being investigated, as the intensity of the diffracted x-rays from a given mass of mineral will vary considerably with particle size. Standards necessary to quantitatively examine dust extracts from tissue specimens are particularly difficult to produce because they have to be reduced to a very fine and narrow particle size range. This means that the standard specimens have to be ground very finely which can adversely affect the crystallinity of the sample [88] and interfere with the accuracy of the mineral determination. It has been shown [30,31] that estimation of quartz levels in dust samples can be severely influenced by the variation in particle size of the mineral with an estimated detection level falling from 100 to 60% with a change in mean particle size from 1.9 to 0.5 μm. Changes were also noted as the mean particle size of quartz increased from 2 to 15 μm, with estimations of the mineral being enhanced by approximately 20%. Diffractometer results can also be influenced by the way in which specimens are prepared for x-ray diffraction analysis. Many minerals, especially those with a platelike structure, produce enhanced reflections when the particles are deposited as an oriented layer as compared to a layer of randomly oriented particles. Perhaps the most serious factor affecting the use of x-ray diffractometry for quantitative analysis, however, is the variation in intensity of reflections that always exist between samples of the same mineral obtained from different geological sources [89]. It is necessary therefore to obtain some chemical information from the sample to help confirm diffractometer results.

Figures 3 and 4 illustrate the form of the results that can be expected from the x-ray examination of bulk samples of dust extracted from lung tissue. Figure 3a is an electron micrograph of the inorganic residue of a dust sample produced by the digestion of a tissue specimen from a case of coal workers' pneumoconiosis. The preparation involved the use of glacial acetic acid and ammonium acetate with the residue being finally ashed in an oxygen plasma ashing unit to remove all carbonaceous material. Figure 3b is a picture of the x-ray powder photograph obtained from the final residue illustrated by Figure 3a, while Figure 3c is a corresponding x-ray diffractometer trace obtained from the material. Similarly, Figure 4a is an electron micrograph of the dust residue extracted and prepared as previously, but from a case of pneumoconiosis which occurred in the china clay industry. Figures 4b and 4c are the corresponding x-ray powder photograph and diffractometer trace obtained from this sample. An examination and measurement of the powder x-ray films from both specimens revealed that the x-ray patterns were very similar. There are distinct

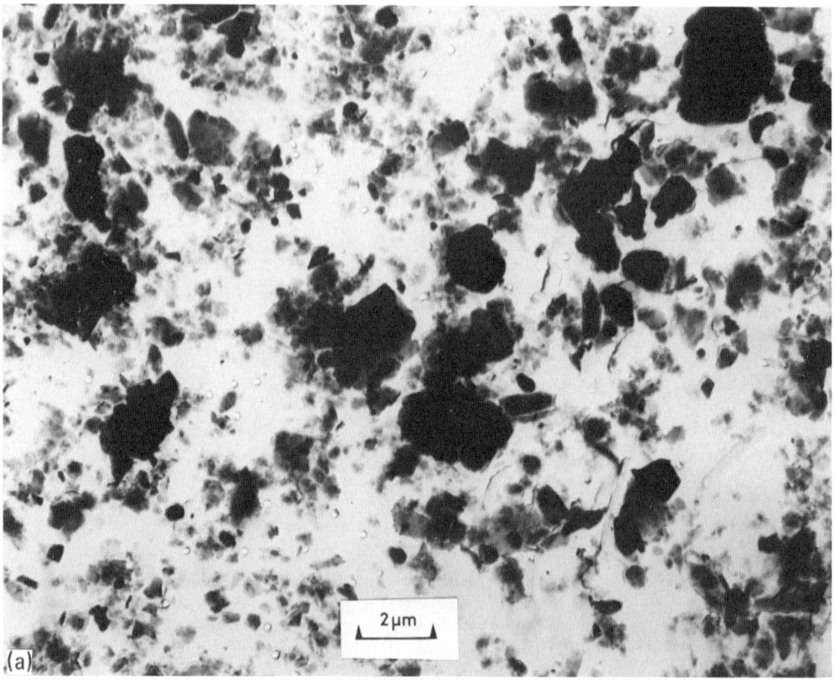

Figure 3a Electron micrograph of a dust extract from a case of coal workers' pneumoconiosis.

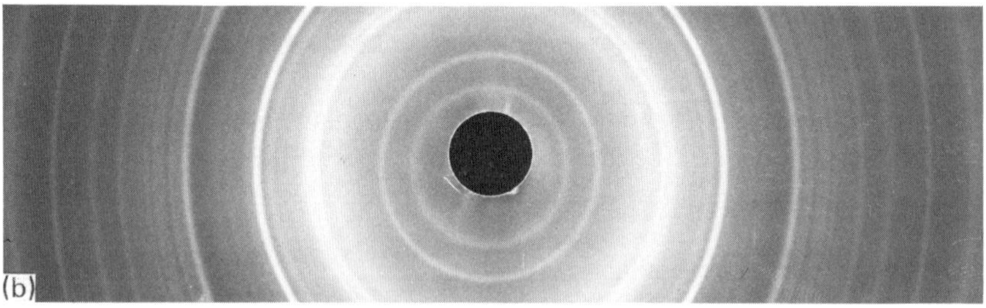

Figure 3b X-ray powder photograph of the extract.

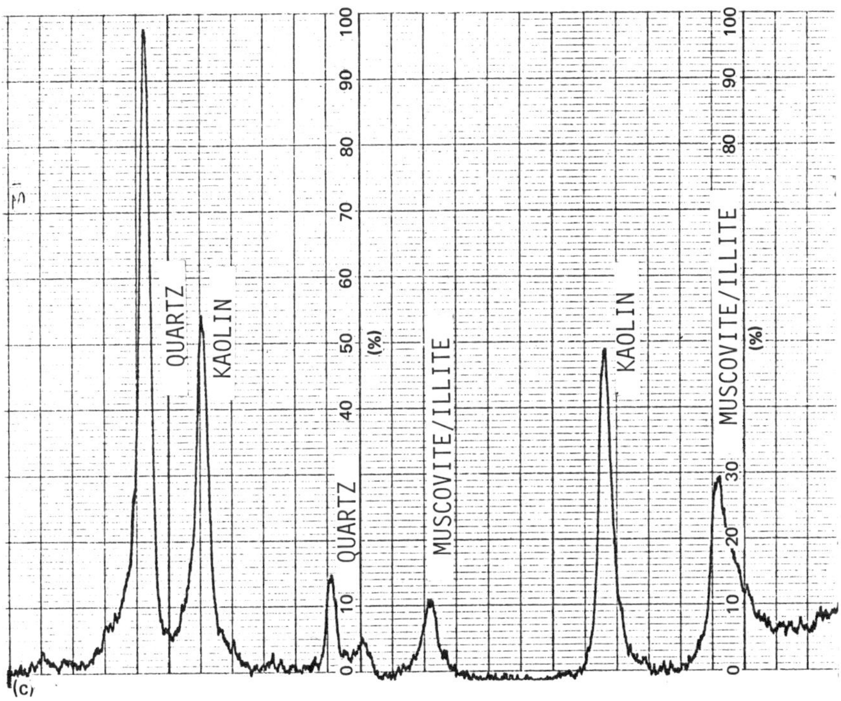

Figure 3c X-ray diffractometer trace also obtained from the extract.

intensity differences occurring between corresponding reflections in the two photographs which indicate that although both samples contain the same type of minerals, the relative proportions of each mineral in the samples were different, the major minerals identified being kaolin, quartz, and muscovite. This quantitative difference is highlighted by a comparison of the diffractometer traces in which the peaks corresponding to the minerals which have been identified from the x-ray powder photographs have been labeled. The composite nature of the x-ray result for both dust extracts can be observed from a comparison of the x-ray reference data and the calculated data from the dust residues. Although the diffractometer traces obtained from the two dust residues indicate that there are quantitative mineralogical compositional differences, the information contained in the traces cannot be used to produce actual figures of the composition because of the inability to prepare suitable standards. In the x-ray powder photographs the presence of some minor mineral components such as rutile have also been indicated by the measurement of the

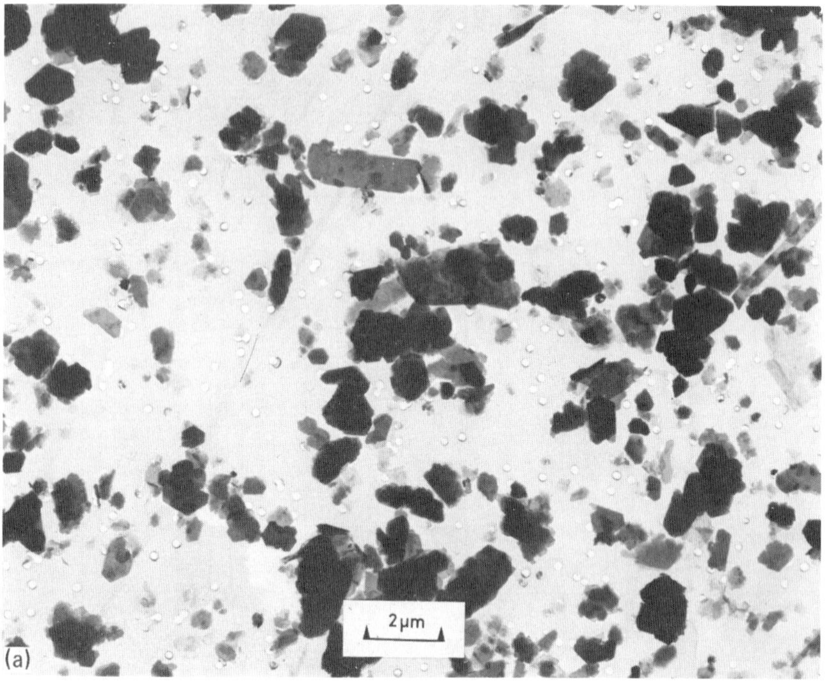

Figure 4a Electron micrograph of a dust extract from a case of kaolin pneumoconiosis.

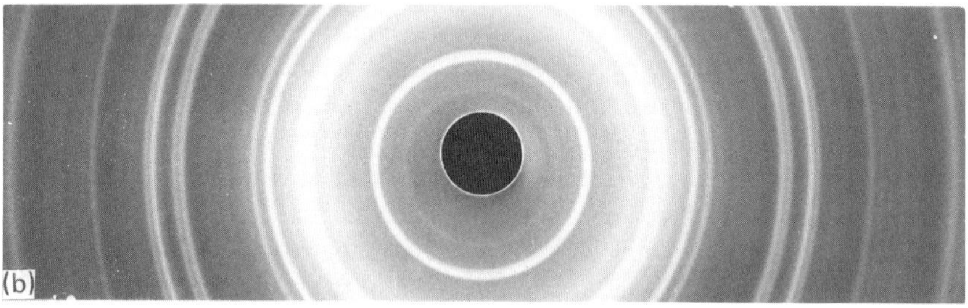

Figure 4b X-ray powder photograph of the extract.

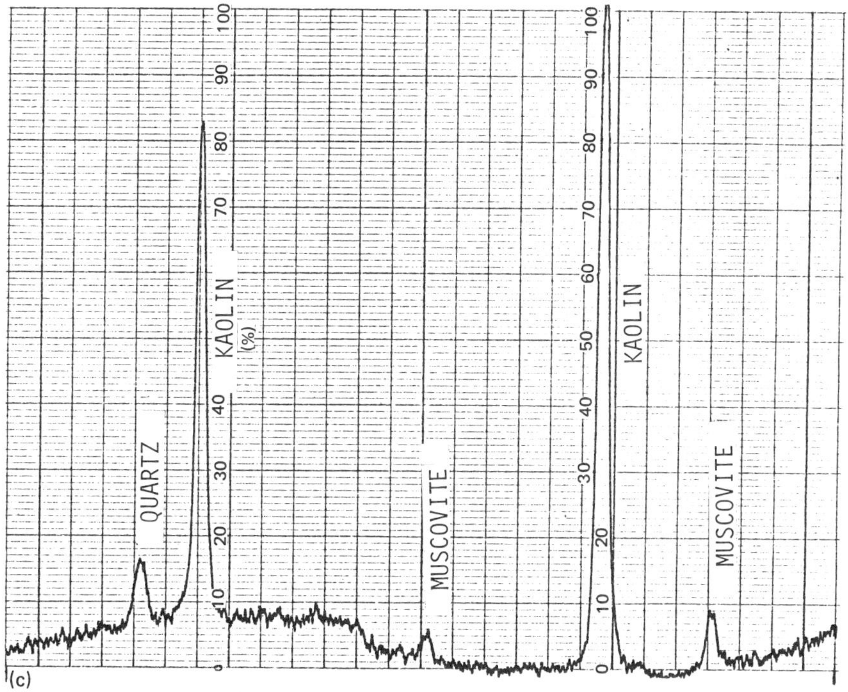

Figure 4c X-ray diffractometer trace also obtained from the extract.

diffraction patterns. These components can only be verified by a chemical analysis of the dust as should the major components also. There are some differences other than the relative peak heights to be observed between the two diffractometer traces, one of these being the difference in the shapes of the first peak corresponding to the major reflection for muscovite on each of the traces. The peak shape on the trace from the coal pneumoconiosis case is indicative of the presence of illite as well as muscovite. These two minerals are very similar both in chemistry and structure and further information, mainly chemical, would be required to confirm the presence of illite; determination of the proportions of each mineral present would be extremely difficult.

The x-ray diffraction results for the two examples illustrated by Figures 3 and 4 have shown that as such x-ray techniques are useful as a means of confirming the presence of major crystalline phases in a sample and indicating the possible presence of minor phases. Confirmatory results using another analytical procedure would be necessary to substantiate the results obtained from the x-ray data.

C. Electron Optical Techniques

The first applications of electron optical equipment in dust research was in the early 1950s when the first commercial transmission electron microscopes (TEM) were employed to produce a more accurate description of the size and shape of dust particles [90,91]. The TEM was initially very limited in its analytical capabilities, however, to a morphological examination of dust material, together with the ability to produce electron diffraction patterns from crystalline phases which could give information about the structure and possible identity of certain particles, and several attempts were made at this stage to employ the TEM for particle identification [48,92-96]. As the TEM was developing a parallel development was taking place with electron optical equipment using finely focused electron beams in a scanning and fixed mode to produce electron optical images of surfaces and also to generate x-rays characteristic of the elements contained within the irradiated surface. The analysis of such x-rays with suitable x-ray spectrometers to yield quantitative chemical information resulted in the production of the electron probe microanalyzer, while scanning electron microscope instruments were developed to examine surfaces. The scanning electron microscope (SEM) provided much more detail of the surface of dust particles but did not possess the image resolution and operating advantages of the TEM. However, specimen preparation was claimed to be easier to perform for an SEM [97,98]. Recently, electron microscope manufacturers have produced combined transmission and scanning microscopes so that dust samples can be examined in either mode with all the advantages of the transmission microscope with its high resolution and diffraction capabilities. Figure 5 illustrates the images of particles that can be produced in such a machine, the switch from one mode to another being performed in seconds.

The electron probe microanalyzer has been employed in several dust research investigations [35-37,41], and it was demonstrated that quantitative information could be obtained from single dust particles using such equipment [99-101]. These instruments, however, do not possess the image resolution and operating advantages of the TEM, while the area of analysis is limited approximately to a circle 1 μm in diameter. With most electron probe equipment the visual examination of dust samples is limited to the use of an optical microscope so that the finer particles cannot be observed and therefore cannot be analyzed. The preparation of dust particles on flat solid substrates for analysis also introduced difficulties as the electron beam often interacted with the substrate beneath the particles producing additional x-ray information which was superimposed on that being obtained from the particle making an accurate analysis of the particle extremely difficult to perform. As particles could be most accurately studied in a TEM it was only natural that researchers involved in such studies should want to analyze the ultrafine features which they ob-

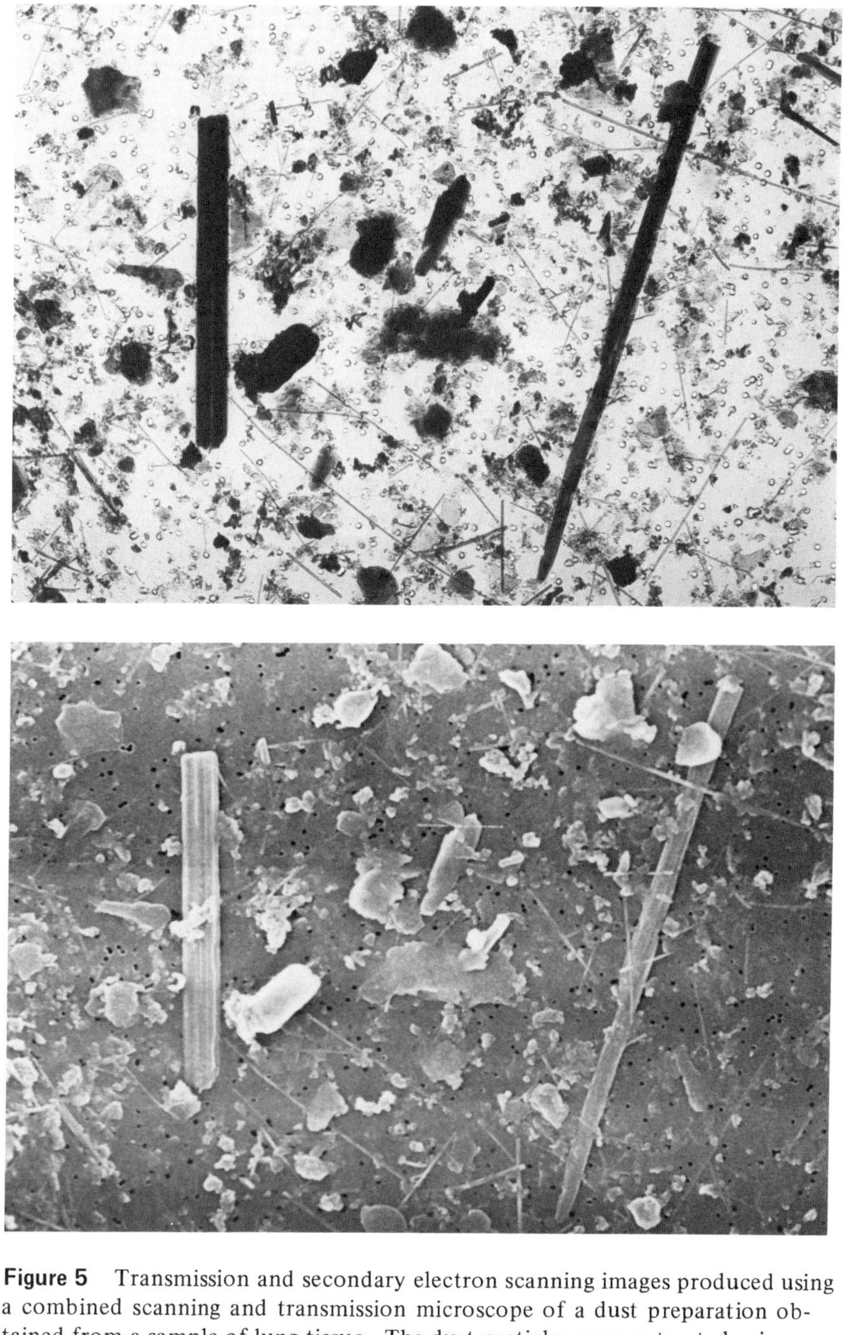

Figure 5 Transmission and secondary electron scanning images produced using a combined scanning and transmission microscope of a dust preparation obtained from a sample of lung tissue. The dust particles were extracted using a sodium hypochlorite digestion procedure and prepared on a 0.2 μm Nucleopore filter which was subsequently carbon coated and prepared for examination.

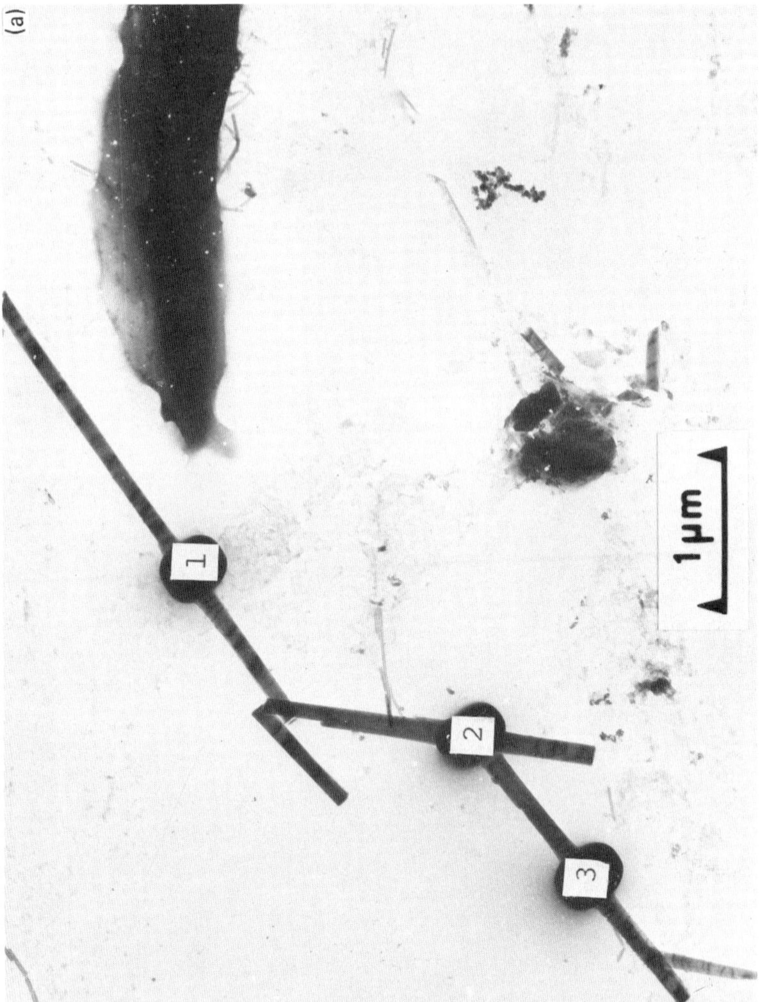
(a)
1
2
3
1 µm

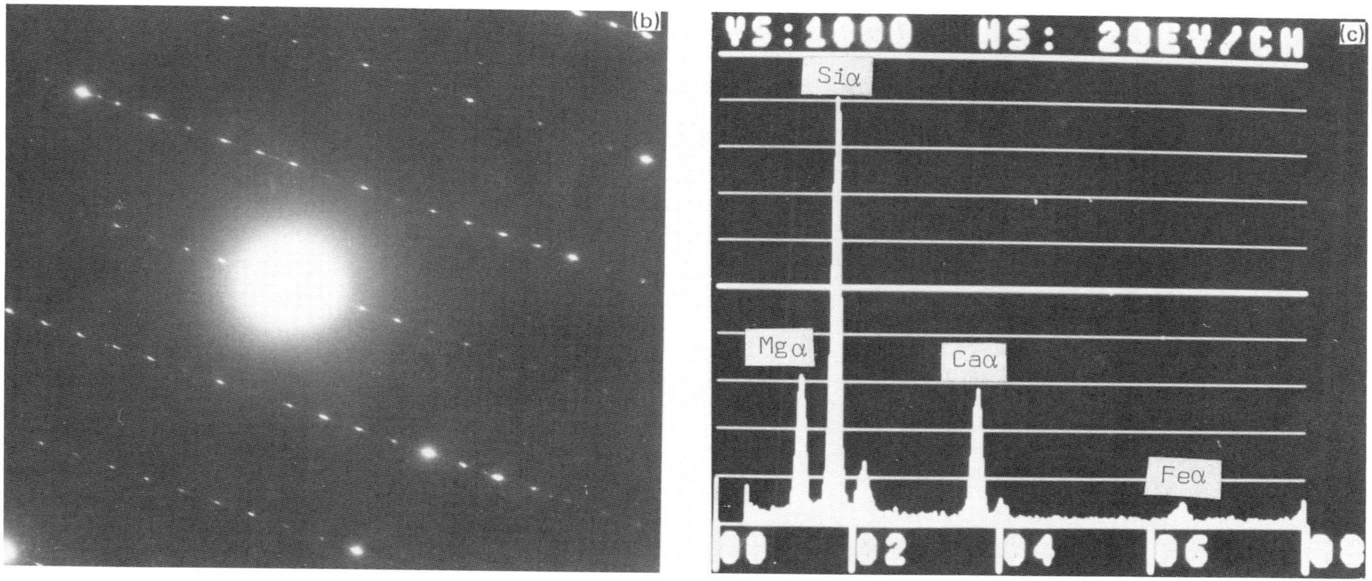

Figure 6 Electron micrograph of mineral fibers detected in an ashed histologic section of lung tissue together with an illustration of the type of selected area electron diffraction pattern and energy-dispersive x-ray spectrum obtained from each of the three analysis points labeled.

served, and this resulted in the combination of x-ray spectrometry with the TEM and also the SEM. The first TEM equipment fitted with multicrystal spectrometers provided some useful information concerning the chemical composition of dust particles from lung tissue [102], but it was tedious to use as only one or two elements at a time could be measured, and before this equipment could be refined x-ray technologists produced a new form of solid-state x-ray spectrometer which when combined with the TEM and the SEM gave comparable results to the crystal spectrometer microscope combinations. This development also allowed research workers to obtain the simultaneous analysis of many elements. It was also found that existing designs of microscope could be readily modified to accept this type of equipment, which is referred to as the energy-dispersive x-ray spectrometer. The operating characteristics and theory of the energy-dispersive and crystal or wavelength dispersive spectrometers have been extensively described [103-105] while their merits for analysis on both TEM and SEM instruments have also been detailed [106]. At the present time, although the experience in dust analysis on either form of electron microscope is limited, most researchers now appear to prefer the combination of the TEM and energy-dispersive x-ray equipment, and it has been demonstrated to be a most versatile and accurate tool for the examination of dust particles whether from biological air or water samples [47,49-51,107-113]. Quantification and identification of the various components of a dust can be obtained with such equipment from only microgram amounts of material while the technique is also nondestructive [114]. The advantages of the TEM and energy-dispersive x-ray equipment combination are described by Figure 6 in which the fibrous particles illustrated by the electron micrograph have been analyzed by focusing the electron beam in the positions labelled 1, 2, and 3. At each position an x-ray spectrum of the type illustrated was produced indicating that each particle contained the same proportion of magnesium, calcium, iron, and silicon. Also from each position labeled, a diffraction pattern of the type shown was also obtained indicating that the fibers were crystalline. From such diffraction patterns it is possible to calculate certain crystallographic information which can be used as confirmation of the identity of the particular mineral. In the case of the selected area diffraction pattern contained in Figure 6 the spacing normal to the lines of diffraction spots represents one crystallographic axial dimension of the fibers while the spacing between spots along the lines represents a second dimension. This technique of selected area electron diffraction cannot be used to uniquely distinguish between certain minerals, but in conjunction with the microchemical information illustrated by the x-ray spectrum in Figure 6 it can provide a unique identification. The combined information from a TEM and energy-dispersive x-ray spectrometer combination as electron diffraction information cannot be obtained with an SEM.

Some recent publications [115-117] have stated that the use of selected area electron diffraction patterns generated from particles in the TEM is the most reliable way of confirming the identity of the particles. This is performed by obtaining good diffraction patterns for two different orientations of the particle with respect to the electron beam and accurately measuring them for comparison with standard patterns generated by a computer in which has been stored unit cell data of the minerals likely to occur in the sample. This technique is obviously time consuming and is subject to considerable error as not all particles when subjected to this form of analysis will give patterns suitable for interpretation and from some larger particles it is impossible to produce a diffraction pattern at all. It would appear that selected area electron diffraction when it is applied is only suitable as a means of confirming the identity of the various minerals encountered in a sample while the use of single-particle x-ray analysis is much more convenient as a method of distinguishing between mineral types and a means of preliminary identification, it is also much simpler to perform.

The qualitative nature of the results that can be obtained from an analytical TEM is illustrated by Figure 7, which is a montage of an electron micrograph of a dust sample extracted from a specimen of lung tissue and also three photographs of x-ray spectra obtained from the analysis of single dust particles observed in the electron micrograph and labeled A, B, and C. It can be seen that spectrum A contains peaks labeled magnesium and silicon of approximately equal height, this spectrum being obtained from the very fine long fiber labeled A. This fiber can be seen to be one of many with similar size characteristics, and they are fibers of the asbestos mineral chrysotile. Spectrum B has been obtained from the fibrous particle labeled B which has a larger diameter than fiber A, and in the x-ray spectrum generated from this particle we can see major peaks corresponding to the elements magnesium, silicon, and calcium; this is a fiber of tremolite. The third x-ray spectrum, C, obtained from the particle labeled C, contains major peaks for silicon and iron together with a minor peak for magnesium. This spectrum is characteristic of the asbestos mineral amosite. The three x-ray spectra can be seen to be very different in character and when they are generated from single fibers in the sample can be used to "fingerprint" and distinguish between particles of different types. Selected area diffraction patterns obtained from representative fibers in the sample can be used to confirm the presence of the particular mineral species present which have been indicated by the microchemical analysis results, and these minerals can be more firmly established by subjecting the sample to an x-ray diffraction examination.

An example of such an application is illustrated by Figure 8 which contains a further electron micrograph of the dust extract used as an illustration of Figure 4 to demonstrate the application of x-ray techniques. In this illustration individual particles have been subjected to microprobe analysis and three chemical types have been established. These are illustrated by the three energy-dispersive x-ray spectra. An examination of these results reveals that three predominant minerals are contained in the sample which correspond to the minerals

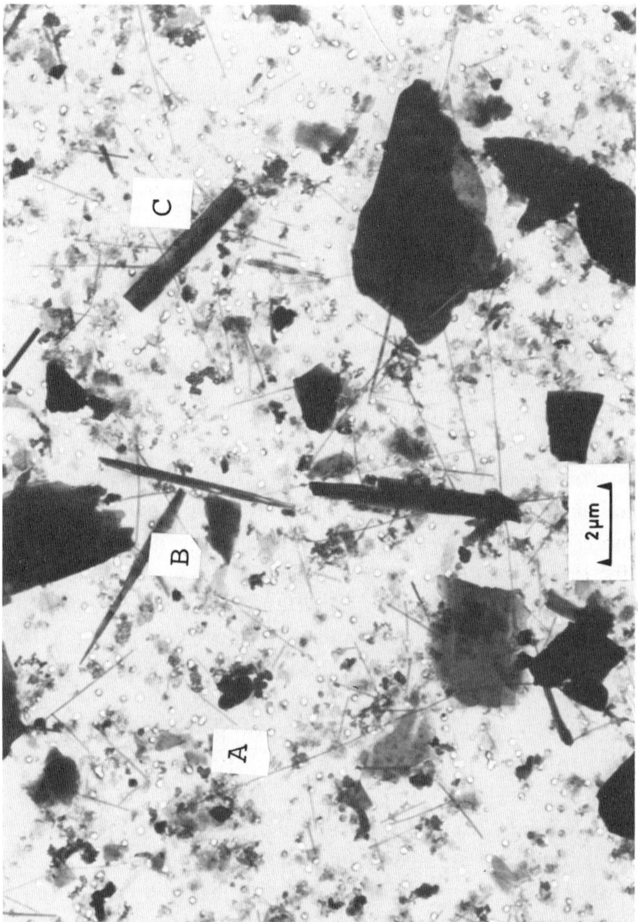
C
B
A
2µm

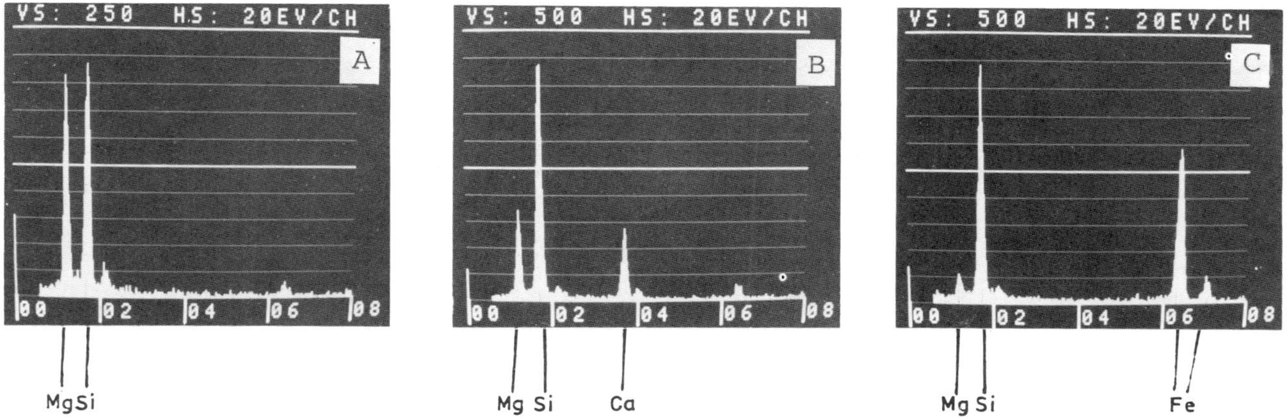

Figure 7 Electron micrograph of a dust extract from a lung tissue specimen obtained from a mesothelioma case together with illustrations of the energy-dispersive x-ray spectra obtained from the three fiber types labeled in the micrograph.

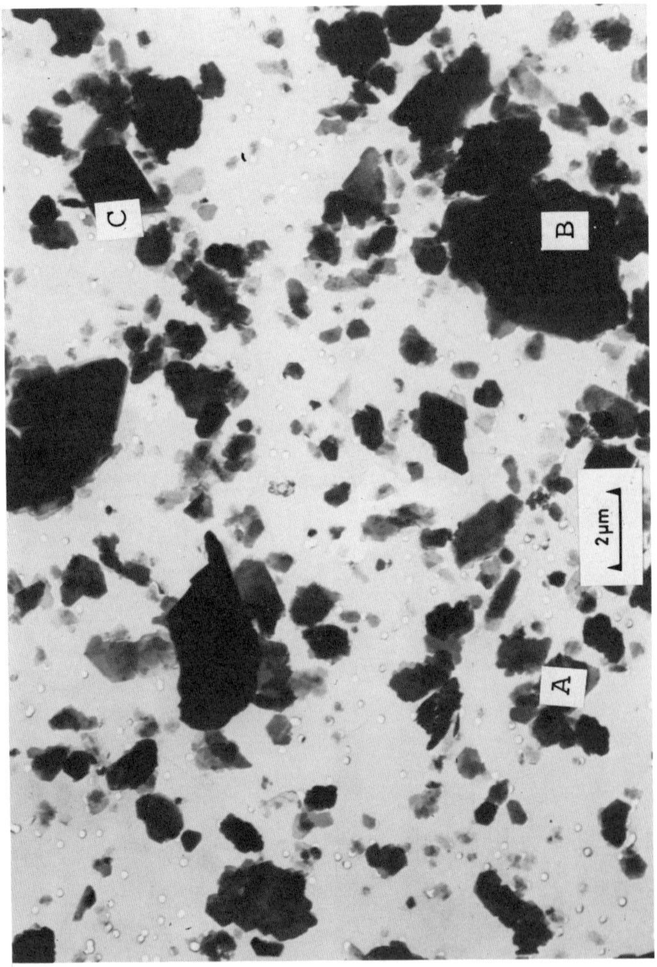
C
B
A
2 µm

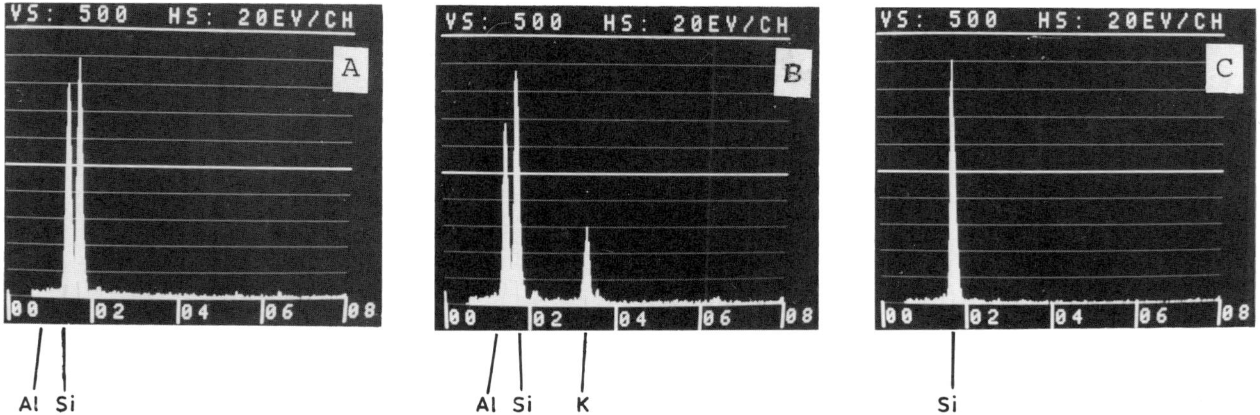

Figure 8 Electron micrograph of a dust extract from a case of kaolin pneumoconiosis together with illustrations of the energy-dispersive x-ray spectra obtained from particles of the three major mineral components of the dust labeled in the micrograph.

kaolin, muscovite, and quartz. Reference to the x-ray data contained in Figure 4 obviously confirms this finding.

D. Other Analytical Techniques

Many other analytical techniques have been applied to study dust particles extracted from lung tissue specimens or to examine individual particles directly in thin sections of tissue. Infrared spectroscopy is one such technique which is very suitable for routine analyses of dust extracts and can be used for both quantitative and qualitative determinations [118]. This technique has been employed to study quartz levels in dust extracts from cases of coal workers' pneumoconiosis and has also been investigated as a possible technique for the determination of asbestos in lung tissue samples [119]. Milligram quantities of dust are normally required for analysis, and the technique has a detection limit of between 10 and 20 μg of any specific material. As with the x-ray diffraction techniques, infrared analysis relies upon having good reference data available for identification purposes while the technique is normally only applied to the determination of single components in a sample. The infrared spectra of many minerals greatly resemble each other, and interferences are very common so that the interpretation of data obtained from dust samples of unknown mixtures of minerals can be extremely difficult and a second analytical technique may be required to help in the interpretation of results. Where overlap of spectra does occur the technique becomes difficult to employ for quantification. It is also known that samples of the same mineral from different geological sources and possessing small differences in chemistry will produce infrared spectra in which the intensity and position of adsorbtion bands will vary. Another disadvantage of the technique is that it is destructive.

Differential thermal analysis is another important mineral technique which can be used to detect and quantify the presence of specific minerals in dust samples. It is not sensitive enough, however, to detect microgram quantities of material and also requires relatively large quantities of sample in order to be employed. It also is a destructive technique.

The magnetic properties of mineral particles and their behavior in magnetic fields have been extensively studied as means of identifying and quantifying the presence of specific minerals in dust samples extracted from lung tissue specimens. Magnetic measurements of pulmonary tissues for contaminants [120,121] have been suggested as a means of estimating quantities of ferromagnetic material in disease situations arising from industrial occupations such as arc welding. The use of magnetic fields to orient dust particles so that they scatter light in a particular fashion has also been suggested as a means of identifying and quantifying certain mineral types such as asbestos [122]. These novel techniques have yet to be shown to have any practical application, however.

A very well established and sophisticated analytical technique which has been shown to have a very useful and practical application is that of ion microprobe mass analysis. This technique has been used [42–44] to demonstrate the presence of single particles containing high levels of beryllium in tissue sections and also to estimate the amount of the element in a given volume of tissue. Another very sophisticated analytical instrument, namely the laser microprobe has also been employed [123,124] in a similar role to study beryllium in fibrotic tissue samples from the lung. The ion probe and laser microprobe are both very specialized and expensive items of equipment which at present can only be justified for specialized investigative purposes.

The bulk chemical analysis of dust samples extracted from lung tissue by wet chemical techniques has been employed extensively in the past but is not recommended in the manner in which it was originally performed. The analysis of dust fractions or solutions prepared from dust samples with equipment such as the atomic adsorbtion spectrophotometer and the more sophisticated plasma optical spectrometer can, however, provide valuable information which can help to interpret analytical results obtained by other techniques such as x-ray diffraction and analytical electron microscopy. The use of nondestructive techniques such as x-ray fluorescence and γ-ray spectroscopy can also be extremely useful in collecting chemical information where samples need to be retained for further analysis.

The investigation of dust deposited and retained in lung tissues can be approached in many ways with the aid of many different analytical techniques. The success and value of such investigations, however, lies in the careful preparation of the tissue samples and the correct selection of analytical procedures necessary to produce the results required to qualify and quantify the various components of the dust being investigated.

V. Summary

The history of the investigation of dust deposits in lung tissue specimens is closely linked to the availability and development of analytical techniques. At the start of the century, using crude extraction procedures, optical microscopy in combination with wet chemical analysis methods were employed to examine large samples of dust, often from whole lungs, to produce only very limited information. With modern research equipment, however, it is possible to study in detail the chemistry, structure, and morphology of individual dust particles and with careful application to extend this examination to large numbers of particles so that complete samples can be characterized. It is apparent that no single analytical technique is sufficient to fully characterize a dust sample and that careful combinations of techniques will normally be required in most investigations [125]. Careful specimen preparation is necessary to ensure that the results obtained are not modified in any way.

The aim of any study of lung dust is to provide information which can be correlated with the pathology and progression of a disease and the environmental and occupational history of the patient. More often the emphasis in such studies is placed upon identification of only a single constituent of the dust and much valuable information is overlooked. The scope of some investigations has been dictated solely by the availability of certain items of analytical equipment, and their inadequacies in supplying the information required has often not been recognized.

Very careful planning and experimental design are required before embarking upon an investigation, and all techniques and procedures to be employed should be thoroughly tested so that results can be qualified statistically before publication. Other investigators may then repeat and perhaps improve upon past techniques. It will also allow them to compare their experimental results with those in the literature.

There are many recognized occupational diseases arising from the inhalation and retention of dust particles in the lungs and many unsolved problems facing the pathologists involved in the study of such diseases. It is obvious that a more concerted and accurate study of particles involved in such disease situations is required in order to establish the role of the various constituents of these dusts in the precipitation and progression of such diseases.

References

1. Wagner, J. C., C. A. Sleggs, and P. Marchand, Diffuse pleural mesothelioma and asbestos exposure in the North Western Cape Province, *Br. J. Ind. Med.*, **17**:260–271 (1960).
2. Watkins-Pitchford, W., and J. Moir, On the nature of the doubly-refracting particles seen in microscopic sections of silicotic lungs, *Rep. S. African Inst. Med. Res.*, **1**(September):000–000 (1916).
3. Watson, H. H., Dust sampling investigations, *Rep. I.M.M. Meeting*, November (1936).
4. Salazer, A., and L. Silverman, A new method for the detection of free silica in industrial dusts, *J. Ind. Hyg. Toxicol.*, **25**(4):000–000 (1943).
5. Irwin, D. A., The histological demonstration of siliceous material by microincineration, *Can. Med. Assoc. J.*, **31**:135 (1934).
6. Belt, T. H., A. A. Ferris, and E. J. King, The silicotic nodule in human experimental silicosis: A comparative study, *J. Pathol. Bacteriol.*, **51**(2): 263 (1940).
7. Gross, P., M. L. Westrick, and J. M. NcNerny, Silicosis the topographic relationship of mineral deposits to histologic structures, *Am. J. Pathol.*, **32**(4):739 (1956).

8. Jones, W. R., Silicotic lungs: The minerals they contain, *J. Hyg.*, **33**(3): 000 (1933).
9. Haldane, J. B. S., Contribution to discussion of paper by W. R. Jones, *TIMM*, **43**:387 (1934).
10. Faulds, J. S., E. J. King, and G. Nagleschmidt, Dust content of lungs of coal workers from Cumberland, *Br. J. Med.*, **16**:43 (1959).
11. King, E. J., and T. H. Belt, The silica content of tissues with and without silicotic lesions, *J. Pathol. Bacteriol.*, **51**(2):269 (1940).
12. King, E. J., B. A. Maguire, and G. Nagleschmidt, Further studies of the dust in lungs of coal workers, *Br. J. Med.*, **13**:9 (1956).
13. Nagleschmidt, G., D. Rivers, and E. J. King, Dust and collagen content of lungs of coalworkers with P.M.F., *Br. J. Ind. Med.*, **20**:181 (1963).
14. McDonald, G., and A. P. Piggott, Two cases of acute silicosis, *Lancet*, **2**: 846 (1930).
15. MacLaughlin, A. I. G., Pneumoconiosis in foundry workers, *Br. J. Tuberc. Dis. Chest*, **51**:000 (1957).
16. MacLaughlin, A. I. G., and H. E. Harding, Pneumoconiosis and other causes of death in iron and steel foundry workers, *A.M.A. Arch. Ind. Health*, **00**:350 (1956).
17. Meiklejohn, A., and W. W. Jones, The effect of the use of calcined alumina in china biscuit plating on the health of workmen, *J. Hyg. Toxicol.*, **30**(3):000 (1948).
18. Stewart, W., Estimation of silica in lung tissues, *Birmingham Med. Rev.*, **8**: 000 (1933).
19. Thomas, R. W., Silicosis in the ball-clay and china clay industries, *Lancet*, **1**:133 (1952).
20. Badham, C., and H. B. Taylor, The lungs of coal, metalliferous and sandstone minerals and other workers in N.S. Wales. *Annual Report of the Department of Public Health, New South Wales*, 1936.
21. Durkan, T. M., The determination of free silica in industrial dust, *J. Ind. Hyg. Toxicol.*, **28**(5):217 (1946).
22. S. R. Haythorn, and F. A. Taylor, Experimental silicosis produced with the ash from human silicotic lungs, *Am. J. Pathol.*, **21**:000 (1945).
23. Hale, L. W., J. Gough, E. J. King, and G. Nagleschmidt, Pneumoconiosis of kaolin workers, *Br. J. Ind. Med.*, **13**:251 (1956).
24. King, E. J., B. D. Stacey, P. F. Holt, D. M. Yates, and D. M. Pickles, The colorimetric determination of silicon in the microanalysis of biological material and mineral dusts, *Analyst*, **80**(951):441 (1955).
25. Fauls, J. S., and G. Nagleschmidt, The dust in the lungs of hematite minerals from Cumberland, *Ann. Occup. Hyg.*, **4**:255 (1962).
26. Berkelhamer, L. H., X-ray diffraction—An important tool in pneumoconiosis research, *J. Ind. Hyg. Toxicol.*, **23**:000 (1941).
27. Sweany, H. C., R. Klaas, and G. L. Clark, The detection of crystalline silica in lung tissue by x-ray diffraction analysis, *Radiology*, **31**(3):299 (1938).

28. Jephcott, C. M., W. M. Gray, and D. A. Irwin, A study of the crystalline siliceous material present in silicate lungs by the x-ray diffraction method, *Can. Med. Assoc. J.*, **38**:209 (1938).
29. Gordon, R. L., O. G. Griffin, and G. Nagleschmidt, The quantitative determination of quartz by x-ray diffraction, *Res. Rep. Safety Mines,* **52**: 000 (1952).
30. Gordon, R. L., and G. W. Harris, Geiger-Muller counter equipment for quantitative x-ray diffraction analysis of powders, *Res. Rep. Safety Mines,* **138**:000 (1956).
31. Gordon, R. L., and G. W. Harris, Effect of particle size on the quantitative determination of quartz by x-ray diffraction, *Nature,* **175**:1135 (1955).
32. Nagleschmidt, G., Inter-laboratory trials on the determination of quartz in dusts of respirable size, *Analyst,* **81**:210 (1956).
33. Rivers, D., M. E. Wise, and E. J. King, Dust content, radiology and pathology in simple pneumoconiosis of coalworkers, *Br. J. Ind. Med.,* **17**:87 (1960).
34. Pimental, J. C., R. Avila, and A. G. Laurenco, Respiratory disease caused by synthetic fibers: A new occupational disease, *Thorax,* **30**:204 (1975).
35. Berry, J. P., P. Henoc, P. Galle, and R. Poriente, Pulmonary mineral dust, *Am. J. Pathol.,* **83**(3):427 (1976).
36. Stettler, L. E., D. H. Broth, and G. R. Mackay, Identification of stainless steel welding fume particulates in human lung and environmental samples using electron probe microanalysis, *Am. Ind. Hyg. Assoc. J.,* **38**(2):76–82 (1977).
37. Ferrin, J., J. R. Coleman, S. Davis, and B. Morehouse, Electron microprobe analysis of particles deposited in lungs, *Arch. Environ. Health,* **00**: 113 (1976).
38. Brody, A. R., and M. D. Craighead, Cytoplasmic inclusions in pulmonary microphages of cigarette smokers, *Lab. Invest.,* **32**:125 (1975).
39. Goni, J., G. Remond, M. C. Journant, J. Bignon, G. Bonnaud, and I. Bravet, Present possibilities of identification of ferruginous bodies in human lung using the scanning electron microscope, *Rev. Tuberc. Pneumol.,* **36**(8):1223 (1972).
40. Greaves, H., Energy dispersion x-ray analysis by scanning electron microscopy for measuring cellular elemental composition in bacterial cells, *Appl. Microbiol.,* **27**(3):609 (1974).
41. Bonfield, W. G., A. J. Tousimis, J. C. Hagerty, and T. R. Padden, Electron probe analysis of human lung tissues. In *X-ray and Electron Probe Analysis in Biochemical Research.* Edited by New York, Plenum Press, 1969, pp. 000–000.
42. Abraham, J. L., Recent advances in pneumoconiosis: The pathologists role in etiologic diagnosis. In *The Lung.* Edited by W. T. Thurlbeck and M. Abell. Baltimore, Williams & Williams Co., 1978, pp. 000–000.
43. Abraham, J. L., R. Rossi, and R. M. Wagner, Ion microprobe mass analysis of beryllium in situ in human lung: preliminary results. In *Scanning Electron Microscopy,* Vol. 2. Edited by O. Jahari. Chicago, I.I.T. Research Institute, 1976, p. 501.

44. Abraham, J. L., and T. A. Whatley, Ion microprobe analysis of beryllium-containing particles in situ in human lungs, *Fed. Proc.*, **36**:1090 (1977).
45. Abraham, J. L., R. M. Wagner, K. Miyai, R. Bollock, and P. J. Friedman, Choice of imaging modes in S.E.M. study of respirable radiographic contrast medium: Tantalum particles in the lung. In *Scanning Electron Microscopy*, Vol. 2. Edited by O. Jahari. Chicago, I.I.T. Research Inst., 1976, p. 691.
46. Frazer, F. W., and C. B. Belcher, Quantitative determination of the mineral matter content of coal by a radiofrequency-oxidation technique, *Fuel*, **52**:000 (1973).
47. Pooley, F. D., Electron microscope characteristics of inhaled chrysotile asbestos fiber, *Br. J. Ind. Med.*, **29**:146 (1972).
48. Pooley, F. D., P. D. Oldham, Um Chang-Hyun, and J. C. Wagner, The detection of asbestos in tissues. In *Proceedings of the International Conference on Pneumoconiosis*. Edited by Johannesburg, Oxford University Press, 1969, pp. 108–116.
49. Langer, A. M., I. B. Rubin, J. Selikoff, and F. D. Pooley, Chemical characterization of uncoated asbestos fibers from the lungs of asbestos workers by electron microprobe analysis, *J. Histochem. Cytochem.*, **20**(9):735 (1972).
50. Pooley, F. D., Asbestos fiber in the lung and mesothelioma, *Acta Pathol. Microbiol. Scand. [A]*, **81**:390 (1973).
51. Pooley, F. D., An examination of the fibrous mineral content of asbestotic lung tissue from the Canadian chrysotile mining industry, *Environ. Res.*, **12**:281 (1976).
52. Matsudo, H., N. M. Hodgkinson, and A. Tanaka, Japanese gastric cancer, *Arch. Pathol.*, **97**:366 (1974).
53. Suzuki, Y., S. Aita, T. Hoshino, and H. Iwata, Identification of submicroscopic asbestos fibrils in tissue by analytical electron microscopy, *Geol. News*, **12e**:No. 2 (1972).
54. Suzuki, Y., and J. Chung, Structure and development of the asbestos body, *Am. J. Pathol.*, **55**:79–107 (1969).
55. David, J. M. G., The ultrastructure of asbestos bodies from human lung, *Br. J. Exp. Pathol.*, **45**:642–646 (1964).
56. Guest, L., The recovery of dust from formalin-fixed pneumoconiotic lungs: A comparison of the methods used at S.M.R.E., *Ann. Occup. Hyg.*, **19**:37–47 (1976).
57. Bergman, I., Determination of coal in formalin-fixed pneumoconiotic lungs, *Anal. Chem.*, **38**(3):441–444 (1966).
58. Whitewell, F., J. Scott, and M. Grimshaw, Relationships between occupations and asbestos-fibre content of the lungs in patients with pleural mesothelioma, lung cancer and other diseases, *Thorax*, **32**:477 (1977).
59. Ashcroft, T., and A. G. Heppleston, The optical and electron microscopic determination of pulmonary asbestos fiber concentration and its relation to the human pathological reaction, *J. Clin. Pathol.*, **26**:224 (1973).

60. Gold, C., The quantitation of asbestos in tissue, *J. Clin. Pathol.*, **21**:537 (1968).
61. Langer, A. M., I. J. Selikoff, and A. Sastre, Chrysotile asbestos in the lungs of persons in New York City, *Arch. Environ. Health,* **22**:348 (1971).
62. Nenadic, C. M., and J. V. Crable, Enzymatic digestion of human lung tissue, *Am. Ind. Hyg. Assoc. J.*, **00**:81–86 (1970).
63. Gross, P., J. Tuma, and R. T. D. De Treville, Fibrous dust particles and ferruginous bodies, *Arch. Environ. Health,* **21**:38–46 (1970).
64. Gross, P., L. J. Cralley, J. M. G. Davies, R. T. P. De Treville, and J. Tuma, A quantitative study of fibrous dust in the lungs of city dwellers. In *Inhaled Particles III,* Vol. II. Edited by W. H. Walton. Old Woking, Surrey, England, Unwin Brothers, The Gresham Press, 1971, pp. 671–681.
65. Smith, M. J., and B. Naylor, A method for extracting ferruginous bodies from sputum and pulmonary tissue, *Am. J. Clin. Pathol.,* **68**:250–254 (1972).
66. Gross, P., R. A. Harley, J. M. G. Davies, and L. J. Cralley, Mineral fiber content of human lungs, *Am. Ind. Hyg. Assoc. J.*, **00**:148–151 (1974).
67. Gross, P., R. T. P. De Treville, L. J. Cralley, and J. M. G. Davis, Pulmonary ferruginous bodies, *Arch. Pathol.,* **85**:539–546 (1968).
68. Gross, P., J. Tuma, and R. T. P. De Treville, Unusual ferruginous bodies, *Arch. Environ. Health,* **22**:534–537 (1971).
69. Utidjian, M. D., P. Gross, and R. T. P. De Treville, Ferruginous bodies in human lungs, *Arch. Environ. Health,* **17**:327–333 (1968).
70. Sebastien, P., M. A. Billon, X. Janson, G. Bonnaud, and J. Bignon, Use of the transmission electron microscope for the measurement of asbestos contamination, *Arch. Mal. Profess. Med. Travail Séc. Social (Paris),* **39**(4–5):229–248 (1978).
71. Bignon, J., P. Sebastien, and A. Gaudichet, Measurement of Asbestos Retention in the Human Respiratory System Related to Health Effects. *National Bureau of Standards (U.S.) Special Publication No. 506,* 1978, pp. 95–118.
72. Jaunarajs, K. L., and R. S. Liebling, The digestion of lung tissue for mineral dust recovery, *Am. Ind. Hyg. Assoc. J.*, **33**:535 (1972).
73. Cunningham, H. M., and R. D. Pontefract, Penetration of asbestos through the digestive tract of rats, *Nature,* **243**:352 (1973).
74. Henderson, W. J., D. M. D. Evans, J. D. Davies, and K. Griffiths, Analysis of particles in stomach tumours from Japanese males, *Environ. Res.*, **9**: 240–249 (1975).
75. Henderson, W. J., and K. Griffiths, Identification of talc particles in ovarian tissue, *Gynecol. Malig.*, **00**:225–240 (1975).
76. Stewart, I., Selected thoughts on asbestos quantification, *Proceedings of the FDA Symposium on Electron Microscopy of Microfibers.* HEW Publication No. (FDA) 77-1033, August 1976, p. 93.
77. Nagleschmidt, G., and E. J. King, Isolation and identification of minerals in lung residues and airborne dusts from coal mines, *Biochem. J.*, **35**: 152–158 (1941).

78. Kerr, P. F., *Optical Mineralogy*. McGraw-Hill, New York, 1977.
79. Maclaughlin, A. J. G., E. Rogers, and K. C. Dunham, Talc pneumoconiosis, *Br. J. Ind. Med.*, **6**:184 (1949).
80. McCrone, W. C., Identification of Asbestos by Polarized Light Microscopy. *National Bureau of Standards (U.S.) Special Publication No. 506,* November, 1978, pp. 235–248.
81. McCrone, W. C., and L. McCrone, Light microscopy of microfibers—uses and limitations. In *Symposium on Electron Microscopy of Microfibers.* HEW Publication No. (FDA) No. 77-1033, August, 1976, pp. 37–43.
82. Azaroff, L. V., and M. J. Buerger, *The X-ray Powder Method.* New York, Mc-Graw-Hill, 1958.
83. Le Bouffant, L., Investigation and analysis of asbestos fibers and accompanying minerals in biological materials, *Environ. Health Perspect.,* **9**: 149 (1974).
84. Rickards, A. L., Estimation of true amounts of chrysotile asbestos by x-ray diffraction, *Anal. Chem.,* **44**:1872 (1972).
85. Crable, J. V., Quantitative determination of chrysotile, amosite and crocidolite by x-ray diffraction, *Am. Ind. Hyg. Assoc. J.,* **27**:293 (1966).
86. Miller, A., A. S. Teirstein, M. E. Bader, R. A. Bader, and I. J. Selikoff, Talc pneumoconiosis, *Am. J. Med.,* **50**:395 (1971).
87. Rohl, A. N., and A. M. Langer, Identification and quantification of asbestos in talc, *Environ. Health Perspect.,* **9**:95–109 (1974).
88. Langer, A. M., M. S. Wolf, A. N. Rohl, and I. J. Selikoff, Variation of properties of chrysotile asbestos subjected to milling, *J. Toxicol. Environ. Health,* **4**:173–185 (1978).
89. Haartz, J. C., B. A. Lange, R. G. Draftz, and R. F. Scholl, Selection and Characterization of Fibrous and Nonfibrous Amphiboles for Analytical Methods Development. *National Bureau of Standards (U.S.) Special Publication No. 506,* November, 1978, pp. 295–312.
90. Cartwright, J., and J. W. Skidmore, The measurement of size and concentration of airborne dusts with the electron microscope, *Res. Rep. Safety Mines,* **79**:000 (1973).
91. Cartwright, J., G. Nagleschmidt, and J. W. Skidmore, The study of air pollution with the electron microscope, *Q. J. R. Met. Soc.,* **82**:82 (1956).
92. Pooley, F. D., and W. J. Henderson, Replication of the particle surface as an aid to identification, *Proc. R. Soc. Med. (Part 3),* **1**:169 (1966).
93. Pooley, F. D., The use of the electron microscope as a tool in mining research, *Mining Eng.,* **00**:321 (March 1968).
94. Timbrell, V., F. D. Pooley, and J. C. Wagner, Characteristics of respirable asbestos fibers. In *Proceedings of the International Conference on Pneumoconiosis.* Edited by Johannesburg, Oxford University Press, 1969, p. 65.
95. Miller, A., A. M. Langer, A. S. Teirstein, and I. J. Selikoff, "Nonspecific" interstitial pulmonary fibrosis, *N. Engl. J. Med.,* **292**(2):91 (1975).
96. Fondimore, A., J. Desbordes, and J. Tayot, An unusual case of talc asbestosis, *Anal. Anat. Pathol. (Paris),* **20**(1):277 (1975).

97. Davies, J. M. G., S. T. Beckett, E. Bolton, P. Collings, and A. P. Middleton, Mass and number of fibers in the pathogenesis of asbestos related lung disease in rats, *Br. J. Cancer,* **37**:673 (1978).
98. Bignon, J., J. Goni, G. Bonnaud, M. C. Journant, G. Dufour, and M. C. Pinchon, Incidence of pulmonary ferruginous bodies in France, *Environ. Res.,* **3**:430 (1970).
99. White, E. W., P. J. Denny, and S. M. Irving, Quantitative microprobe analysis of microcrystalline powders. In *The Electron Microprobe.* Edited by T. D. McKinley, K. F. Heinrich, and D. B. Wittry. New York, John Wiley, 1966, pp. 791–804.
100. Mellors, R. C., K. G. Carroll, and T. Solberg, Quantitative analysis of Ca/P molar ratios in bone tissue with the electron probe. In *The Electron Microprobe.* Edited by T. D. McKinley, K. F. J. Heinrich, and D. B. Wittry. New York, John Wiley, 1966, p. 834.
101. Rubin, I. B., and C. J. Maggiore, Elemental analysis of fibers by means of electron probe techniques, *Environ. Health Perspect.,* **9**:81–94 (1974).
102. Stumphius, J., and P. B. Myer, Asbestos bodies and mesothelioma, *Ann. Occup. Hyg.,* **11**:283 (1968).
103. Cooke, C. J., and P. Duncombe, *Fifth International Conference on X-ray Optics and Micro-analysis, Tubingen.* Edited by G. Mollenstadt and K. H. Gaulker. Berlin, Springer Verlag, 1968, pp. 245–247.
104. Duncumb, P., Precipitation studies with EMMA—a combined electron microscope and x-ray analyzer. In *The Electron Microprobe.* Edited by T. D. McKinley, K. F. Heinrich, and D. B. Wittry. New York, John Wiley, 1966, pp. 000–000.
105. Gedcke, D. A., The Si(Li) x-ray energy analysis system: operating principles and performance, *X-ray Spectrom.,* **1**:129–141 (1972).
106. Russ, J. C., X-ray spectrometry on the electron microscope, *X-ray Spectrom.,* **2**:11–14 (1973).
107. Pooley, F. D., Methods for assessing asbestos fibers and asbestos bodies in tissue by electron microscopy. In *Biological Effects of Asbestos.* Edited by Lyon, Publisher, 1973, p. 50.
108. Langer, A. M., and Pooley, F. D., Identification of single asbestos fibers in human tissue. In *Biological Effects of Asbestos.* Edited by Lyon, Publisher, 1973, p. 119.
109. Langer, A. M., A. D. Mackler, and F. D. Pooley, Electron microscopical investigation of asbestos fibers, *Environ. Health Perspect.,* **9**:139 (1974).
110. Pooley, F. D., The identification of asbestos dust with an electron microscope, *Ann. Occup. Hyg.,* **18**:181 (1975).
111. Pooley, F. D., The use of the analytical electron microscope in the analysis of mineral dusts, *Philos. Trans. R. Soc. Lond. [A],* **286**:625 (1977).
112. Lorimer, G. W., and P. E. Champness, Combined electron microscopy and analysis of orthopyroxene, *Am. Mineral,* **58**:243–248 (1973).
113. Rowse, J. B., W. B. Jepson, A. T. Bailey, N. A. Climpson, and P. M. Soper, Composite elemental standards for quantitative electron microscope microprobe analysis, *J. Phys. E. Sci. Instrum.,* **7**:512–514 (1974).

114. Rickards, A. L., Estimation of submicrogram quantities of chrysotile asbestos by electron microscopy, *Anal. Chem.*, **45**:809 (1973).
115. Lee, R. J., Computerized SAED and the electron optical identification of particulates. In *Proceedings of the FDA Symposium on Electron Microscopy of Microfibers.* HEW Publication No. (FDA) 77–1033, August 1976, p. 60.
116. Lally, J. S., and R. J. Lee, Computer indexing of electron diffraction patterns including the effect of lattice symmetry. In *Electron Microscopy and X-ray application to Environmental and Occupational Health Analysis.* Edited by P. A. Russell and A. E. Hutchins. Ann Arbor, Michigan, Ann Arbor Science Publishers Inc., 1978, pp. 169–174.
117. Lee, R. J., J. S. Lally, and R. M. Fisher, Identification and Counting of Mineral Fragments. *National Bureau of Standards (U.S.) Special Publication No. 506,* November, 1978, pp. 387–402.
118. Dodgson, J., and W. Whittaker, The determination of quartz in respirable dust samples by infrared spectroscopy (the potassium bromide disk method), *Ann. Occup. Hyg.*, **16**:373 (1973).
119. Heidermanns, G., G. Reidiger, and A. Schütz, The determination of asbestos in respirable industrial and lung dusts, *Staub-Reinholt,* **36**(3): 107 (1976).
120. Cohen, D., Ferromagnetic contamination in the lungs and other organs of the human body, *Science,* **180**:745–748 (1973).
121. Kalliomäki, P. L., P. Korp, T. Katila, P. Mäkipää, P. Saar, and A. Tossavainen, Magnetic measurements of pulmonary contamination, *Scand. J. Work Environ. Health,* **4**:232 (1976).
122. Timbrell, V., Magnetic separation of respirable asbestos fibers, *Filtration Separation,* **14**:241–242 (1977).
123. Prine, J. R., S. F. Brakeshoulder, D. E. McVean, and F. R. Robinson, Demonstration of the presence of beryllium in pulmonary granulomas, *Am. J. Clin. Pathol.,* **45**:448–454 (1966).
124. Robinson, F. R., S. F. Brakeshoulder, A. A. Thomas, and J. Cholak, Microemission spectro-chemical analysis of human lungs for beryllium, *Am. J. Clin. Pathol.,* **49**:821–825 (1968).
125. Langer, A. M., and F. D. Pooley, Identification of single asbestos fibers in tissue. In *Proceedings of the International Conference on Biological Effects of Asbestos.* Edited by P. Bogouski, et al. Lyon, IARC, 1974, p. 199.

11

Mechanisms of Fibrogenesis

ERIC D. BATEMAN, ROBERT J. EMERSON, and PETER COLE

Cardiothoracic Institute
Brompton Hospital
London, England

I. Introduction

For many years research in the field of pulmonary disease has been concerned with mechanisms by which fibrosis occurs in the lung. Workers in the field of occupational medicine have shared this interest because of the large number of fibrogenic agents encountered in industrial or work-related environments.

Fibrosis can be considered in the first instance as an advantageous host response. Its value in repair of traumatic or destructive lesions such as cavitating pneumonias is obvious. Less obvious is the advantage of the fibrogenetic response in trapping and incarcerating foreign particles and organisms which gain access to the lungs from the external environment. This is required when such "first-line" pulmonary defenses as cough, phagocytosis by macrophages, and clearance via the mucociliary apparatus have failed. Such failure may be due to physical or chemical properties of a particle (e.g., asbestos) or in the case of an organism (e.g., *Mycobacterium tuberculosis*), to its relative resistance to bactericidal defenses.

The lung is a distinctive organ in two respects. One, by virtue of its large "external" gas exchange surface area which is exposed to the atmosphere, and its large "internal" surface or vascular bed exposed to blood-borne agents, the possibility of fibrogenic agents reaching and interacting with lung tissue is great. Two, whereas in most organs fibrosis is well tolerated and is beneficial as a method of healing and repair, in the lung a relatively small amount of fibrous tissue is associated with considerable impairment of pulmonary function leading to significant morbidity and mortality. The gas-exchanging property of the lung is dependent on the preservation of a thin membrane for diffusion of gases, an intact vascular bed, and normal ventilatory mechanics (including compliance); since fibrosis disrupts all of these, it has an early and often disastrous effect on lung function.

As will become apparent when considering recent improvements in techniques for studying fibrogenetic mechanisms, the development of fibrosis in the lung cannot be thought of as a single process, but rather as the final common pathway of many biological responses to various insulting agents.

An increasing variety of ways are being defined in which fibrous tissue can be laid down, and it is becoming apparent that most agents act in more than one way to produce fibrosis. For this reason, fibrosis which is unhelpful to the host should be considered to be the result of an imbalance between biosynthetic and degradative processes influencing the metabolism of collagen (Fig. 1).

While considerable research has been directed toward elucidating the factors stimulating fibroblasts and collagen synthesis, less has been done to gain an understanding of the regulatory processes by which tissue destruction occurs in disease. It seems a paradox that the early lesions of several conditions which lead to fibrosis are associated with destruction or disruption of connective tissue. Gross [1] has demonstrated that the alveolar stromal destruction and cellular necrosis which occur in various pathological states may occur independently of one another. Alveolar stromal destruction has been shown in experimental tuberculous chronic fibrosing pneumonitis [1], particularly in proximity to giant cells, and tissues staining positively for both reticulin and collagen are affected. Similar features have also been found in the lungs of rabbits exposed to ozone, and in radiation pneumonitis [1].

The characteristic histologic features of early stromal destruction (which are best shown before collagenous fibrosis is established) have been outlined by Gross [1] It is argued that, because fibrosing conditions may end in the production of a honeycomb lung or similar lesions, it is reasonable to assume that dissolution of parenchymal tissue also plays a part, together with the traction on airspaces produced by surrounding fibrosis.

The Pi^{zz} phenotype provides a further example of the close relationship between the tendency to develop fibrosis and connective tissue destruction. This genetic predisposition to both infantile cirrhosis [2] and the early onset of lower zone emphysema related to tobacco smoke may reflect a common defect in these persons. Inadequate protection of tissues by plasma inhibitors of neutral proteases (including elastase and collagenase) released from polymorphonuclear leukocytes (PMN) and macrophages occurs. Since the PMN has a central

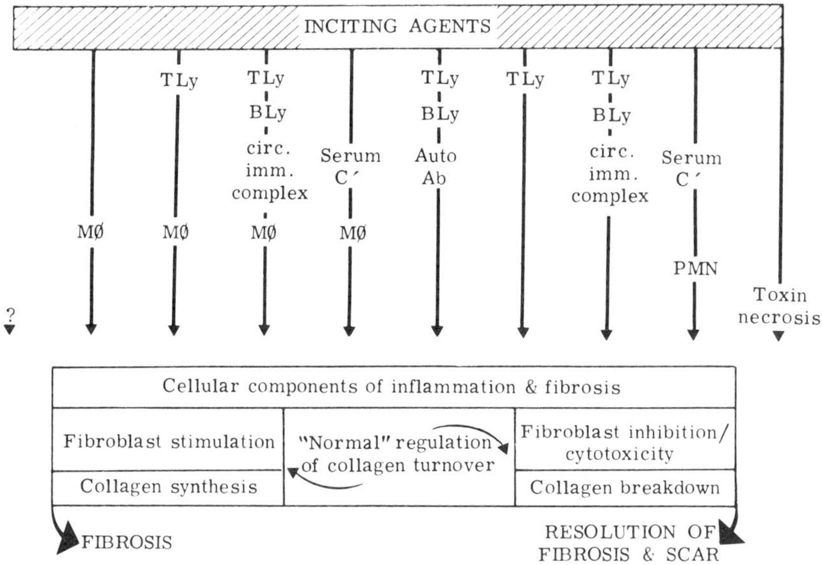

Figure 1 Mechanisms of fibrogenesis.

role in acute inflammatory processes and the macrophage is recognized as being important in fibrotic processes, it is of interest that their combined role produces these two pathological processes in the same host.

Pulmonary fibrosis should therefore be considered to be more than a simple increase of collagen in the lungs. In fact, as will be discussed, lung collagen may not be measurably increased, but rather altered in distribution, fibril configuration, or collagen type [3]. There is also an increase in cellular components and other connective tissue elements. The general features of the cells involved have been extensively reviewed [4,5], but their functional role in fibrogenetic mechanisms will be discussed in various parts of this chapter. Because an understanding of fibrosis requires some knowledge of the connective tissue elements involved, an outline of their structure and metabolism, and of methods for their detection and measurement will be given. This provides a basis for discussion of the known mechanisms of fibrosis and of models useful for research in this field.

II. Materials

A. Collagen

Three connective tissue elements provide the structural support of the lung. These are collagen, elastic fibers, and proteoglycans. Of these, collagen is the most plentiful, comprising 15-20% of the alveolar dry weight and 60-70% of the total interstitial connective tissue [6].

The primary structure of collagen, referred to as tropocollagen, is made up of three polypeptide chains, called α chains, each containing approximately 1100 amino acids, which are coiled in such a manner as to form a triple-helical configuration.

The major amino acids of the polypeptide chains that make up the tropocollagen molecule are glycine, proline, and lysine, the glycine moiety occurring at every third position of the peptide. Two amino acids, hydroxyproline and hydroxylysine, are important constituents of the collagen molecule and until recently were thought to be unique to collagen. However, it has been demonstrated that elastin, the Clq component of complement, and the tail structure of acetylcholinesterase also contain hydroxyproline [7]. When the polypeptide is formed it usually consists of the 1100 amino acids repeating themselves as tripeptide units of $(\text{x-y-glycine})_n$, the amino acids in the x-y position most commonly being proline-hydroxyproline and lysine-hydroxylsine.

Types

Table 1 summarizes the molecular structure and some features of the five varieties of collagen that occur in the lung.

Synthesis

A simplified scheme of the steps involved in the synthesis of collagen is presented in Figure 2.

As with other proteins, the initial step is the transcription of the genetic code for collagen to messenger RNA (mRNA) within the nucleus of the cell. This mRNA diffuses into the cytoplasm and attaches to ribosomes and translation occurs. The newly formed protein (pro-α-chain) undergoes a number of important posttranslational modifications. These are hydroxylation, glycosylation, and eventually triple-helix formation. The triple-helical protein formed in this way is procollagen, which has peptide extensions at the amino- and carboxyl-terminal ends. It was originally thought that the function of these was to aid in the formation of the triple-helical structure, but other important functions are now being proposed for these extensions [7]. These include the inhibition of the formation of premature fibril formation; a helper role in the assembly of pro-α chains and fibrils; and, following their cleavage from the procollagen molecule, action as a feedback control mechanism for the synthesis of new collagen [7].

Hydroxylation of proline and lysine commences at the amino-terminal end, as the pro-α chain enters the cisternae of the endoplasmic reticulum, and continues along the polypeptide. The hydroxylation of these amino acids requires specific enzymes and the presence of ferrous ions, ascorbic acid, α-keto-

Table 1 Summary of Types, Molecular Structure, and Distinguishing Characteristics of Lung Collagen

Type	Distribution in lung	Molecular structure	Characteristics	Cell responsible for synthesis
I	Bronchi Blood vessels Interstitium	$[\alpha 1(I)]_2\alpha 2$	High tensile strength; low content of hydroxylysine	Fibroblast type I epithelial
II	Cartilagenous tissue Trachea, Bronchi	$[\alpha 1(II)]_3$	No prominent fibrils, associated with proteoglycans, high content of hydroxylysine	Chondrocytes
III	Interstitium	$[\alpha 1(III)]_3$	High content of hydroxyproline Contains cysteine Extremely insoluble due to disulfide bonds	Fibroblast type I epithelial
IV	Basement membrane	$[\alpha 1(IV)]_3$	High content of hydroxylysine Contains cysteine Large amount of carbohydrate residues 3-Hydroxyproline	Epithelial Endothelial
V	Basement membrane	$\alpha A \alpha B$	Similar to type IV	Epithelial Endothelial

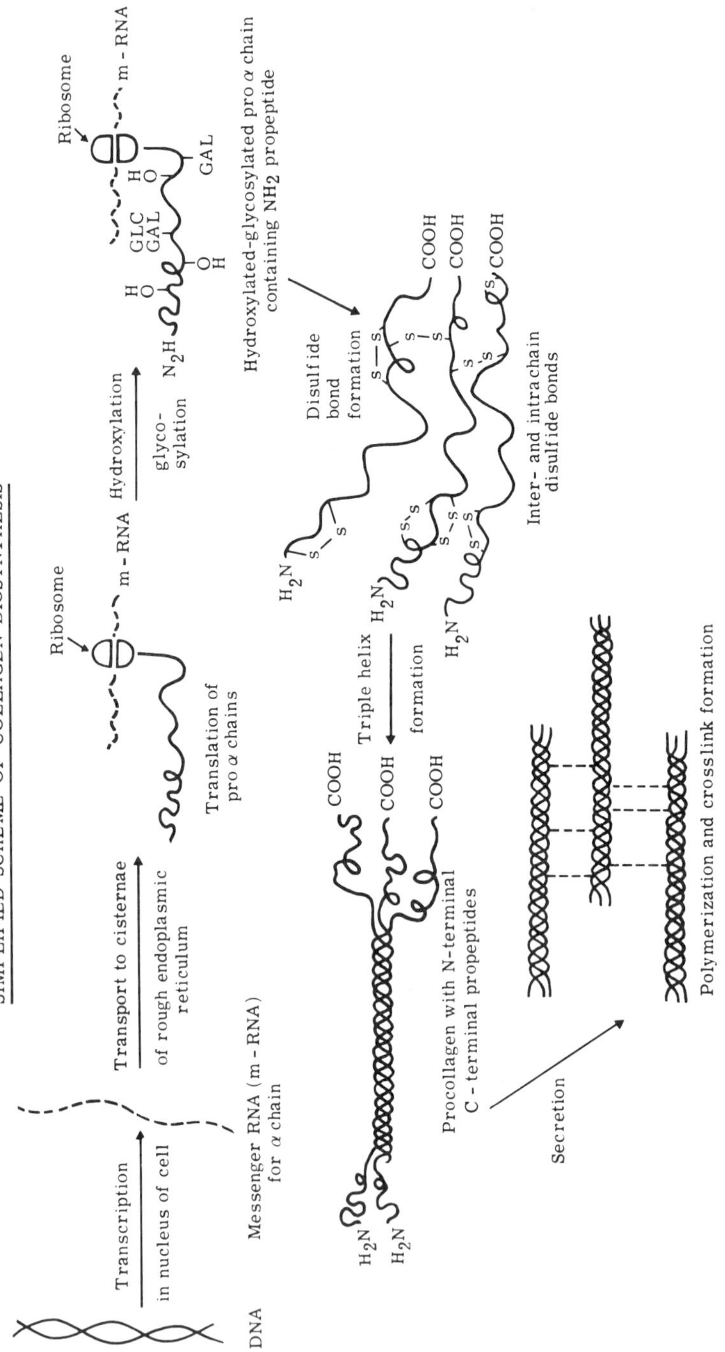

Figure 2 Simplified scheme of collagen biosynthesis.

glutarate, and oxygen as cofactors in the reaction. These enzymes, prolylhydroxylase and lysylhydroxylase, have been the subject of considerable study, and many details of the requirements for their activity are known [8,9]. They exert an important intracellular control on the rate of collagen biosynthesis, although it is not known whether they do so together or by independent mechanisms [10]. Hydroxylation of proline is essential for the formation of a stable triple helix. The levels of these enzymes have been observed to change in disease. A 3- to 10-fold increase in prolylhydroxylase has been noted in experimental fibrosis and granulomas [7].

In anoxic states the incorporation of amino acids into α chains is unaltered, but the amount of hydroxylated procollagen is reduced [7]. The hydroxylation of this procollagen can be completed when the required oxygen tension for hydroxylation enzyme activity is reached.

Deficiency of vitamin C (ascorbic acid) as occurs in scurvy also results in reduced hydroxylation of α chains and procollagen, and ultimately in the cessation of procollagen synthesis, explaining the deficiency of fibrillar collagen in this disease [7].

Glycosylation is the next posttranslational step and takes place within the cisternae of the rough endoplasmic reticulum. This involves the addition of galactose and glucose to the hydroxylysine residues. This too requires specific enzymes, and will only occur prior to triple-helix formation.

The formation of the triple helix requires the establishment of disulfide bonds within and between the peptide extensions of the three pro-α chains, the presence of hydroxyproline within the chains, and the correct association of the latter.

Secretion

Control of the rate of procollagen secretion is dependent on the formation of triple-helical procollagen. If this process is prevented by arresting hydroxylation or disulfide bond formation, the synthesis of pro-α chains continues for a short time and then slows while the accumulated pro-α chains are secreted slowly as a nonhelical functionless protein.

Tropocollagen and Microfibril Formation

In the extracellular space, specific proteases cleave the amino- and carboxyl-terminal groups of the procollagen molecule, forming tropocollagen. Molecules of tropocollagen have the propensity to associate to form microfibrils provided that the extracellular milieu is suitable. Such microfibrils are in the form of a left-handed superhelix, comprising five molecules of tropocollagen, each overlapping its nearest neighbor by 234 amino acid residues. Microfibrils are microscopically indistinguishable from those of mature fibers, but they lack tensile strength which is achieved by stabilizing covalent crosslinks within and between tropocollagen molecules.

Degradation

It has been shown by Bradley et al. [11] that there is continuous synthesis of collagen in the normal adult rabbit lung, yet the net concentration of collagen does not change. Therefore, degradation of collagen must occur. Compared with other proteins, collagen has a relatively low rate of turnover, possibly because the triple-helical form is extremely resistant to proteolytic enzyme degradation at physiological pH.

Four enzymes of the neutral proteinase class are capable of degrading the triple-helical structure of collagen: bacterial collagenase, vertebrate collagenase, cathepsin B1, and collagenolytic cathepsin [12]. Vertebrate collagenase cleaves collagen at a glycine-leucine or glycine-isoleucine bond, situated one-quarter the length of the molecule from the C-terminal portion [12]. This yields two helical fragments, an N-terminal TC^A fragment, and a smaller C-terminal TC^B fragment, which unlike their parent tropocollagen are denatured under physiological conditions.

Catabolism of collagen can be considered to occur in three separate stages. First, the fibroblast is capable of controlling the amount of collagen that leaves the cell. This is achieved by rapid degradation of newly synthesized pro-α chains within the fibroblast.

Since these have a nonhelical configuration, they are a suitable substrate for a variety of lysosomal enzymes which reduce them to small peptides or amino acids. This mechanism is of interest because the rapid degradation is of sufficient order to influence the total quantity of collagen in an organ as it involves a large proportion of collagen synthesized [13], and because intracellular degradation is not a usual mechanism for the regulation of quantity of proteins with extracellular functions.

Second, the extracellular catabolism of collagen can take two forms. Helical tropocollagen molecules are split by collagenases as described above. Insoluble fibrils, composed of multiple crosslinked tropocollagen molecules, are split into fibril fragments (TC^A and TC^B linked by intermolecular crosslinks) by collagenase. This collagenase activity on intact fibers occurs when the enzyme is secreted on the fiber by macrophages, polymorphonuclear leukocytes, and even bacteria.

Several factors have an influence on collagen degradation.

1. Conditions which stimulate the production and release of collagenase. For example, mechanisms have been described in vitro whereby inflammatory cells (macrophages and lymphocytes) can be induced to release soluble factors which stimulate production and release of collagenase from PMN and macrophages [14]. The observation that total hydroxyproline in guinea pig lungs falls during the early phase of a chronic inflammatory response suggests that this mode of increase

Table 2 Collagen Content of Lungs from SPF Guinea Pigs Treated With *M. tuberculosis* or Asbestos[a]

Time (weeks)	Control	*M. tuberculosis*[b]	Asbestos[c]
2	19.43 ± 1.58	6.08 ± 0.30	6.68 ± 0.23
4	30.38 ± 4.35	8.03 ± 0.68	11.70 ± 2.40
6	27.76 ± 3.46	17.48 ± 4.35	25.72 ± 3.68

[a]Collagen was determined by measuring the hydroxyproline content of acid-extractable autoclavable collagen. Hydroxyproline values were multiplied by 7.5 for conversion to collagen. The values represent the mean and standard deviation of three lungs for each group at each time point and are expressed in milligrams.
[b]A 0.1 ml dose of a suspension of 1.0 x 10^7 viable organisms per milliliter (strain H37Ra) was injected subcutaneously in both right and left inguinal regions.
[c]Animals inhaled chrysotile A (UICC reference sample) for two 8-hr periods. The asbestos concentration was approximately 5000 fibers per ml^3 of air.

of collagenase may occur in vivo (Table 2) (R. J. Emerson, unpublished data, 1979).

2. Conditions which reduce the local concentration or compete for the binding sites on serum inhibitors. Serum α_2-macroglobulin is the major inhibitor for almost all known proteases acting at a neutral pH, and blocks nearly all animal collagenases by an almost irreversible binding under physiological conditions [15].
3. The susceptibility of collagen to collagenase degradation has been shown to be influenced by its anatomic location, the age of the tissue, its degree of crosslinkage, and the tissue complexity. The latter refers to the effects of ground-substance components such as proteoglycans which, by their close association with collagen fibers, may reduce the rate of collagenolysis [12]. As a result of this, factors and enzymes unrelated to collagenase (e.g., hyaluronidases), which regulate the rates and types of proteoglycan accumulation, will also influence collagen degradation. In addition, rates of collagenolysis depend upon collagen type, types I, II, and III being degraded at markedly different rates by collagenases [12].
4. Higher tissue temperature such as occurs in inflammation also increases the rate of collagenolysis [12].

In the third stage of collagen catabolism the TC^A, TC^B, and fibril fragments produced by collagenase activity are phagocytosed by the macrophage and digested in its phagolysosome by the action of collagenolytic cathepsins (which act at acid pH), such as cathepsin B^1 and other proteolytic enzymes.

The study of collagen at the molecular level following insults which lead to fibrosis is only beginning. The effects of insult on types of collagen produced, changes in rates of synthesis and degradation, and possible alteration in the structure of the molecule require further investigation.

Measurement

Histochemical Staining Histochemical staining of tissue sections is a rapid and simple screening method for studying collagen. It gives only an approximate indication of quantity and cannot distinguish specific collagen types. Several connective tissue stains have been described, and each has its own sensitivity and specificity for connective tissue components. The basis for the tissue affinity of each is often an ill-understood physicochemical reaction. These methods are fully described in such texts as that of Pearse [16]. However, a few points are particularly pertinent to the study of fibrosis. The methods in common usage are Weigert van Gieson's (and other modifications of the resorcinol-fuchsin technique useful in distinguishing collagen from elastic fibers and other tissue constituents), Masson's trichrome, Gomori's aldehyde-fuchsin trichrome, and silver impregnation methods. As a general principle none of these detects all the collagen present in a tissue when compared with collagen immunofluorescence and electron microscopy, and this can result in an underestimation of collagen, particularly in the early stages in experimental models. The silver impregnation method is most useful in the latter circumstance as it appears to have a particular affinity for newly formed "immature" collagen. None of these methods stains collagen alone. Thus, Masson's trichrome is useful for detection of early fibrosis because of its sensitivity, but also stains other free proteins such as cell debris and inflammatory exudate. Finally, little is known of the changes in staining affinity of collagen which occur in disease.

"Reticulin" is a histopathological term applied to fibers of connective tissue which are argyrophilic (i.e., stain black with silver impregnation), usually appear delicate and branching, stain only faintly red with van Gieson's stain, and are isotropic under polarized light [16]. It is sometimes implied that reticulin is noncollagenous but, while this might be true in respect of its histologic and staining characteristics, biochemically and on electron microscopy it appears to be collagen [17]. However, there are extractable components of reticulin which are noncollagenous [18] but their exact nature has not been determined. Some fibers adopt the staining characteristics of collagen after a time, possibly because of maturation. Until this occurs, however, an increase of argyrophilic fibers may be the only light microscope feature of developing fibrosis.

Electron Microscopy Electron microscopy (EM) is particularly useful in the study of collagen in fibrogenesis because it provides specific identification of collagen fibers. These are recognized by their cross striations at 67 nm intervals, a feature found in fibrils with a diameter of over 20 nm but not in fibrils less than 10 nm in diameter. Specific types of collagen can also be distinguished but only when EM is combined with ferritin-labeled anticollagen antibodies [19]. Transmission EM allows definition of the packing of collagen polymers into fibers, as well as fibroblast morphology, but scanning electron microscopy is required to define the three-dimensional structure and spatial relationships of the various components in the tissue.

Immunofluorescent Identification While biochemical analysis allows *quantitation of the relative proportions* of the different collagen types within a tissue sample, the relative amounts obtained with different extraction methods may not be uniform, and total extraction is never achieved. Furthermore, in most tissues localization is not possible except in structures with fairly uniform anatomic composition such as intervertebral disk or articular cartilage.

With advances in isolation and purification of different types of collagen and procollagen, and their precise immunochemical characterization, it has been possible to produce in animals type-specific antibodies to these molecules. Following immunoabsorption on purified immobilized antigen (or similar methods) these antibodies may be sufficiently specific for use in indirect immunofluorescent studies of human or animal tissues [20]. The antibodies have partial species specificity, but if used in higher concentration antibodies to bovine collagen can detect human collagen. The immunohistochemical method has advantages over biochemical analysis. It is considerably more sensitive and therefore allows precise *anatomic localization* of even fine fibers of collagen within tissues, which are well outside the range of biochemical detection.

Useful information relevant to fibrogenesis has been obtained from immunohistochemical localization of collagen types.

Age-related changes in types of collagen occur in human skin, the ratio of type III to type I decreasing with age. These changes have been confirmed using immunofluorescent techniques by Nowack et al. [21], who also demonstrated that in both human embryonic and adult tissue the fine network of reticular fibers consists of a mixture of type III collagen and procollagen molecules. The persistence of extracellular type III procollagen into adult life may indicate functional significance. In contrast very little type I procollagen is detectable in normal adults, except in the stratum papillare of skin [20] and the liver capsule [21].

A knowledge of the normal adult collagen and procollagen components of tissues allows detection of changes in disease. For example, Wick et al. [20] studied liver biopsies from patients with liver diseases associated with fibrosis, and was able to assess rate as well as site of collagen synthesis. The increased production of type I procollagen was preceded by a rise in type III procollagen. Scanning fluorescence analysis with computerized evaluation of the results is being tested as a way of quantitating fluorescence in tissue sections [20].

Fibroblasts can in a sense be regarded as a *single cell type* whose product may vary in response to different influences. Using simultaneous double labeling with rhodamine-labeled anti-type I and fluorescein-labeled anti-type III collagen antibodies, Gay et al. [22] showed that human embryonic skin fibroblasts are capable of simultaneous synthesis of both these collagen types. The factors governing the type of collagen synthesized by a particular fibroblast are not known, but Müller et al. [23] showed that chondrocytes in tissue culture could be induced to change from producing type II collagen to type I by changing the culture conditions.

"Invading" fibroblasts synthesize type III collagen *in the early stages of tissue repair.* This has been observed in human and experimentally induced liver cirrhosis [20], in wound healing in children, and in early atherosclerotic intimal fibrosis. This increase in type III collagen might have functional relevance because type I and type III collagen, besides having different structural properties, also have different biochemical properties. Type III collagen is a more potent inducer of platelet aggregation than type I [24] and has a greater susceptibility to degradation by proteolytic enzymes. The implications of these and other differences between type I and type III collagen have yet to be shown. They suggest, however, that type III collagen may be remodeled, and even totally resorbed, more easily than type I collagen either spontaneously or as a response to treatment.

Studies of collagen types in lung tissues using indirect immunofluorescent techniques have recently been performed by Bateman et al. (unpublished data, 1979). Fetal and adult lung samples were examined for the *normal appearances and distribution* of collagen types. These features were contrasted with appearances in lung specimens from cases of silicosis and cryptogenic fibrosing alveolitis (CFA). In areas of established fibrosis which were relatively acellular and in which collagen fibers were closely packed (e.g., the center of silicotic nodules), type I predominated almost to the exclusion of type III. In sites at which fibroblasts and inflammatory cells were present, indicating the development of new fibrous tissue, a striking increase in the amount of type III collagen was noted. The clinical course and response to treatment of CFA is being correlated (Bateman et al., unpublished data, 1979) with increases in type III collagen in lung biopsy specimens. This more refined technique of collagen localization has yet to be applied to other types of occupational lung fibrosis, but promises to throw more light on fibrogenetic mechanisms.

Biochemical Estimations *Extraction:* Collagen is extracted with a neutral salt solution (e.g., 1.0 M NaCl –50 mM Tris, pH 7.4) or 0.5 M acetic acid and the yield of collagen can be increased by limited proteolytic enzyme digestion with pepsin [25].

Separation: Differential salt precipitation of the extracted collagen is used to separate various collagen types in partially purified form [25].

Analysis: The measurement of *hydroxyproline* quantitates lung collagen. This may be expressed as total collagen per lung or lobe. Alternatively, concentration per unit dry weight, wet weight, or per unit mass of some other lung constituent such as DNA may be used. However, these latter parameters all increase during inflammation, therefore; concentration expressed as such may be misleading [26].

Ion exchange chromatography and polyacrylamide gel electrophoresis are used to characterize the types of collagen extracted, and can also be used to obtain information about the frequency and nature of crosslinks [27]. *Cyanogen bromide* cleaves extracted collagen at predictable sites, and the resulting peptides can be characterized further by one of the above methods [27].

Radioisotopes are useful for determining the rates of collagen and non-collagen protein synthesis. The majority of studies have used pulse labeling techniques, which are subject to error because of reutilization of isotope [28]. Therefore, it is possible that these studies have underestimated the true rates of turnover. A recent method employing a continuous infusion of radioisotope over a fixed period of time may allow more accurate measurement of the in vivo rate of collagen synthesis [28].

Lung explant cultures, perfused lungs, fibroblast cultures, and cell-free systems are useful for in vitro analysis of collagen turnover. The advantages and disadvantages of these methods have recently been reviewed by Hance and Crystal [6].

B. Elastic Fibers

Elastic fiber [29] is the term applied to a mixture of two biochemically distinct connective tissue elements, microfibrils and elastin, which were once thought to have a precursor-product relationship. Several differences between the composition and properties of these constituents have been defined [29]. Elastin has an amorphous appearance at the limits of electron microscope resolution, whereas the microfibril is composed of tubular fibrils 10–12 nm in diameter. Elastin stains with anionic stains (e.g., phosphotungstic acid), are rich in nonpolar amino acids (alanine, valine, leucine, and isoleucine), contain no cysteine or methionine, but possess small amounts of hydroxyproline and crosslinks of desmosine, isodesmosine, and lysinonorleucine. Elastin is derived from tropoelastin which is synthesized in fibroblasts and smooth muscle cells. In contrast, the microfibril [29] stains with cationic stains (e.g., uranyl acetate or lead citrate), is rich in polar amino acids (e.g., aspartic and glutamic acids), contains cysteine and methionine but no hydroxyproline or crosslinks. The susceptibility of microfibrils to a variety of proteolytic enzymes, including trypsin, chymotrypsin, and pepsin, contrasts with the resistance of elastin to all except elastase [29]. Hydroxylysine is absent from both components, which distinguishes them from collagen. The ratio of amorphous to microfibrillar components in tissues increases with age and, whereas mature elastin has a very slow turnover rate, newly synthesized elastin can be degraded more rapidly.

Elastin, like rubber, has a low Young's modulus and is highly extensible, but has low tensile strength compared with collagen. The significance of these properties to lung mechanics is obvious. Most methods used for quantitation of elastic fibers are based on their relative insolubility. Uncrosslinked tropoelastin is more soluble, however, and some is lost during extraction.

Changes in elastin content of tissues which occur in the course of disease have been little studied, but its concentration, like that of proteoglycans and collagen, has been shown to increase in some animal models of pulmonary fibrosis [30].

C. Proteoglycans

Proteoglycans [31] form part of the amorphous matrix (ground substance) of the interstitial spaces of the lung. Seven types of proteoglycans have been described, and all comprise a protein linked covalently to glycosaminoglycan (GAG), a complex polysaccharide. The proteoglycans include hyaluronic acid, chondroitin sulfate, heparin, heparan sulfate, and keratan sulfate. The last of these is confined to cartilage of the tracheobronchial tree and heparin is found in mast cells, but the remainder occur in the interstitial space. No stains are specific for GAG but it may be demonstrated by the periodic acid-Schiff reaction and toluidine blue for light microscopy, and by ruthenium red for electron microscopy. Fibroblasts, endothelial cells, chondrocytes, and possibly epithelial cells synthesize GAG [31]. Proteoglycans may have an important influence on rate of collagen degradation, but their other functions in the lung in health and disease are not understood.

III. Mechanisms and Methods In Vitro

As is evident from Fig. 1, there are many recognized interactions between agents and different cells which can result in fibrosis. To understand these mechanisms a knowledge of the biological characteristics of both agent and cell types is required, but such detail is beyond the scope of this chapter. Instead we have selected examples from the many in vitro test systems available in order to demonstrate aspects of these mechanisms, and where possible the etiological agents which trigger these events are mentioned.

A. Agent-Fibroblast Direct Interactions

Most mechanisms described involve the mediation of cells such as mononuclear cells or lymphocytes for fibroblast stimulation. However, direct contact between inhaled mineral dust and fibroblasts in the interstitial tissues does occur and studies have been performed in vitro to assess the results of such interactions.

Richards and associates have performed several such experiments [32-34]. It has been shown that lung fibroblasts cultured in vitro and exposed to coal, glass, and quartz did not stimulate collagen production, whereas UICC Rhodesian chrysotile asbestos did [32]. Further studies in vitro have shown that chrysotile asbestos induces changes in fibroblast morphology [35] and biochemistry, including an alteration in the ratio of hyaluronic acid to chondroitin sulfate in the culture medium, and the alteration in the pattern of protein production associated with cell growth [33]. All commercial preparations of asbestos were shown to have these effects on fibroblast collagen production to varying degrees, chrysotile producing the greatest "biological reactivity" in cultures, followed by anthophyllite, then amosite and crocidolite [32]. A similar order of reactivity was found by Harington et al. [36] and Desai et al. [37] in tests of asbestos-induced hemolysis. However, when the dose of asbestos is increased above a critical level (50 μg/ml culture medium), the stimulation is replaced by a depression of collagen levels [34]. Finally, when lung fibroblasts were exposed to small quantities of chrysotile asbestos during 37 passages in vitro, a situation thought to be closer to in vivo events, considerable enhancement of their capacity to synthesize and/or deposit collagen is observed [38].

Properties of Fibroblasts

Increasingly, fibroblasts are recognized as having other biological activities besides their main function of collagen synthesis. Appreciation of these other properties is necessary to understand their interactions with other cells, and their role in the "last step" of inflammatory reactions—accumulation of fibroblasts and the elaboration of collagen and proteoglycans. *Fibroblasts are motile* and migrate in vivo and in vitro under the influence of chemotactic factors [39]. In vitro assays to quantitate fibroblast chemotaxis have been devised, and at least three different factors which are chemotactic for fibroblasts have been described.

1. A 22,000 MW protein released from antigen- or mitogen-stimulated T lymphocytes, called lymphocyte-derived chemotactic factor for fibro-

blasts (LDCFF) [40], which has different molecular characteristics from other known lymphokines, which may play a role in fibrogenesis.

2. Human dermal fibroblasts are strongly attracted by types I, II, and III collagen, peptides from degraded collagen (including α chains and small peptides split off by bacterial collagenase), and synthetic tripeptides and dipeptides [41]. In the course of inflammation when new collagen is being laid down, these products are generated and could be expected to provide chemotactic stimulus for fibroblasts from surrounding tissues.
3. A fragment from the fifth component of the complement system, which is generated by activation of the classic and alternative pathways, has been shown to be chemotactic for fibroblasts [41]. C5a is the most potent complement-derived peptide for neutrophil and monocyte chemotaxis, but the fibroblast chemotactic fragment is larger and thus distinct. On this basis, since many events in the inflammatory response to inhaled occupational dusts are capable of activating the complement system, some degree of fibroblast chemotaxis is likely to ensue.

It has not been determined whether these fibroblast chemotactic factors derived from lymphocytes, collagen degradation, and complement are also capable of stimulating fibroblasts to secrete collagen and proteoglycans, but there are several other mechanisms by which newly arrived fibroblasts might be stimulated. These will be described in the sections which follow.

A second property of the fibroblast is its *phagocytic function* [42]. Endocytosis of collagen fragments by human gingival fibroblasts has been observed in vitro [42]. This implicates the fibroblast in the process of collagen resorption and remodeling which occurs in both normal and pathological states, and also provides a mechanism whereby the fibroblast, by producing collagen degradation products, can generate chemotactic fragments. That the fibroblast is able to degrade collagen intracellularly is known from the work of Bienkowski et al. [13], who demonstrated intracellular degradation of newly synthesized collagen by fibroblasts in culture. In rabbit lung explants, 30–40% of newly synthesized collagen is degraded within minutes of its synthesis [43]. This method of collagen breakdown is probably of less importance than the extracellular varieties which have already been discussed.

B. Agent-Macrophage-Fibroblast Interactions

Silica-Induced Fibrosis

This is the principal mechanism by which silica is thought to exert its fibrogenicity, and it has been the subject of extensive research. Early theories of the action of silica included the "solubility theory" postulated by Kettle [44]. It was considered that free silica, which gradually passed into solution in tissue fluids, produced silicic acid which was the fibrogenic agent. This theory was discarded when it became clear that the fibrogenetic potential of different forms of free silica bore little relationship to differences in solubility [45], and when Curran and Rowsell [46] demonstrated that silica, enclosed in a semipermeable diffusion chamber implanted in the peritoneal cavity of mice, did not result in fibrosis—in spite of the fact that silicic acid was able to diffuse freely out of the chamber. This finding lent support to the theories that a silica-cell interaction was required for the fibrogenetic effect to occur. Current concepts of silica fibrogenicity have arisen from a better understanding of the interaction of silica with the macrophage, information mainly derived from in vitro experiments.

Properties of Silica Silica (silicon dioxide) occurs in several forms, but the main crystalline varieties, quartz, tridymite, and cristobalite, are all highly cytotoxic to macrophages in culture and fibrogenetic in experimental animals [47]. Stishovite is the exception as it is neither cytotoxic to macrophages in vitro nor fibrogenetic in animals [45]. The others increase in fibrogenicity and cytotoxicity from quartz glass (vitreous silica) through quartz and cristobalite to tridymite [48]. A basic difference between stishovite and the other crystalline types is its octahedral structural form. It appears that the tetrahedral form, as in the other types, is necessary for the fibrogenetic activity of silica [49].

Effects of Silica on Cell Membranes Silica particles have been shown to have two types of cytotoxic effects on macrophages. A *rapid cytotoxicity*, which is produced by relatively large amounts of silica added to a serum-free culture, and a delayed cytotoxicity observed in serum-containing macrophage cultures using moderate doses of silica [48]. Both varieties result from the interaction of the particles with membranes. Early cytotoxicity occurs when silica interacts with the plasma membrane, resulting in increase in permeability, release of both lysosomal and cytoplasmic enzymes into the medium, and signs of cell death within an hour of exposure to silica. This is the same mechanism by which silica produces hemolysis, and can be inhibited by coating the silica particles with phosphatidylcholine or protein, or by the presence of poly-2-vinylpyridine-1-oxide (PVPNO) [48].

Delayed silica cytotoxicity occurs 2-6 hr after the particles coated with protein are ingested by the macrophage. Lysosomes surround the phagosome containing silica, fuse with it, and release their enzymes into it [47]. These digest away the protein coat, exposing the silica surface, which can then interact with the lysosomal membrane. Increased permeability of the lysosomal membrane ensues and lysosomal enzymes leak into the cytoplasm, as has been shown by histochemical stains [47]. The liberation of lysosomal enzymes results in cell death and disintegration, and the silica is released. The particles are then reingested by other macrophages and the process may be repeated many times. This variety of cytotoxicity can also be greatly reduced by poly-2-vinylpyridine-1-oxide, if the polymer is given at approximately the same time as the silica. The macrophages phagocytose both silica and polymer, and when the protein coat is digested the silica becomes coated by the nondegradable polymer within the secondary lysosome [47].

A more comprehensive review of the mechanisms by which silica damages cell membranes has recently been published [48]. Additional information has come from the work of Depassé [50] who demonstrated an interaction of the $-N(CH_3)_3{}^+$ groups of membranes and the surface of silica, and from that of Gabor et al. [51] who presented support for the lipoperoxidase hypothesis of silica effect on cell membranes. According to the latter theory silica enhances lipid peroxidation in cell membranes, and macrophages isolated from quartz-treated guinea pigs show higher levels of peroxides. In an extension of this study it was found that α-tocopherol (vitamin E) treatment of experimental animals receiving quartz significantly moderated the fibrotic response. This was associated with a parallel decrease of lipid peroxides and hydroxyproline in the lungs. This protective effect was thought to be due to the antioxidant effect of α-tocopherol.

Theory of Silica-Induced Fibrogenesis The interaction of silica and macrophages forms the first essential part of the "two-stage" theory of silica-induced fibrogenesis suggested by Allison et al. [47] in which silica affects the macrophage in such a way that a factor or factors are released which stimulate collagen biosynthesis by fibroblasts.

Several lines of evidence have been put foward to support this theory, but it has proved difficult to isolate the macrophage factor(s) which stimulates fibroblasts. Some support for the two-stage theory came from the work of Allison et al. [52] in experiments using diffusion chambers limited by Millipore filters implanted in mouse peritoneum. These experiments have not been published in full, but their observations included the following: unstimulated mouse peritoneal cells alone, or silica alone, within the chamber, produced only a "slight reaction" which was no different from that elicited by chambers containing saline solution. By contrast, the combination of small amounts of silica and peritoneal cells produced fibrosis of parietal and visceral peritoneum. Larger amounts ($> 50\ \mu g$) of silica which resulted in cell death of most of the macrophages in the chamber produced a lesser reaction.

Bateman and colleagues [53], using modified diffusion chambers limited by Nuclepore membrane of pore diameter 0.05 μm, have obtained significantly different results. The smaller pore size was used to prevent the escape from the chamber of the particulate Dorentrup No. 12 quartz used in these experiments, and to prevent cell contact by cytoplasmic processes through the membrane filter pores. Sizing of this grade of quartz was performed by Griffiths and colleagues (personal communication, 1979) using electron microscopy, and whereas more than 75% of particles were less than 0.8 μm in diameter (the pore size used in Allison's experiments) only 10.7% were less than 0.2 μm. Direct cell contact was shown to be absent by electron microscopy, and this confirmed the findings of others [54]. The opposite has been observed with Millipore nitrocellulose membranes which, because of their spongy three-dimensional structure, permit cytoplasmic ingrowths and direct contact through the membrane. The exclusion of this cell contact is important when confirmation of diffusible macrophage products or factors is sought. Using this modified diffusion chamber three observations were made:

1. Silica alone in the chamber produced no significant fibrosis.
2. Unstimulated mouse peritoneal macrophages alone caused a mild but significant fibrotic response on the outer surface of the diffusion chamber filter.
3. The combination of silica and peritoneal macrophages failed to produce fibrosis over a range of silica from 20 μg per 10^6 macrophages to as little as 5 μg per 10^6 macrophages. The presence of lymphocytes did not appear to influence this result. The reason for this result is the rapid cytotoxic effect of silica even at this low concentration, such that insufficient numbers of macrophages survive for long enough to produce fibrogenetic factor(s) in sufficient amounts, and for adequate duration, to produce fibrosis. This was confirmed by very low viable cell counts at 2 weeks compared with identical experiments performed with asbestos where fibrosis was produced and viable cell counts of up to 25% were observed at this time point.

These results highlight the difference between silica and asbestos. There is no definite evidence that their fibrogenetic effect is exerted via the same fibrogenetic factor(s), but neither is there reason to suspect a difference. However, asbestos is less cytotoxic for macrophages and its presence can be tolerated for longer, thus allowing a more prolonged stimulation of the macrophage, which in turn can produce or release fibrogenetic factor(s) for a longer period. Unlike the situation in vivo, the diffusion chamber has a nonreplaceable pool of macrophages, so any fibrosis observed is the result of fiber interactions with only one generation of macrophages. Silica, therefore, appears to require a large continuous recruitment of macrophages for its effect [55]. In addition, the fibrosis produced in this model by asbestos was maximal at 2-4 weeks and then resolved completely over the next 2 months, suggesting that a sustained production of fibrogenetic factor(s) is required for chronic and progressive fibrosis. This is achieved in vivo, as silica and asbestos are able to react with successive generations of macrophages over many years.

Investigation of Macrophage Fibrogenetic Factor(s) Another direction which investigation of fibrogenetic factor(s) from macrophages has taken arose from the work of Heppleston and Styles [56] who observed that homogenates of rat peritoneal macrophages which had ingested silica were able to increase collagen biosynthesis in chick tibia fibroblast cultures. Many similar experiments have been performed by the same authors and by other workers [55,57,58], but interpretation of some of the results has been difficult. Apparently conflicting results may be due to the inherent problems of in vitro systems and the many nonspecific factors which can influence collagen biosynthesis in fibroblast cultures [52,57]. In addition, the choice of species from which effector and target cells were obtained may explain some differences. Burrell and Anderson [58], using rabbit alveolar macrophage and human fibroblasts, achieved similar results to Heppleston and Styles, whereas Harington et al. [57] showed an inhibitory effect of suspensions of hamster macrophage extracts on collagen synthesis in hamster fibroblast cultures.

Aalto et al. [59] have extended this area of research by employing a variety of target fibroblast systems and by fractionating silica-treated macrophages, and medium from macrophage cultures, to isolate macrophage fibrogenetic factor(s). The fibroblast systems include:

1. Granulation tissue slices which contain cells in their natural environment, but which have problems of restricted access for substances in the medium and a limited cell life.
2. Fibroblasts cultured from granulation slices which are thought to represent cells involved in the repair process, with all the synthetic activity that this involves.
3. Preparations of polysomes isolated from granulation tissue which are capable of protein synthesis. Polysome preparations have the disadvantage of greater variability than do the first two systems.

In experiments involving fractionation of the homogenate of silica-stimulated macrophages by differential centrifugation, these workers were able to demonstrate that the active fraction resided in the 20,000 *g* supernatant. Furthermore, the 7000/500 *g* sediment of the homogenate from normal macrophages could be induced to produce a stimulatory factor by incubating it with silica, and this factor could then be separated by repeat centrifugation, when it appeared in the 20,000 *g* supernatant. Isolated in this way it stimulated collagen synthesis in tissue slices, as measured by ratio of radiolabeled proline to hydroxyproline incorporated into protein, as well as some DNA synthesis [59].

Since the majority of lysosomes are disrupted during the process of freezing and thawing involved in the cell fractionation the macrophage factor was thought not to be liberated hydrolytic enzyme. Another macrophage factor, found in the 100,000 *g* supernatant of homogenate derived from the cytosol fraction, was of interest because it caused a depression of collagen synthesis in tissue slices.

The medium from macrophage cultures has more recently been found to be a "cleaner" source of the stimulatory silica macrophage factor, as is also the medium from human peripheral blood monocytes and malignant histiocytes cultured in the presence of silica [59]. Repeated gel filtration chromatography of this medium yielded a homogeneous protein of 14,300 MW which increased the incorporation of tritiated proline and tritiated thymidine into cultured granuloma cells [59]. The effect of silica on the macrophage is thought by these authors to involve a reduction of macrophage ribonuclease (RNase) activity [60]. This effect is the opposite of its influence on most other hydrolytic enzymes during the process of macrophage stimulation. It is of interest that a similar decrease in acid ribonuclease occurs during phytohemagglutinin (PHA) stimulation of lymphocytes, when RNA accumulates [61]. This macrophage RNA could be the fibroblast stimulating factor, which stabilizes polysomes of fibroblasts and increases collagen and noncollagen protein synthesis, including DNA [60].

Further support for these theories was obtained in granulomas produced by sponge containing silica particles and macrophages. Decrease in RNase activity in the developing granulation tissue, and increase in the number of polysomes and in collagen synthesis occurred [62]. The exact relationships and relative importance of the RNase changes, nucleic acid production, and collagen synthesis have yet to be determined, and the answers to these questions will probably be relevant to understanding fibrogenesis induced by other agents.

Macrophage Replenishment All the fibrogenetic mechanisms discussed have stressed the necessity of continuous local replacement of macrophages. Heppleston [55] has studied the mechanism of macrophage replenishment in silica-treated experimental animals, and has put forward the view that this process depends on stimulation of the marrow by a lipid component, probably derived from type II alveolar cells or from silica-bearing macrophages, or both. In support of this theory, lipids of cellular and bacterial origin have been shown to cause increased alveolar macrophage migration [63] and phagocytosis (as measured by clearance of an intravenously administered carbon suspension) [64]. Heppleston [55] examined the kinetics of the rat mononuclear phagocytic system (MPS) by injecting radiolabeled thymidine in vivo, and examining cell suspensions of marrow from these animals. The assessment of phagocytic ability and cell size thus obtained allowed identification of promonocytes and monocytes. It was shown that the intravenous (IV) administration of the lipid fraction of lungs with silica-induced lipoproteinosis, greatly reduced the cell cycle time of the promonocytes, suggesting an augmented proliferation. On the basis of separate experiments in mice [55], comparing cell kinetics of interstitial monocytes from areas of lung containing silica with those from parts which did not, decreased mitotic activity was found in the silica-containing parts and this was considered to be the result of too rapid a migration of these cells into alveoli for cell division to occur. It was concluded that the local response to silica is an acceleration of monocyte emigration from blood vessels to alveoli rather than local proliferation, and therefore that the more important source of incoming macrophages is the bone marrow.

Asbestos-Related Fibrosis

Effect of Asbestos on Cell Membranes The mechanism of interaction of asbestos with cytoplasmic and lysosomal membranes is different from that of silica [34,48] and is thought to be the result of surface magnesium groups on the fibers which interact electrostatically with sialic acid groups on glycoproteins in the membrane. These glycoproteins, which are usually able to migrate within the membrane, are immobilized in the area of contact with the fiber. This aggregation of proteins forms ion-conducting channels which permit the efflux of potassium and influx of sodium ions and water, resulting in osmotic lysis of the cell. This theory is supported by the observation that prior treatment of the cell membranes with neuraminidase, which removes sialic acid residues, or treatment of the asbestos with agents which preferentially chelate magnesium, inhibits hemolysis [36]. There is still some doubt, however, as to whether surface magnesium ions are the correct explanation for the observed effects of asbestos, an alternative being the surface charge (zeta potential) which is the result of several components of the fiber. Dispersion of fiber in water containing surface-active agents such as acid, and coating the fibers with the lung surfactant component dipalmitoyl lecithin, affects this potential. Light and Wei [65] demonstrated a close correlation between the zeta potentials of several asbestos types and their in vitro hemolytic activity. In a third area of research on asbestos-cell membrane interactions, the observation has been made that following asbestos exposure changes in membrane glycolipids and glycoproteins occur [66]. Since these effects are not immediate but occur several hours after exposure to asbestos, they are probably the result of an inhibition of the metabolism of these compounds. The glycolipid changes, which included a decrease in longer and a concomitant increase in shorter glycolipids, were different for the three types of asbestos tested, and correlated with the relative cytotoxicity of the different types.

Asbestos-Macrophage Interaction Allison [48] showed by electron microscopy that small particles of asbestos were phagocytosed by macrophages, and remained in phagocytic vesicles and secondary lysosomes for several hours. Only after one or more days were some fibers seen free within the cytoplasm, presumably as a result of lysosomal membrane lysis. This corresponds to the *delayed cytotoxicity* of silica but is a slower process with asbestos. A much more *rapid cytolysis* occurs if protein is absent from the culture medium, and this early cytotoxicity is greatest in respect of chrysotile and less in respect of amosite and anthophyllite [48]. This form of cytolysis probably has little relevance in vivo. Often fiber shape and size allow only incomplete ingestion by macrophages, and this allows a more prolonged interaction with plasma membranes of one or more cells [48]. Fibers of less than 5 μm are completely ingested, intermediate fibers (5-20 μm) are only occasionally taken up by one macrophage but large fibers (greater than 30 μm) are never totally ingested. Cells may envelop such long fibers at each end, but some of the fiber remains in an extracellular position. Asbestos also differs from silica in that it induces selective release of lysosomal hydrolases without cell death [67]. This enzyme release is dose related in the range of 1-100 μg/ml, commences within 5 hr of exposure [48], and increases for more than 24 hr.

Chrysotile asbestos fibers in microgram amounts have recently also been shown to be capable of activating the alternative pathway of complement in vitro (Saint-Remy, personal communication, 1979) and, since macrophages can synthesize some of the protein components of the complement system, this presents a possible additional mechanism of asbestos-induced fibrogenesis.

Theory of Asbestos-Induced Fibrogenesis The results of experiments with asbestos in diffusion chambers, which have already been mentioned, confirmed that macrophages are required for fibrosis, and provided evidence that asbestos fibrogenicity, like that of silica, operates via a two-stage mechanism. The first is the fiber-macrophage interaction, and the second a macrophage-fibroblast interaction. It is thought that during the first phase prolonged stimulation of macrophages in relation to, or containing, asbestos fibers results in chronic lysosomal enzyme release. At least three ways are recognized whereby the second stage, macrophage-fibroblast interaction, might occur, and two of these involve lysosomal enzymes. These enzymes might have a direct effect on fibroblasts, or fibroblast stimulation might result from products of tissue destruction or mediators released from the inflammatory response. Lysosomal enzymes can cause tissue damage by degrading components of connective tissues, cell membranes, pulmonary surfactant, and proteins of the complement system. In this way other systems become involved which can influence fibroblast activity. Third, it is possible that other macrophage factor(s) like the non-lipid macrophage factor described with silica may be produced in response to asbestos exposure.

In some dust diseases, immunological factors undoubtedly play a part (e.g., berylliosis and silicosis), but evidence in asbestos-induced fibrosis suggests that these contribute no more than a possible adjuvant effect. Evidence for this will be presented in Section IV.B.

C. Antigen-Lymphocyte-Macrophage-Fibroblast Interactions

The lymphocyte plays a key role in the pathogenesis of granulomata, chronic inflammation, and fibrosis which is associated with *delayed hypersensitivity* to an antigen. Stimulation of T lymphocytes results from direct contact with the antigen or from presentation of antigen on macrophage membrane. This results in secretion of lymphokines, and initiates the formation of a hypersensitivity reaction or granuloma at the site of the antigenic stimulus. Lymphocytes migrate into established areas of chronic inflammation. T lymphocytes are present at the height of the granulomatous reaction, while in the chronic stage an equal number of B and T cells are noted [68]. Little is known about the relative proportions of effector, helper, and suppressor T cells, effector and suppressor B cells, and antibody-forming plasma cells at various stages, but they may be critical to the outcome of the reaction. Sensitized T cells secrete migration-inhibiting lymphokines and chemotactic factors which induce differentiation, multiplication, and mobilization of monocytic, myelocytic, and lymphocytic cells from the bone marrow. These cells reach the site of the antigen, and extravasation may occur via the direct effect of the lymphokine on vascular endothelium, or through chemical mediators (e.g., kinins, histamine, prostaglandins, and so on). Incoming macrophages become activated by lymphokines and carry out their functions of phagocytosis and degradation. Increased endocytic activity can result in the release of lysosomal enzymes which enhance chemotaxis, but on the other hand may cause tissue damage. Lymphotoxins have also been described which damage "innocent bystander" cells [69]. Fibroblast cultures, in common with several other cell types, are a source of colony-stimulating factor/macrophage growth factor (CSF/MGF), a sialoglycoprotein of MW 70,000 [70]. This factor stimulates human bone marrow cells to form colonies of granulocytes, mononuclear phagocytes, or mixtures of the two, and also acts on colony-forming cells in other sites, e.g., alveolar spaces and pleural exudates, causing monocyte proliferation [70]. In this way fibroblasts augment the cellular response in fibrosis.

Factors Acting on Fibroblasts

Antigenic stimulation of lymphocytes has been shown to result in the release of lymphokines which cause fibroblasts to proliferate and produce collagen [71].

Cell-free supernatants from nonstimulated lymphocytes do not have this effect [71]. However, Johnson and Ziff [72] in experiments similar to those mentioned above, demonstrated that cell-free culture supernatants from mitogen-stimulated lymphocytes produced a lymphotoxin which inhibits proliferation of W1-38 fibroblasts and causes their death. However, the remaining viable cells show enhanced collagen synthesis. The discrepancies between these experiments may be explained by the different fibroblast lines and different culture conditions employed. Wahl et al. [14] observed that lymphokine treatment of macrophages results in secretion of collagenase-like enzyme. By this means the lymphocyte may play a role in the regulation of collagen resorption.

Autoantibodies to Collagen

The sequence involving lymphocyte and macrophage in fibrogenesis results from stimulation by a specific antigen, e.g., beryllium or organic dust. In certain circumstances host antigens may provoke such reactions. Lewis and Burrell [73] demonstrated that antibodies to lung connective tissue could stimulate macrophages to release a collagen-stimulating factor. The latter caused collagen production from fibroblast cultures. The antibody had no direct effect on collagen synthesis. It is not known whether this mechanism is relevant in vivo, but it is important to note that non-organ-specific autoantibodies to connective tissue antigens have been found in human dust-induced disease.

Kravis et al. [74] provided evidence that cell-mediated hypersensitivity to collagen occurs in vivo. They demonstrated that circulating T lymphocytes from patients with pulmonary fibrosis, when exposed to type I collagen in vitro, produce macrophage inhibiting factor (MIF) and cell-mediated lysis of collagen-coated sheep red blood cells. Evidence of cellular sensitization to collagen has been found in rheumatoid arthritis in humans, and in a model of type II collagen-induced arthritis in animals [75].

D. Agent Inflammation and Tissue Injury

Inflammation is a complex tissue response and includes several elements. These are vasodilatation and increased vessel permeability, the extravasation of serum components, fluid, and cells from blood vessels, the local accumulation of cellular elements, and healing and repair. Once the process is initiated by an agent, the stimulus is augmented and maintained by such chemical mediators as histamine, heparin, serotonin, catecholamines, slow-reacting substance of anaphylaxis (SRS-A), prostaglandins, products of the complement, clotting, and kinin systems, as well as lymphokines. Serum kinins have been shown to be involved in both foreign body and hypersensitivity granulomatous inflammation [76]. Anticoagulants have a strongly suppressive effect on delayed hypersensitivity reactions in skin, indicating that components of the coagulation mechanism are involved in such reactions [77]. Prostaglandin E_1 has been shown to inhibit migration inhibition factor production in vitro by sensitized lymphocytes, and this is of interest as prostaglandin E_1 is produced by activated macrophages [78]. Chemotactic influences are derived from many sources. The triggering of the complement system results in the formation of C5a, a potent chemotactic agent, and occurs in response to antigen-antibody complexes, endotoxin, proteolytic enzyme, and macrophage-derived acid proteases [74]. The activation of the fibrinolytic pathway produces plasminogen activator, and the kinin-generating pathway produces kallikrein, both of which possess chemotactic activity for mononuclear cells. Furthermore, the plasmin generated by plasminogen activator is able to generate chemotactic fragments from the C5 component of complement [80].

Polymorphonuclear leukocytes and macrophages are attracted by substances produced during tissue injury such as fibrin [68] and degraded collagen fragments [81]. Various components of neutrophils are also chemotactic for macrophages, including cationic peptides of lysosomal origin [79], components of neutrophil granules [68], and a neutral proteinase [79].

Liquefaction is a common finding in granulomas, nodules, and conglomerate lesions of dust-induced diseases. Degradative enzymes released from inflammatory cells are probably the most important cause of these changes. The variety of circumstances under which lysosomal enzymes are released from macrophages have already been mentioned. These include cell death, "frustrated phagocytosis" [48], reversed endocytosis, lymphokine, and a variety of other stimuli [82]. Cell death may also occur as a result of lymphotoxins [69]. Other aspects of tissue injury influence healing and fibrosis. Platelets have been shown to release factors which are mitogenic for fibroblasts [83], and injury-associated clotting may activate this mechanism. Macrophages may produce fibrogenetic factors in certain conditions such as silicosis. The inflammatory reaction ensures the presence of large numbers of these cells. When systemic monocytopenia is induced by the administration of hydrocortisone and macrophages are eliminated by simultaneous subcutaneous injection of anti-macrophage serum, a marked retardation of wound healing, debridement, fibroblast proliferation, and scar formation is observed [84].

IV. Mechanisms and Methods In Vivo

A. Animal Studies

It is well established that a variety of agents (Table 3) are capable of causing lung damage in animals which may lead to fibrosis. These agents include inorganic dusts, bacteria, radiation, drugs, toxic chemical, and experimentally contrived

Table 3 Animal Models of Fibrosis

Species	Insult	Reference
Mice	Irradiation	Adamson et al. [85]
Mice	Asbestos	Sahu et al. [86]
Rats	$CdCl_2$	Palmer et al. [87]
Rats	Paraquat	Thurlbeck et al. [88]
Rats	Irradiation	Adamson et al. [85]
Rats	Silica	Heppleston [55]
Rats	Asbestos	Miller and Kagan [89]
Hamsters	Bleomycin	Snider et al. [90]
Hamsters	N-Nitroso-N-methylurethane	Ryan [91]
Guinea pig	Asbestos	Holt et al. [92]
Guinea pig	Asbestos	Wagner [93]
Rabbits	BSA, ConA	Willoughby et al. [94]
Rabbits	Bacteria	Harris et al. [95]
Rabbits	Asbestos	Wagner [93]
Dogs	Irradiation	Pickrell et al. [96]
Monkey	Asbestos	Wagner [93]
Baboons	Bleomycin	McCullough et al. [97]

insults such as prepared immune complexes. Despite the volume of research conducted in animals to determine the effects of these agents, surprisingly little is known of the pathogenetic mechanisms underlying these effects in each case.

There are several advantages in the use of animal models for the analysis of mechanisms by which fibrosis occurs (Table 4). Whole animals are capable of a range of host response which might be relevant to humans. The design of the experiment can be manipulated to allow the mechanism in question to be studied. Of the large number of experiments which have been performed in the past, the majority have attempted to assess the fibrogenicity of agents or to reproduce particular disease entities (e.g., asbestosis or extrinsic allergic alveolitis), and have concentrated on histopathological changes, i.e., the results of rather than the basic mechanisms of fibrogenesis. The assessment of mechanisms requires detailed study with as many techniques as possible at frequent intervals both shortly after the insult, and over the subsequent evolution. Most studies have not done this, the common problems being study of the event too long after the insult, or failure to include sufficient time points. To obtain full advantage of the freedom permitted by animal models the study should include an assessment of dose-response relationships and temporal course, with observation of such parameters as collagen synthesis and degradation, enzyme analysis, immunological events, and changes in the serum complement system.

Availability of the lung as an intact organ allows regional differences in pathology to be studied in their natural setting, and even such details as their

Table 4 Animal Models for the Study of Fibrogenetic Mechanisms

Advantages
Provides complete host response
Manipulation of test system (dose-response, time-response, morphology, *and* function, host response)
Allows assessment of whole lung
Large cell quantities obtainable
Inbred strains–elimination of genetic influence
Influences of drugs
Refinement of techniques
Problems
Interspecies comparisons difficult (including with humans)
Available techniques of analysis too insensitive
Expense

effect on gas exchange and lung mechanics to be assessed [90]. This contrasts with the sampling problem attendant to all human studies.

The large cell numbers obtained from these animals can be used for a greater variety of tests in vitro than is permitted by human samples. By using inbred strains of animals the effect of genetic variability encountered in humans, as a result of their "outbred" status, is overcome. This permits conclusions to be drawn from smaller numbers, and the pooling of cells and tissues from small animals. An obvious further advantage of the animal model is the facility of screening for the effects of drugs on fibrogenesis. Finally, techniques can be refined in animals for future use in humans.

Two important limitations of animal studies are that extrapolation between different species, and particularly between animals and humans, may be invalid; furthermore, although methods are improving, they are still too insensitive to permit detailed analysis of some of the complex interactions in the lung. However, systematic studies of the type described above provide much useful information.

Choice of Animal Species

Success or failure in answering an experimental question may depend on the type of animal chosen, because of species variability in response to any given agent. An example of this is the variety of animal responses to asbestos exposure. Vorwald et al. [98] found that guinea pigs developed pulmonary fibrosis and asbestos bodies, rats developed fibrosis but no asbestos bodies, mice formed asbestos bodies but developed no fibrosis, cats developed mild fibrosis but no asbestos bodies, and rabbits showed no response. Therefore, logically the most suitable animal to use when attempting to mimic human asbestosis would be the guinea pig.

Specific Pathogen-Free (SPF) Status of Animals

It is well known that the lung response to various infective agents may be considerably altered by the prior colonization of the animals with various specific pathogens such as mycoplasma. Although it is difficult to find well-attested evidence of such circumstances unequivocally affecting the outcome of fibrogenetic insults, there is a consensus that they do. However, the problems encountered in maintaining animals in this state for long-term experiments are considerable.

Prior Nonspecific Stimulation of the Immune System

Richerson et al. [99] have shown that repeated intravenous injections of heat-killed BCG into rabbits, previously sensitized with Freund's complete adjuvant (FCA), resulted in interstitial pulmonary fibrosis, whereas animals not so sensitized failed to develop fibrosis. The reaction produced was an accelerated granulomatous response which could not be produced by other soluble or particulate antigen (ovalbumin and keyhole limpet hemocyanin). Moore and colleagues [100] obtained similar results; both studies demonstrated that the lesions progressed for a period but subsequently resolved. In a different experiment, SPF guinea pigs, treated with FCA prior to inhalation of asbestos and then infected with mycobacteria, were protected against the fibrosis which occurred in animals treated with asbestos alone (Emerson, unpublished data, 1979). In this experiment, the greatest amount of collagen, measured as hydroxyproline, was found in animals sensitized with FCA and then challenged with mycobacteria. Animals given FCA or mycobacteria alone showed no evidence of fibrosis. A further example of the protective effect of nonspecific host stimulation was the demonstration by Butler [101] that FCA-treated hamsters were protected against the fibrosis induced by paraquat poisoning.

The opposite effect to prior FCA stimulation was observed in experiments by Göthe and Swensson [102]. Intravenous BCG followed by intratracheal installation of fibrogenic dusts produced lung lesions that were more pronounced than those produced by either treatment alone.

Manipulation of Elements of the Immune System

One way of defining the possible role of various elements of the immune system in fibrogenesis is to selectively abrogate such elements in animals and/or passively restore such elements to animals totally deprived of their immune system. Examples of this procedure are the use of T-lymphocyte depleted, B-lymphocyte depleted, macrophage-depleted, and decomplemented mice.

Drugs

Besides having implications for the treatment of fibrosis [103], drugs provide a potentially important tool for dissecting fibrogenetic mechanisms. Some speci-

Table 5 Drugs Affecting Collagen Metabolism

Drug	Mode of action	Reference
d-Penicillamine	Blocks crosslink formation by binding to aldehydes, and at high concentrations chelates copper, inhibiting lysyl oxidase activity	Nimni [104]
β-Aminoproprionitrile	Blocks crosslink formation by interference with lysyl oxidase preventing aldehyde formation	Jackson [105]
Proline analogs	Incorporated into newly synthesized collagen in place of proline, preventing hydroxylation	Prockop et al. [10]
Heparin	Stimulates collagenase production	Sakamoto et al. [106]
Cycloheximide	Increases prolyl-hydroxylase activity; blocks secretion or synthesis of collagenase; inhibits protein synthesis	Levene et al. [107] Wahl et al. [14]
Colchicine	Prevents assembly of microtubules; increases collagenolysis; inhibits collagen synthesis, procollagen secretion, and conversion of procollagen to collagen	Ehrlich et al. [108]

fically affect biosynthetic pathways and thus influence the quantity or nature of collagen produced, others are cytotoxic and deplete cell populations involved in fibrogenetic pathways, and some alter nucleoproteins controlling protein synthesis. Examples of some of these, and their suggested mode of action, are cited in Table 5.

B. Human Studies

Every mechanism observed by in vitro experimentation or in an animal model requires evaluation and confirmation by human studies to be certain of its practical significance in human fibrosis. Since all nonhuman studies have this limitation, the methods of studying and analyzing the disease process in vivo are being continually improved. An example of a recent important milestone in these techniques is the development of small-volume subsegmental bronchoalveolar lavage which, as will be discussed, can be used to obtain information about several cell types at various stages of the disease.

Animal species differ widely in their susceptibility and pattern of response to the same disease-producing agent and, even in those species in which the histopathological result most closely mimics that in humans, different mechanisms might be operating to produce this disease. In addition, the pattern of human disease always involves important modifications resulting from host factors, both genetically determined and acquired (such as smoking and co-existent infections or disease).

Forms of Human Studies

Human studies can take several forms and each has its own value. These are: clinical epidemiological studies (Chapter 13), study of lung biopsy tissue, study of lung cells, and secretions and serological tests.

Lung Biopsy The principal limitation of human studies is difficulty in obtaining adequate and repeated specimens which represent the pathological process in the lung. At present "open" lung biopsies afford the most useful samples for experimental purposes but these can only be done in a minority of patients when warranted by the clinical indication. Drill biopsy and transbronchial biopsy via fibreoptic bronchoscope are more readily performed and carry less morbidity, but they only provide small specimens of tissue, and these are frequently too distorted for critical research assessment. A further advantage of a biopsy taken at formal thoracotomy is the better sample selection which is possible. The worst affected area is not necessarily the most helpful and a more representative sample should be selected. This has been shown in CFA, and whereas the lingula is frequently the most affected part in this disease, a more representative sample is obtained from the area of lung underlying the third and fourth ribs in the midaxillary line [109].

Histologic assessment of the pathology in tissue specimens remains the cornerstone of descriptive research into disease mechanisms, and efforts have been directed as follows:

Identification of factors involved in the *etiology* of disease and in the *quantitation* of dust exposure (See Chapter 10).

Assessment of the variety of *pathological responses* to a single etiological agent, and the severity of these in relation to the quantity and pattern of dust exposure. For example, asbestos can produce a variety of lesions. From animal studies it is known that an early feature of dust exposure is a desquamative alveolar response. A similar reaction has been observed in humans, and, although the usual pattern of disease is a diffuse interstitial fibrosis, several cases of severe desquamative interstitial pneumonia have also been described [110]. From this it is surmised that different modes of presentation of the dust to the lung, or different host factors, activate alternative pathogenetic mechanisms and produce different diseases [55].

Assessment of the pattern and *cellular constituents* of the inflammatory response gives an indication of the cellular mechanisms involved in the fibrosis, and there is value in contrasting the pattern of response to various agents and correlating them with the in vitro characteristics of the agent. An example of this is the presence of plasma cells within the nodules in Caplan's syndrome which are not seen in the other forms of nodular fibrosis such as silicosis [111]. These cells point to a role for antibodies in this condition.

Histologic grading of lung pathology with scoring of such parameters as severity of organ fibrosis, cellular infiltration, and distortion and disruption of airspaces has been used in some lung diseases (e.g., CFA) in an attempt, not only to assess the stage of the disease, but to gain insight into the mechanisms of lung damage [109,112]. As an extension of this, point scores of differential cell counts in intra-alveolar and interstitial sites have been obtained [112], and in some instances comparisons are possible with cell ratios obtained by broncho-alveolar lavage [109]. These semiquantitative methods have not been used to any extent in the assessment of human occupational disease because of the scarcity of biopsy specimens, particularly in the early phases of the disease.

Electron microscopic examination of the lung exposed to toxic occupational agents is particularly useful for determining early cell injuries and detecting etiological agents in disease (see Chapter 10).

A number of *immunofluorescent techniques* have been used in the study of fibrotic lung disease. Normal lung constituents such as collagen and elastin can be demonstrated and semiquantitated, and abnormal accumulation of these and of serum components, such as immunoglobulins, fibrin, and immune complexes, detected [111,113]. Increases in plasma cells producing particular antibody classes can be defined (e.g., in silicotic nodules) [111].

Cells extracted from lung biopsies can be studied in a variety of ways, although their numbers are small, which limits the use of this method. Immediate extraction of lung cells for differential cell counts, studies of lymphocyte subclasses and of macrophage characteristics and function, have been used in a number of lung disorders. Lung biopsies have been put to three other uses:

1. Lung slices have been used to study collagen and proteoglycan turnover in short-term organ culture [6].
2. Alveolar lining cells (types I and II pneumocytes) have been cultured to study in vitro effects of environmental agents such as hyperoxia, ozone, and metals.
3. Cultures of lung fibroblasts have been extensively studied in various in vitro experiments.

Bronchoalveolar Lavage Cells and Fluid The development of human bronchoalveolar lavage has provided a means of access to some of the cells implicated in the fibrogenic process. The advantages of the method are that it is a relatively simple procedure with low morbidity, which can be repeated on several occasions in the same patient, if indicated, to follow the course of the disease, and it provides viable cells in sufficient quantity to perform a variety of functional tests.

The differential cell counts in the recovered fluid closely correlate with the differential counts seen histologically in the alveolar spaces [114], and with those obtained when the cells are extracted from lung biopsy specimens by teasing them apart [109,114,115]. The latter method provides a combination of intra-alveolar and interstitial cells. Caution is required in interpreting alveolar lavage cell ratios because they do not reflect the ratios in lung interstitium [116]. Davis et al. [116] were unable to demonstrate histologically a clear correlation between the percentage of airspace lymphocytes and the degree of interstitial mononuclear cell infiltration. This was presented as evidence that the presence of lymphocytes is not the result of a simple concentration gradient of cells, but rather due to specific stimuli that attract cells to, or retain them in, the various anatomic compartments.

Furthermore, the technique used during lavage can affect the population of cells obtained. Recent work in animals [117] suggests that the cell yield may depend upon the force with which the fluid is introduced, the number of lavage aliquots used, the total lavage volume introduced, and the presence of additives, e.g., Lignocaine. This raises serious problems in interpretation because different workers may recover and test different admixtures of alveolar cells (possibly also of varying maturity). It also highlights the dangers of extrapolating lavage findings to cellular events in the interstitial compartment, which is probably inaccessible to this procedure.

Details of the technique of bronchoalveolar lavage have recently been described [118]. This method is being used extensively in the study of diffuse interstitial lung disease, particularly CFA. There have been few reports of its use in occupational diseases of the lung, other than the hypersensitivity pneumonias [119,120], although the inorganic dust diseases are currently being studied in several centers. For example, a study comparing the cell proportions in lavage fluids from normal controls and patients with asbestos exposure but no fibrosis were similar, but both differed from those from patients with asbestos-induced pulmonary fibrosis [121]. The latter had an increased percentage of polymorphonuclear leukocytes, of a similar order to that in patients with CFA [121].

The fluid recovered by bronchoalveolar lavage is an additional means of gaining information about lung pathology, since it reflects "secretory" activities of the lung (e.g., enzymes), cell functions such as antibody production, and abnormal events such as inflammation and immune complex formation within the lung [122].

Lavage fluid from patients with asbestosis has been shown in one study to have a higher average concentration of albumin, IgG, IgA, and α_1 antitrypsin than that from persons with asbestos exposure without fibrosis, and normal controls [121]. No difference was found for transferrin, C_3, haptoglobin, IgM, and α_2-macroglobulin [121]. The expression of components measured in lavage fluid as concentration fails to take into account the variations in fluid volume recovered from different patients. Several alternative methods have been suggested but each has its problem [123].

Serological Tests Serum factors, antibodies, and other blood tests have been extensively studied in occupational disease because of the ease with which serial blood samples can be obtained, stored, and tested (Chapter 7).

Patterns of Human Response In general, occupational diseases caused by organic inhaled material are mediated by specific immunological mechanisms, whereas those caused by inorganic or mineral dusts are produced by nonspecific but cell-dependent mechanisms.

Mineral dusts are able to produce four basic types of lesion as a consequence of the deposition of the dust on alveolar walls. These are simple aggregation of dust particles and their adherence to the walls of alveoli of respiratory bronchioles, localized cellular reaction without fibrosis in the peribronchiolar region, localized nodular lesions with collagen accumulation, and diffuse alveolar wall fibrosis.

Although these basic categories of reaction hold true for mineral dusts as a group, it is the individual characteristics of the pathology caused by different agents which give pointers to different mechanisms of fibrogenesis.

Human Response to Selected Agents

Silica-Induced Fibrosis There appears to be no simple relationship between the total amount of dust (measured as total mineral dust or silica at postmortem examination) and the severity, or even the presence, of silicotic nodules in the lung. The reaction must therefore be influenced by a number of individual factors, both genetic and acquired, which act together. Several points which bear on this are mentioned below.

1. The lesions are proliferative in that the collagen deposition is out of proportion to the amount of dust present. Furthermore, they progress long after exposure ceases [124]. This continued activity might be due to secondary immunological features which supervene, or it may be due to the tendency for macrophages containing silica to migrate toward existing sites of disease (nodules) where they die and release their silica [124]. The role of macrophages in silica-induced fibrogenesis has been discussed.

2. In a number of patients silicosis has an accelerated course and the nodules are less well defined, extending into the surrounding lung. These have been shown to possess numerous plasma cells containing gammaglobulin [111].
3. In addition, a number of alterations in cell-mediated and humoral immunity have been described in silicosis.

Cell-mediated immunity in silicosis: No specific cell-mediated hypersensitivity to silica has been demonstrated. Recent studies have shown no difference between silicotics and controls in delayed skin responses to four recall antigens, in total lymphocyte numbers, and T- and B-cell percentages in peripheral blood, or in lymphocyte responses to a variety of mitogens [125]. However, lymphocyte responsiveness to suboptimal concentrations of concanavalin A (ConA) was lower in silicotics [125]. In anthrosilicosis, a reduced percentage of T lymphocytes has been reported and in autologous serum there was a reduced transformation of ConA-treated peripheral blood lymphocytes [126].

The influence of silica exposure on human susceptibility to infection, and on severity of lung damage which follows, has long been recognized, and in 1937 Gardner [127] studied silicotics from a variety of industries and found coexistent tuberculosis in 65–75%. Chatgidakis [128] showed a direct correlation between severity of silicosis and the incidence of tuberculosis. Silicosis in sandblasters has been noted to run an accelerated course and result in early fatality, and in these patients an increased incidence of mycobacterial infections (both *Mycobacterium tuberculosis* and low-virulence organisms such as *M. kansasii*) and opportunist fungal infections was found [129]. In animals, silica has been shown to increase the severity of lung damage which occurs in experimental mycobacterial infections [130]. Increased skin sensitivity to tuberculin in silicotics was reported by Vidal et al. [131], but because no distinction was made between cases of PMF and silicotuberculosis (where cavitated and contracted upper lobes are associated with AFB-positive sputum) the results are difficult to interpret. In a study by Schuyler et al. [125], no increase in delayed hypersensitivity to tuberculin was demonstrated.

Increased susceptibility to infection of subjects exposed to silica is at least partially explained by the results of in vivo and in vitro animal experiments concerning the effect of silica on the macrophage system. These include abnormalities of phagocytosis, antigen processing, and effector cell function. Silica is a relatively selective and potent macrophage toxin [47]. Immediately after treatment with silica, mice have an increased susceptibility to *Neisseria gonorrhoea* and *Haemophilus influenza* endotoxins (P. J. Cole and D. Roberts, personal communication, 1979), and to herpes simplex virus infections [137]. These effects are in part related to the transient fall in macrophage numbers which follows silica administration. This fall lasts several days but is followed by a marked increase [133] because of rapid entry of blood monocytes of bone marrow origin. However, longer lasting abnormalities of macrophage function have also been shown in silica-treated animals. Alveolar macrophages from silica-exposed mice have less ability to phagocytose *Escherichia coli* in vitro [134], and both alveolar and splenic macrophages from these animals exhibit decreased capacity to phagocytose antigen, induce splenic plaque-forming cells, and initiate antibody formation when these antigen-primed cells are transferred to irradiated syngeneic hosts. Silica treatment of mice also abrogates their resistance to bone marrow transplantation, and the rejection of skin grafts [125].

Humoral aspects of silicosis: Several abnormal antibodies have been demonstrated in silicotics. These include non-organ-specific lung antibodies, antinuclear antibodies, rheumatoid factor, and also elevated IgG levels.

Burrell and colleagues [135] tested serum from patients with a variety of lung diseases, and demonstrated antibodies to soluble lung antigen extracts using complement fixation tests, and to insoluble extracts using antiglobulin and complement consumption tests. The most significant antibody was directed against insoluble connective tissue elements thought to be to collagen. They were considered to be non-organ-specific in nature because they could be removed by prior absorption with liver and kidney. In later studies of sera from patients with silicosis complicated by PMF, elevated serum IgA levels were found in most cases, and anti-lung reactivity was associated predominantly with this IgA fraction [136]. However, the response to lung was heterogenous in that antibodies of IgG and IgM classes were also found. Increased prevalence of rheumatoid factor has been shown in silicotics [137]. In a study by Pernis [111] presence of rheumatoid factor correlated with severity of radiological changes. Antinuclear antibodies (ANA) were also present in a significant number of silicotics, and in a study of sandblasters with a rapidly accelerating form of disease, 44% had positive ANA (titer of 1:10 or greater) [138]. The ANA were IgG in most cases and were rarely complement fixing (14%). Diffuse nuclear immunofluorescence was the most common pattern seen. In 41%, precipitins to single-stranded DNA (but no LE cells or antibodies to nuclear protein) were found [138].

A further link between humoral mechanisms and silicosis, is the latter's association with the autoimmune diseases systemic lupus erythematosus (SLE) and scleroderma [138].

Development of tissue autoantibodies and their role in disease: Damage to tissues resulting in antigenic alteration and exposure of immunologically competent cells to tissue components which they have previously not met, are two situations thought to favor the production of autoantibodies. However, nonspecific tissue damage, as occurs in any form of chronic destructive lung disease (e.g., sarcoidosis), does not appear to result in an increased prevalence of ANA or rheumatoid factor. Turner-Warwick [137] has suggested that the cytotoxic effects of mineral dusts for macrophages might provide antigen for autoantibody production by causing the chronic liberation of nuclear material. Antibody production could be augmented in various ways:

1. The dust could impair macrophage function and result in poor clearance of potential antigens, increasing their opportunity of interaction with antibody-producing cells.
2. Nuclear material might become more immunogenic as a result of damage by dust or enzymes liberated from macrophages.
3. Molina [139] has suggested that inorganic dusts might act as adjuvants and augment the formation of autoantibodies. This might be achieved by a nonspecific mechanism because adjuvants augment the helper role of T lymphocytes.
4. Suppressor T lymphocytes exert specific feedback control on antibody synthesis by B cells [140], and defective functioning of these cells, as has been described in asbestotics [141] and silicotics [125], would permit autoantibody formation.
5. A nonspecific adjuvant effect might also result from coexistent infections in some instances, e.g., tuberculosis.

With the exception of Caplan's syndrome in coal miners, there is little definite evidence that these antibodies play a significant part in the fibrogenetic process. They may simply be a marker of continuous macrophage and tissue destruction which occurs in response to certain dusts. Other suggested roles for these antibodies are that they might form immune complexes and cause additional tissue damage, or that they might accelerate fibrogenesis once the dust-induced triggering effect has occurred. Long-term follow-up studies of groups with various dust diseases, and controls, are required to ascertain the stage at which autoantibodies appear, the relationship of antibody titers to lung damage, and their behavior after removal of the patients from dust exposure and when disease progresses rapidly.

Asbestos-Related Fibrosis A consistent relationship between estimated dose of asbestos and response has been observed when the parameters for assessment have been symptoms, lung function, and radiographic findings [142,133]. In addition, Ashcroft and Heppleston [144] measured the dose of both coated and uncoated fiber retained in the lung and demonstrated a direct relationship of dose to mild or moderate degrees of fibrosis. The same has been shown in animals [145]. However, progression from moderate to severe fibrosis does not appear to be associated with a further increase in dose, and additional mechanisms may therefore come into play. These could include genetic factors (there is a minor order association of the HLA/B27 gene type with asbestosis) [146], nonspecific inflammation as suggested by Ashcroft and Heppleston [144], or immunological mechanisms related to autoantibodies such as those described below.

Several *immunological abnormalities* have been described in asbestosis. A low total lymphocyte count and reduction in the absolute numbers of T lymphocytes has been observed by several workers [147–149]. Functional abnormalities of lymphocytes have also been observed, including decreased transformation in response to phytohemagglutinin [149,150] (not confirmed in a series by Gaumer et al. [141]), reduced PHA-induced lymphocyte-mediated cytotoxicity [148], and a reduction in suppressor T-cell function [141]. Cutaneous anergy to certain recall antigens and 2,4-dinitrochlorobenzene, described by Kagan et al. [148], was not found in the series of Gaumer et al. [141]. Serum inhibitors of mitogen-induced lymphocyte transformation were detected in several asbestotics [148].

Abnormalities of the humoral immune system have also been described. Polyclonal increase in gammaglobulins, and selective increases in serum IgA, IgG, and IgM [150,151], as well as an increase in serum IgE [149], has been shown in a percentage of asbestotics. Cold-reactive serum lymphocytotoxins were found in the serum of 81% of patients as compared with 21% of controls in one series [149]. Non-organ-specific anti-lung antibodies are present in only a small percentage of patients [152], but increased prevalence of rheumatoid factor (RF) [153] and ANA [151] is a more common finding. Turner-Warwick [151] reported a prevalence of positive RF in 23% and positive ANA in 25% of asbestotics compared with 3% for each in controls with a history of asbestos exposure but normal x-rays. The ANA tended to be of low titer and was often IgM. Prevalence increased with duration of exposure and age of the patient [151,154]. Precipitins to single-stranded DNA were present in some patients with ANA, and a few showed evidence of lymphocyte sensitization to DNA in transformation tests [155]. However, other features often found in SLE, including LE cells, antibodies to nuclear protein, and DNA-binding tests, were negative [155].

Further evidence of humoral immunological disturbances related to asbestos exposure has come from work with experimental animals. Miller and Kagan [156] showed an increased number of IgG receptor sites on alveolar macrophages or rats exposed to crocidolite asbestos in vivo, and in a later study the number of binding sites for complement on these cells was shown to be increased [157]. These alveolar macrophages were also noted to be capable of inducing T-lymphocyte proliferation by two different mechanisms: the first nonspecific binding due to aldehyde-like groups on the macrophage membrane, the second a consequence of specific immunological interaction of T-lymphocyte and antigen molecules on macrophage membrane which was thought to have been altered by asbestos ingestion [158]. The significance of the above findings is not clear and confirmation of some of the findings is awaited.

Asbestos bodies: The relevance of asbestos bodies to the fibrogenetic properties of asbestos have been studied and several important points have emerged. (1) There is some evidence that the coating of a fiber renders it non-fibrogenetic [159]. (2) Only a small (25%), but relatively constant, proportion of asbestos fibers in the lung become coated [144,160], electron microscopy being necessary to obtain a more accurate quantitation of uncoated fibers. (3) Although all asbestos fiber types may become coated in experimental animals, in humans amphibole fibers are more frequently coated than chrysotile fibers, even when both fiber types are present in the lung [144,160]. This may provide a further reason for the greater observed fibrogenicity of chrysotile asbestos as compared with the amphibolites.

Coal and Carbon-Induced Fibrosis *Simple coal worker's pneumoconiosis* is characterized by numerous black dust macules and nodules (2-5 mm in diameter) concentrated around or near respiratory bronchioles.

The extent of the changes correlates well with duration of exposure [161] and dust content of the lung [162]. The total amount of dust in the lungs is considerably more than that found in nodular silicosis, varying from 5 to 88 g, of which only 2% is quartz. Coal and carbon are relatively nontoxic to cells in vitro and in experimental animals they behave as inert dusts, but when quartz is added fibrosis is more pronounced. The combination of silica and coal, however, is less fibrogenetic than the same concentration of silica given alone [163]. Simultaneous administration of PVPNO with quartz causes a further reduction in fibrogenicity, proof of it being a quartz-induced fibrosis [163]. Similarly, in vitro clay and coal in mixed dusts are seen to have a protective effect on the cytotoxicity of quartz [164]. The lack of correlation between cytotoxicity of a mixed dust and its quartz content indicates the importance of other components of the dust [164,165]. This effect is not abolished by thorough washing and appears to be a property of their particulate form. High-rank coals (i.e., with high carbon but low oxygen and volatile contents) such as anthracite result in more pneumoconiosis than low-rank coals [166], but this is thought to relate to their poor clearance from the lung [167] resulting in a larger mass of retained dust.

An increased prevalence (34%) of circulating ANA has been found in coal miners with "simple" pneumoconiosis [168,169], and is more common in complicated cases [168], those with more severe radiographic grades [169] and those exposed to anthracite [168]. These were findings in miners exposed to coal of low silica content.

In *"rheumatoid" coal pneumoconiosis (Caplan's syndrome)* several features besides the presence of numerous plasma cells and lymphocytes in the outer layers of the nodules point to an immunological association of this syndrome: (1) 7S IgG, complement, free IgM, and IgM-containing plasma cells [170] found within the lesion, (2) its occurrence in association with circulating rheumatoid factor (RF) even in the absence of rheumatoid arthritis [171], (3) its presence in lungs with a relatively mild background of coal dust load, and (4) evidence from epidemiological studies of coal workers. Caplan [171] showed a higher prevalence of RF (57% compared with 21%) in coal miners with a typical radiographic appearance of Caplan's nodules than in those with "r" lesions (ILO/UICC classification). Neither group had arthritis. The presence of RF, therefore, seems to modify the tissue response to coal dust. There is however no evidence that coal dust exposure favors the development of RF or rheumatoid arthritis. The prevalence of radiographic features of Caplan's syndrome in coal miners is no greater than the incidence of circulating rheumatoid factor in the general population [172]. Coal dust is known to adsorb proteins in vitro, and Turner-Warwick [137] has suggested that in patients with circulating rheumatoid factor, immune complexes may be deposited on dust and trigger local inflammatory changes.

V. Prediction of Fibrogenicity of Mineral Dusts

While information from human epidemiological studies provides the best evidence for fibrogenicity of new or unknown dusts, the chief concern of occupational medicine is prevention of pathology. There is, therefore, an increasing need for reliable methods of assessing biological activity of mineral dusts for the purpose of predicting their fibrogenicity. This topic was considered in detail at a recent International Workshop on the In Vitro Effects of Mineral Dusts (Cardiff, 1979) [173], and for a more complete review of methods currently employed, the reader is referred to the proceedings of this meeting.

Test samples of dust should routinely be submitted to two groups of experiments. First, *animal experiments which provide in vivo evidence of fibrogenicity*. These take two forms: (1) inhalation studies, which mimic the normal route of administration to human lungs, but are costly and do not allow precise quantitation of dose, and (2) experiments involving the intratracheal instillation of suspensions of dust in which the dose delivered is controlled. The second group comprises *in vitro tests which assess the biological activity of dusts,* and includes tests of hemolysis, and macrophage (or equivalent cell-line) [165] cytotoxicity tests. The purpose of these tests is to provide quick, easy, and inexpensive methods of studying and comparing large numbers of potentially harmful dusts, in order to select those which might be fibrogenetic. Results usually do not indicate the mechanisms whereby the fibrogenicity is exerted in vivo, particularly in the case of the hemolytic tests and tests using macrophage-like cell lines. Some information provided by in vitro experiments with dust and macrophages, however, may be relevant in vivo, as has already been discussed.

The methods of collection and handling of dust samples prior to testing can influence the results obtained, and no single sample can be considered representative of a particular mine or even seam of ore [165].

Dust presented to cell test systems exerts its activity by a variety of mechanisms, but the particle surface characteristics seem to be very important. In the case of asbestos, magnesium content and/or surface charge is important [34,65], and, for silica, the tetrahedral crystalline structural unit [49] has been shown to be necessary for its fibrogenetic effect. The nonfibrogenic aluminium silicates have striking absorptive surface properties and give misleading results in these tests [164]. Because of diversity of particle shape and size, simple comparison of the effects of an equal mass of test samples is inadequate, and the use of particle numbers which takes into account size of particle is more appropriate. The surface area of samples, fiber diameter distribution, and absorptive properties for methylene blue, protein, or paraquat have all been used in an attempt to achieve a basis for comparison of dusts [174].

The cytotoxic effect of dust on red cells is observed as hemolysis, but the definition of cytotoxicity as applied to the macrophage or macrophage-like cell lines is not as simple. Since the latter (e.g., P388D_1 derived from mouse lymphoma) are capable of proliferation, the first toxic effect might be cytostasis—an inhibition of cell division [165]. In macrophages, "cytotoxicity" is most often considered to be cell death, and this can be assessed in various ways, the most simple and possibly the most reliable test being inability to exclude trypan blue dye. However, other methods have been used to assess the toxic effects of dust on macrophages, including release of lysosomal enzymes and lactic dehydrogenase, phospholipid metabolism, triphenyltetrazolium chloride reduction (TTC-RA), oxygen utilization, and lactate production [164,165,174].

The most profitable approach to predicting fibrogenicity might be the use of a combination of tests, some of which assess properties of the fiber, and others which measure their effects on macrophages. For example, Timár et al. [174] used the serum protein and methylene blue absorption tests, the release of LDH from macrophages, and the TTC-RA method, and were able to predict which pattern of tissue reaction would occur in vivo: foreign body reaction, focal storage reaction, or focal fibrosis. Use of the hemolytic test alone is helpful only if negative; that is, the dust is unlikely to be fibrogenetic. It should be emphasized that the purpose of these tests is to assess biological aggressiveness, and they do not indicate mechanisms by which fibrosis may occur.

VI. Conclusion

The production of fibrous tissue is a normal biological response, vital for the maintenance of structural integrity (particularly of tissues such as great vessels and joints which are subjected to continual distortion and stress) and for protection, e.g., for walling off abscesses or harmful foreign bodies.

In this chapter we have concentrated on mechanisms whereby some inorganic agents produce fibrosis, because more is known about them and because their mode of action appears to be less complex than that of the inhaled organic materials. Both these categories of dust, however, share several mechanisms, although the relative importance of each varies. The same is true of individual dusts or agents, and one of the immediate aims of research should be to determine which of the many mechanisms described are the main ones in each case.

In this way it may become possible to design treatment to exploit differences between mechanisms—preventing fibrosis while preserving a degree of normal collagen turnover and repair.

Drugs which affect the quality of collagen produced (e.g., BAPN) intervene too late in the fibrotic process and affect all tissues, therefore having dangerous side effects. Anti-inflammatory drugs are useful in disease with a prominent inflammatory component (e.g., farmer's lung) but have little effect on other dust diseases. Possibilities for the future include the use of drugs which affect specific cells or prevent the action of mediators which influence fibroblasts. It is of considerable interest in this context that Aalto and colleagues have produced antibodies to fibrogenetic factor isolated from silica-treated macrophages [62].

Finally, there is a need for improved methods of studying collagen content and turnover in vivo, particularly in human lung disease. An increase in total collagen content, rate of synthesis, and degradation has been found in some animal models [96], but in most only total content or rate of synthesis has been measured [6,30]. All three parameters are required to assess the fluctuations of collagen, and to be certain whether collagen accumulation is the result of increased synthesis or decreased degradation. Total collagen content has rarely been measured in human disease, and synthetic rates only assessed to a limited degree in lung explant cultures [6]. A method of assessing changes in collagen turnover during development of human lung disease is not yet available, and urgently required to add to the understanding of this fundamental aspect of fibrosis.

References

1. Gross, P., The morphology of alveolar tissue destruction, *Br. J. Exp. Pathol.*, **59**:395–400 (1978).
2. Sharp, H. L., R. A. Bridges, W. Krivit, and G. F. Freier, Cirrhosis associated with α_1-antitrypsin deficiency: A previously unrecognized inherited disorder, *J. Lab. Clin. Med.*, **73**:934–939 (1959).

3. Seyer, J. M., E. T. Hutcheson, and A. H. Kang, Collagen polymorphism in idiopathic chronic pulmonary fibrosis, *J. Clin. Invest.*, **57**:1498–1507 (1976).
4. Hocking, W. G., and D. W. Golde, The pulmonary-alveolar macrophage, *N. Engl. J. Med.*, **301**:580–587, 639–645 (1979).
5. Kuhn, C., The cells of the lung and their organelles. In *The Biochemical Basis of Pulmonary Function.* Edited by R. G. Crystal. New York, Marcel Dekker, 1976, pp. 3–48.
6. Hance, A. J., and R. G. Crystal, Collagen. In *The Biochemical Basis of Pulmonary Function,* Vol. 2. Edited by R. G. Crystal. New York, Marcel Dekker, 1976, pp. 215–271.
7. Grant, M. E., and D. J. Prockop, The biosynthesis of collagen, *N, Engl. J. Med.*, **286**:194–199, 242–249, 291–300 (1972).
8. Cardinale, G. J., and S. Udenfriend, Prolyl hydroxylase, *Adv. Enzymol.*, **41**:245–300 (1974).
9. Popenoe, E. A., and R. B. Aronson, Partial purification and properties of collagen lysine hydroxylase from chick embryos, *Biochem. Biophys. Acta,* **258**:380–386 (1972).
10. Prockop, D. J., K. I. Kivirikko, L. Tuderman, and N. A. Guzman, The biosynthesis of collagen and its disorders, *N. Engl. J. Med.*, **301**:13–23, 77–85 (1979).
11. Bradley, K. H., S. D. McConnell, and R. G. Crystal, Lung collagen composition and synthesis: Characterization and changes with age, *J. Biol. Chem.*, **249**:2674–2683 (1974).
12. Harris, E. D., and S. M. Krane, Collagenases, *N. Engl. J. Med.*, **291**:557–563, 605–609, 652–664 (1974).
13. Bienkowski, R. S., B. J. Baun, and R. G. Crystal, Fibroblasts degrade newly synthesized collagen within the cell before secretion, *Nature,* **276**:413–416 (1978).
14. Wahl, L. M., S. M. Wahl, S. E. Mergenhagen, and G. E. Martin, Collagenase production by lymphokine-activated macrophages, *Science,* **187**:261–263 (1975).
15. Werb, Z., M. C. Burleigh, A. J. Barrett, and P. M. Starkey, The interaction of α_2 macroglobulin with proteinases, binding and inhibition of mammalian collagenases and other metal proteinases, *Biochem. J.*, **139**:359–368 (1974).
16. Pearse, A. G. E., In *Histochemistry: Theoretical and Applied,* Third ed. Edinburgh, Churchill Livingstone, 1968, pp. 214–230.
17. Huang, T. W., Chemical and histochemical studies on human alveolar collagen fibres, *Am. J. Pathol.*, **86**:81–93 (1977).
18. Pras, M., and L. E. Glynn, Isolation of a non-collagenous reticulin component and its primary characterization, *Br. J. Exp. Pathol.*, **54**:449–456 (1973).
19. Olsen, B. R., and D. J. Prockop, Ferritin-conjugated antibodies used for labelling of organelles involved in the cellular synthesis and transport of procollagen, *Proc. Natl. Acad. Sci. USA*, **71**:2033–2037 (1974).

20. Wick, G., Immunofluorescence with specific antisera to collagen and procollagen as a new diagnostic tool. In *Collagen-Platelet Interaction.* Proceedings of the first Munich Symposium on Biology of Connective Tissue held in Munich, July 19–20, 1976. Edited by H. Gastpar, K. Kühn, and R. Marx. Stuttgart, F. K. Schattauer Verlag, 1978, pp. 181–185.
21. Nowack, H., S. Gay, G. Wick, U. Becker, and R. Timpl, Preparation and use in immunohistology of antibodies specific for type I and type III collagen and procollagen, *J. Immunol. Methods,* **12**:117–124 (1976).
22. Gay, S., G. R. Martin, P. K. Müller, R. Timpl, and K. Kühn, Simultaneous synthesis of types I and III collagen by fibroblasts in culture, *Proc. Natl. Acad. Sci. USA,* **73**:4037–4040 (1976).
23. Müller, P., C. Lemmon, S. Gay, K. von der Mark, and K. Kühn, Biosynthesis of collagen by chondrocytes in vitro. In *Extracellular Matrix Influences on Gene Expression.* Edited by H. C. Slavkin and R. C. Greulich. New York, Academic, 1975, pp. 293–302.
24. Hughes, J. F., B. Herion, B. Nusgens, and Ch. M. Lapiere, Type III collagen and probably not type I collagen aggregates platelets, *Thromb. Res.,* **9**:223–231 (1976).
25. Madri, J. A., and H. Furthmayr, Isolation and tissue localization of type AB_2 collagen from normal lung parenchyma, *Am. J. Pathol.,* **94**:323–330 (1979).
26. Crystal, R. G., J. D. Fulmer, W. C. Robert, M. L. Moss, B. R. Line, and H. V. Reynolds, Idiopathic pulmonary fibrosis—clinical, histological, radiographic, physiologic, scintigraphic, cytologic and biochemical aspects, *Ann. Intern. Med.,* **85**:769–788 (1976).
27. Lapière, C. M., and B. Nusgens, Collagen pathology at the molecular level. In *Biochemistry of Collagen.* Edited by G. N. Ramachandran and A. H. Reddi. New York, Plenum, 1976, pp. 377–447.
28. Laurent, G. J., M. P. Sparrow, P. C. Bates, and D. J. Millward, Collagen content and turnover in cardiac and skeletal muscles of the adult fowl and changes during stretch-induced growth, *Biochem. J.,* **176**:419–427 (1978).
29. Ross, R., The elastic fibre: A review, *J. Histochem. Cytochem.,* **21**:199–208 (1973).
30. Starcher, B. C., C. Kuhn, and J. E. Overton, Increased elastin and collagen content in the lungs of hamsters receiving an intratracheal injection of bleomycin, *Am. Rev. Respir. Dis.,* **117**:299–305 (1978).
31. Silbert, J. E., Biosynthesis of mucopolysaccharides and protein-polysaccharides. In *Molecular Pathology of Connective Tissues.* Edited by R. Perez-Tamayo and M. Rojkind. New York, Marcel Dekker, 1973, pp. 323–353.
32. Hext, P. M., and R. J. Richards, Biochemical effects of asbestiform minerals on lung fibroblast cultures, *Br. J. Exp. Pathol.,* **57**:281–285 (1976).
33. Richards, R. J., and T. G. Morris, Collagen and mucopolysaccharide production in growing lung fibroblasts exposed to chrysotile asbestos, *Life Sci.,* **12**:441–451 (1973).

34. Richards, R. J., and F. S. Wusteman, The effects of silica dust and alveolar macrophages on lung fibroblast grown in vitro, *Life Sci.,* **14**:355–364 (1974).
35. Richards, R. J., and F. Jacoby, Light microscope studies on the effects of chrysotile asbestos and fibreglass on the morphology and reticulin formation of cultured lung fibroblasts, *Environ. Res.,* **11**:112–121 (1976).
36. Harington, J. S., K. Miller, and G. MacNab, Haemolysis by asbestos, *Environ. Res.,* **4**:95–117 (1971).
37. Desai, R., P. M. Hext, and R. J. Richards, The prevention of asbestos-induced haemolysis, *Life Sci.,* **16**:1931–1938 (1975).
38. Hext, P. M., J. Hunt, K. S. Dodgson, and R. J. Richards, The effects of long-term exposure of lung fibroblast strains to chrysotile asbestos, *Br. J. Exp. Pathol.,* **58**:160–167 (1977).
39. Kang, A., Fibroblast activation, *J. Lab. Clin. Med.,* **92**:1–2 (1978).
40. Postlethwaite, A. E., R. Snyderman, and A. H. Kang, The chemotactic attraction of human fibroblasts to a lymphocyte-derived factor, *J. Exp. Med.,* **144**:1188–1203 (1976).
41. Postlethwaite, A. E., J. M. Seyer, and A. H. Kang, Induction of fibroblast chemotaxis by type I, II and III collagens, and collagen-degradation peptides, *Proc. Natl. Acad. Sci. USA,* **75**:871–875 (1978).
42. Yajima, T., Phagocytosis of collagen by human gingival fibroblasts, *J. Dent. Res.,* **56**(10):1271–1277 (1977).
43. Bienkowski, R. S., M. Cowan, J. A. McDonald, and R. G. Crystal, Degradation of newly synthesized collagen, *J. Biol. Chem.,* **253**:4356–4363 (1978).
44. Kettle, E. H., Experimental silicosis, *J. Ind. Hyg. Toxicol.,* **8**:491–495 (1926).
45. Brieger, H., and P. Gross, On the theory of silicosis III, *Arch. Environ. Health,* **15**:751–757 (1967).
46. Curran, R. C., and E. V. Rowsell, The application of the diffusion chamber technique to the study of silicosis, *J. Pathol. Bacteriol.,* **76**:561–568 (1958).
47. Allison, A. C., J. S. Harington, and M. Birbeck, An examination of the cytotoxic effects of silica on macrophages, *J. Exp. Med.,* **124**:141–154 (1968).
48. Allison, A. C., Mechanisms of macrophage damage in relation to the pathogenesis of some lung diseases. In *Lung Biology in Health and Disease,* Vol. 5, *Respiratory Defence Mechanisms* (Part II). Edited by J. D. Brain, D. F. Proctor, and L. M. Reid. New York, Marcel Dekker, 1977, pp. 1075–1102.
49. Chao, E. C. T., J. J. Fahey, and J. Littler, Stishovite, SiO_2, a very high pressure new mineral from Meteor Crater, Arizona, *J. Geophys. Res.,* **67**:419–421 (1962).
50. Depasse, J., Mechanism of the haemolysis by colloidal silica. In *The In Vitro Effects of Mineral Dusts.* Edited by R. C. Brown, M. Chamberlain, R. Davies, and I. P. Gormley. London, Academic, 1980, pp. 125–130.

51. Gabor, S., Z. Anca, E. Zugravu, M. Ciugudeanu, and B. Böhm, In vitro and in vivo quartz-induced lipid peroxidation. In *The In Vitro Effects of Mineral Dusts.* Edited by R. C. Brown, M. Chamberlain, R. Davies, and I. P. Gormley. London, Academic, 1980, pp. 131–137.
52. Allison, A. C., I. A. Clark, and P. Davies, Cellular interactions in fibrogenesis, *Ann. Rheum. Dis.,* **36**:Suppl. 8-13 (1977).
53. Bateman, E. D., R. J. Emerson, and P. Cole, The use of diffusion chambers to examine the biological effects of mineral dusts. In *The In Vitro Effects of Mineral Dusts.* Edited by R. C. Brown, M. Chamberlain, R. Davies, and I. P. Gormley. London, Academic, 1980, pp. 289–296.
54. Wartiovaara, J., S. Nordling, E. Lehtonen, and L. Saxen, Transfilter induction of kidney tubules: Correlation with cytoplasmic penetration into Nucleopore filters, *J. Embryol. Exp. Morphol.,* **31**:667–682 (1974).
55. Heppleston, A. G., Cellular reactions with silica. In *Biochemistry of Silicon and Related Problems.* Edited by G. Bendz and I. Lindquist. New York, Plenum, 1978, pp. 357–379.
56. Heppleston, A. G., and J. A. Styles, Activity of a macrophage factor in collagen formation by silica, *Nature,* **214**:521–522 (1967).
57. Harington, J. S., M. Ritchie, P. C. King, and K. Miller, The in vitro effects of silica-treated hamster macrophages on collagen production by hamster fibroblasts, *J. Pathol.,* **109**:21–37 (1973).
58. Burrell, R., and M. Anderson, The induction of fibrogenesis by silica-treated alveolar macrophages, *Environ. Res.,* **6**:389–394 (1973).
59. Aalto, M., and E. Kulonen, Fractionation of connective tissue-activating factors from the culture medium of silica-treated macrophages, *Acta Pathol. Microbiol. Scand. [C],* **87**:241–250 (1979).
60. Aho, S., and E. Kulonen, Effect of silica-liberated macrophage factors on protein synthesis in cell-free systems, *Exp. Cell. Res.,* **104**:31–38 (1977).
61. Green, R. C., Changes in acid ribonuclease and other acid hydrolases during lymphocyte stimulation, *Exp. Cell. Res.,* **110**:215–223 (1977).
62. Kulonen, E., M. Alto, S. Aho, P. Lehtinen, and M. Potila, The SiO_2-liberated fibrogenic macrophage factors with reference to RNA. In *The In Vitro Effects of Mineral Dusts.* Edited by R. C. Brown, M. Chamberlain, R. Davies, and I. P. Gormley. London, Academic, 1980, pp. 281–287.
63. Tainer, J. A., S. R. Turner, and W. S. Lynn, New aspects of chemotaxis. Specific target-cell attraction by lipid and lipoprotein fractions of *Escherichia coli* chemotactic factor, *Am. J. Pathol.,* **81**:401–408 (1975).
64. Conning, D. M., and A. G. Heppleston, Reticuloendothelial activity and local particle disposal, *Br. J. Exp. Pathol.,* **47**:388–400 (1966).
65. Light, W. G., and E. T. Wei, Surface charge and a molecular basis for asbestos toxicity. In *The In Vitro Effects of Mineral Dusts.* Edited by R. C. Brown, M. Chamberlain, R. Davies, and I. P. Gormley, London, Academic, 1980, pp. 139–145.
66. Newman, H. A. I., Y. A. Saat, and R. W. Hart, Putative effects of chrysotile, crocidolite and amosite on the surface membrane glycolipids and glycoproteins. In *The In Vitro Effects of Mineral Dusts.* Edited by R. C. Brown, M. Chamberlain, R. Davies, and I. P. Gormley. London, Academic, 1980, pp. 147–157.

67. Davies, P., A. C. Allison, J. Ackerman, A. Butterfield, and S. Williams, Asbestos induces selective release of lysosomol enzymes from mononuclear phagocytes, *Nature,* **251**:423–425 (1974).
68. Boros, D. L., Granulomatous inflammations, *Prog. Allergy,* **24**:183–267 (1978).
69. Granger, G. A., and T. W. Williams, Lymphocyte cytotoxicity in vitro. Activation and release of a cytotoxic factor, *Nature,* **218**:1253–1254 (1968).
70. Stewart, C. C., and H. Lin, Macrophage growth factor and its relationship to colony stimulating factor, *J. Reticuloendothel. Soc.,* **23**:269–285 (1978).
71. Wahl, S. M., L. M. Wahl, and J. B. McCarthy, Lymphocyte-mediated activation of fibroblast proliferation and collagen production, *J. Immunol.,* **121**:942–946 (1978).
72. Johnson, R. L., and M. Ziff, Lymphokine stimulation of collagen accumulation, *J. Clin. Invest.,* **58**:240–253 (1976).
73. Lewis, O. M., and R. Burrell, Induction of fibrogenesis by lung antibody-treated macrophages, *Br. J. Ind. Med.,* **33**:25–28 (1976).
74. Kravis, C. T., A. Ahmed, T. Brown, J. D. Fulmer, and R. G. Crystal, Pathogenic mechanisms in pulmonary fibrosis. Collagen-induced migration inhibition factor production and cytotoxicity mediated by lymphocytes, *J. Clin. Invest.,* **58**:1223–1232 (1976).
75. Trentham, D. E., R. A. Dynesius, R. E. Rocklin, and J. R. David, Cellular sensitivity to collagen in rheumatoid arthritis, *N. Engl. J. Med.,* **299**:327–332 (1978).
76. Boros, D. L., and H. J. Schwartz, Effect of carrageen on the development of hypersensitivity (*Schistosoma mansoni* egg) and foreign body (divinylbenzene co-polymer beads and bentonite) granulomas, *Int. Arch. Allergy Appl. Immunol.,* **48**:192–201 (1975).
77. Cohen, S., B. Benacerraf, R. T. McCluskey, and Z. Ovary, Effect of anticoagulants and delayed hypersensitivity reactions, *J. Immunol.,* **98**:351–358 (1967).
78. Gordon, S., M. A. Bray, and J. Morley, Control of lymphokine secretion by prostaglandins, *Nature,* **262**:401–402 (1976).
79. Snyderman, R., and S. E. Mergenhagen, Chemotaxis of macrophages. In *Immunobiology of the Macrophage.* Edited by D. S. Nelson. New York, Academic, 1976, p. 323.
80. Gallin, J. I., and A. P. Kaplan, Mononuclear cell chemotactic activity of kallikrein and plasminogen activator and its inhibition by C1 inhibitor and α_2 macroglobulin, *J. Immunol.,* **113**:1928–1934 (1974).
81. Houck, J. C., and C. Chang, The chemotactic properties of the products of collagenolysis, *Proc. Soc. Exp. Biol. Med.,* **138**:69–75 (1971).
82. Allison, A. C., and P. Davies, Increased biochemical and biological activities of mononuclear phagocytes exposed to various stimuli, with special reference to secretion of lysosomal enzymes. In *Mononuclear Phagocytes in Immunity, Infection and Pathology.* Edited by R. van Furth. Oxford, Blackwell, 1975, p. 487.

83. Rutherford, R. B., and R. Ross, Platelet factors stimulate fibroblasts and smooth muscle cells quiescent in plasma serum to proliferate, *J. Cell. Biol.*, **69**:196 (1976).
84. Leibovich, S. J., and R. Ross, The role of the macrophage in wound repair. A study of hydrocortisone and antimacrophage serum, *Am. J. Pathol.*, **78**:71-100 (1975).
85. Adamson, I. Y. R., D. H. Bowden, and J. P. Wyatt, A pathway to pulmonary fibrosis: An ultrastructural study of mouse and rat following radiation to the whole body and hemithorax, *Am. J. Pathol.*, **58**:481–498 (1970).
86. Sahu, A. P., R. K. S. Dogka, R. Shanker, and S. H. Zaidi, Fibrogenic response in murine lungs to asbestos, *Exp. Pathol.*, **11**:21–24 (1975).
87. Palmer, K. C., G. L. Snider, and J. A. Hayes, An association between alveolar cell proliferation and interstitial fibrosis following acute lung injury, *Chest*, **69**:Suppl. 2, 307–309 (1976).
88. Thurlbeck, W. M., and S. M. Thurlbeck, Pulmonary effects of paraquat poisoning, *Chest*, **69**:Suppl. 2, 276–280 (1976).
89. Miller, K., and E. Kagan, The in vivo effects of asbestos on macrophage membrane structure and population characteristics of macrophages: A scanning electron microscope study, *J. Reticuloendothel. Soc.*, **20**: 159–171 (1976).
90. Snider, G. L., B. R. Celli, R. H. Goldstein, J. J. O'Brien, and E. C. Lucey, Chronic interstitial pulmonary fibrosis produced in hamsters by endotracheal bleomycin-lung volumes, volume-pressure relations, carbon monoxide uptake and arterial blood gas studies, *Am. Rev. Respir. Dis.*, **117**:289–297 (1978).
91. Ryan, S. F., Experimental fibrosing alveolitis, *Am. Rev. Respir. Dis.*, **105**:776-791 (1972).
92. Holt, P. F., J. Mills, and D. K. Young, Experimental asbestosis in the guinea pig, *J. Pathol. Bacteriol.*, **92**:185–195 (1966).
93. Wagner, J. C., Asbestosis in experimental animals, *Br. J. Ind. Med.*, **20**: 1-12 (1963).
94. Willoughby, W. F., J. E. Barbaras, and R. Wheelis, Immunologic mechanisms in experimental interstitial pneumonitis, *Chest*, **69**:Suppl. 2, 286–294 (1976).
95. Harris, J. O., D. Bice, and J. E. Salvaggio, Experimental granulomatous pneumonitis: bronchopulmonary response to *Micropolyspora faeni* in rabbits, *Chest*, **69**:Suppl. 2, 287–288 (1976).
96. Pickrell, J. A., C. T. Schnizlein, F. F. Hahn, M. B. Snipes, and R. K. Jones, Radiation-induced pulmonary fibrosis: Study of changes in collagen constituents in different lung regions of beagle dogs after inhalation of beta-emitting radionuclides, *Radiat. Res.*, **74**:363–377 (1978).
97. McCullough, B., J. F. Collins, W. G. Johanson, and F. L. Grover, Bleomycin-induced diffuse interstitial pulmonary fibrosis in baboons, *J. Clin. Invest.*, **61**:79–88 (1978).

98. Vorwald, A. J., T. M. Durkan, and P. C. Pratt, Experimental studies of asbestosis, *Arch. Ind. Hyg.,* **3**:1–43 (1951).
99. Richerson, H. B., J. J. Seidenfield, H. V. Ratajeyak, and D. W. Edwards, Chronic experimental interstitial pneumonitis in the rabbit, *Am. Rev. Respir Dis.,* **117**:5–13 (1978).
100. Moore, V. L., and Q. N. Myrvik, Relationship of BCG-induced granuloma formation in rabbit lungs: Effect of cortisone acetate, *Infect. Immunol.,* **7**:764–770 (1974).
101. Butler, C., Pulmonary interstitial fibrosis from paraquat in the hamster, *Arch. Pathol.,* **99**:563–567 (1975).
102. Göthe, C. J., and A. Swensson, Effect of BCG on lymphatic lung clearance of dusts with different fibrogenicity, *Arch. Environ. Health,* **20**: 579–585 (1970).
103. Hall, D. A., Synergistic effect of age and corticosteroid treatment on connective tissue metabolism. In *Symposium on the Fibrotic Process.* Edited by M. I. V. Jayson. *Ann. Rheum. Dis. (Suppl. 2),* **36**:58–62 (1977).
104. Nimni, M. E., Penicillamine and collagen metabolism. In *Fundamental Studies on Penicillamine for Rheumatoid Diseases.* Proceedings of the Second Bertine Koperberg Conference held in Oosterbeck, the Netherlands, September 14–15, 1978. Edited by T. E. W. Feltkamp. *Scand. J. Rheum. (Suppl. 28),* 1978, 71–77.
105. Jackson, D. S., Nitriles, penicillamine and substituted prolines. In *Symposium on the Fibrotic Process.* Edited by M. I. V. Jayson. *Ann. Rheum. Dis. (Suppl. 2),* **36**:63–64 (1977).
106. Sakamoto, S., P. Coldhaber, and M. J. Clincher, Mouse bone collagenase. The effect of heparin on the amount of enzyme released in tissue culture and on the activity of the enzyme, *Calcif. Tissue Res.,* **12**:247–258 (1973).
107. Levene, C. I., J. J. Aleo, C. J. Prynne, and C. J. Bates, The activation of protocollagen proline hydroxylase by ascorbic acid in cultured 3T6 fibroblasts, *Biochem. Biophys. Acta,* **338**:29–35 (1974).
108. Ehrlich, H. P., R. Ross, and P. Bornstein, Effect of antimicrotubular agents on the secretion of collagen. A biochemical and morphological study, *J. Cell. Biol.,* **62**:390–405 (1974).
109. Haslam, P. L., C. W. G. Turton, B. Heard, A. Lukoszek, J. V. Collins, A. J. Salsbury, and M. Turner-Warwick, Bronchoalveolar lavage in pulmonary fibrosis: Comparison of cells obtained with lung biopsy and clinical features, *Thorax,* **35**:9–18 (1980).
asbestos exposure: The correlations between progression rates and steroid response, *Thorax,* in press (1979).
110. Corrin, B., and A. B. Price, Electron microscopic studies on desquamative interstitial pneumonia associated with asbestosis, *Thorax,* **27**:324–331 (1972).
111. Pernis, B., Silicosis. In *Textbook of Immunopathology,* Vol. 1. Edited by P. A. Miescher and H. J. Müller-Eberhardt. New York, Grune and Stratton, 1968, pp. 293–301.

112. Davis, G. S., A. R. Brody, and J. E. Craighead, Analysis of airspace and interstitial mononuclear cell populations in human diffuse interstitial lung disease, *Am. Rev. Respir. Dis.*, **118**:7–15 (1978).
113. Turner-Warwick, M., P. Haslam, and J. Weeks, Antibodies in some chronic fibrosing lung conditions. II. Immunofluorescent studies, *Clin. Allergy*, **1**:209–219.
114. Davis, G. S., A. R. Brody, J. N. Landis, W. G. B. Graham, J. E. Craighead, and G. M. Green, Quantitation of inflammatory activity in interstitial pneumonitis by bronchofiberscopic pulmonary lavage, *Chest*, **69**:265–274 (1976).
115. Haslam, P. L., A. Lukoszek, A. J. Salsbury, A. Dewar, J. V. Collins, and M. Turner-Warwick, Bronchoalveolar lavage fluid cell counts in cryptogenic fibrosing alveolitis, and their relation to therapy, *Thorax*, **35**:328–339 (1980).
116. Davis, G. S., A. R. Brody, and J. E. Craighead, Analysis of airspace and interstitial mononuclear cell populations in human diffuse interstitial lung disease, *Am. Rev. Respir. Dis.*, **118**:7–15 (1978).
117. Holt, P. G., Alveolar macrophages. III. Studies on the mechanism of inhibition of T cell proliferation, *Immunology*, **37**:437–445 (1979).
118. Cole, P. J., C. W. G. Turton, H. C. Lanyon, and J. V. Collins, Bronchoalveolar lavage for the preparation of free lung cells: Technique and complications, *Br. J. Dis. Chest*, **74**:273–278 (1980).
119. Reynolds, H. Y., J. D. Fulmer, J. A. Kazmierowski, W. C. Roberts, M. M. Frank, and R. G. Crystal, Analysis of cellular and protein content of broncho-alveolar lavage fluid from patients with idiopathic pulmonary fibrosis and hypersensitivity pneumonia, *J. Clin. Invest.*, **59**:165–175 (1977).
120. Weinberger, S. E., J. A. Kelman, N. A. Elson, R. C. Young, H. Y. Reynolds, J. D. Fulmer, and R. G. Crystal, Bronchoalveolar lavage in interstitial lung disease, *Ann. Intern. Med.*, **89**:459–466 (1978).
121. Bignon, J., K. Atassi, M. C. Jaurand, P. Geslin, and R. Solle, Cellular and protein content analysis of bronchoalveolar lavage fluid from patients with idiopathic pulmonary fibrosis and asbestosis, *Am. Rev. Respir. Dis.*, **117**:Suppl. 57 (1978).
122. Low, R. B., G. S. Davis, and M. S. Giancola, Biochemical analysis of bronchoalveolar lavage fluids of healthy human volunteer smokers and non-smokers, *Am. Rev. Respir. Dis.*, **118**:863–875 (1978).
123. Stockley, R. A., M. Mistry, A. R. Bradwell, and D. Burnett, A study of plasma proteins in the solphase of sputum from patients with chronic bronchitis, *Thorax*, **34**:777–782 (1979).
124. Heppleston, A. G., The disposal of dust in the lungs of silicotic rats, *Am. J. Pathol.*, **40**:493–506 (1962).
125. Schuyler, M., M. Ziskind, and J. E. Salvaggio, Cell-mediated immunity in silicosis, *Am. Rev. Respir. Dis.*, **116**:147–151 (1977).
126. Dauber, J. H., D. R. Finn, and R. P. Daniels, Immunologic abnormalities in arthrosilicosis, *Am. Rev. Respir. Dis.*, **113**:Suppl. 94 (1976).

127. Gardner, L. W., The significance of the silicotic problem. In *Proceedings of the Third Symposium on Silicosis.* Edited by B. E. Kuechle. Trudeau Sch. Tuberculosis, Saranac Lake, New York, 1937.
128. Chatgidakis, C. F., Silicosis in South African white gold miners, *Med. Proc.,* **9**:383–392 (1963).
129. Bailey, W. C., M. Brown, H. A. Buechner, H. Weill, H. Ichinose, and M. Ziskind, Silico-mycobacterial disease in sandblasters, *Am. Rev. Respir. Dis.,* **110**:115–125 (1974).
130. Policard, A., C. Gernez-Rieux, A. Tacquet, J. C. Martin, B. Devulder, and L. Le Bouffant, Influence of pulmonary dust load on the development of experimental infection by *Mycobacterium kansasii, Nature,* **216**:177–178 (1967).
131. Vidal, J., F. B. Michel, and J. C. Marty, Allergie tuberculinique et candidinique des mineurs de charbon, *Rev. Tuberc. Pneumol. (Paris),* **32**:507–523 (1968).
132. du Buy, H., Effect of silica on virus infections in mice and mouse tissue culture, *Infect. Immunol.,* **11**:996–1002 (1975).
133. Pearsall, N. N., and R. S. Weiser, The macrophage in allograft immunity. I. Effects of silica as a specific macrophage toxin, *J. Reticuloendothel. Soc.,* **5**:107–120 (1968).
134. Miller, S. D., and A. Zarkower, Alteration of murine immunologic responses after silica dust inhalation, *J. Immunol.,* **113**:1533–1543 (1974).
135. Burrell, R. G., J. P. Wallace, and C. E. Andrews, Lung antibodies in patients with pulmonary disease, *Am. Rev. Respir. Dis.,* **89**:697–706 (1964).
136. Hagadorn, J. E., and R. Burrell, Lung-reactive antibodies in IgA fractions of sera from patients with pneumoconiosis, *Clin. Exp. Immunol.,* **3**:263–267 (1968).
137. Turner-Warwick, M., Immunology of occupational diseases of the lung. In *Current Topics in Immunology,* Series 10, *Immunology of the Lung.* Edited by J. Turk. London, Edward Arnold, 1978, pp. 209–215.
138. Turner-Warwick, M., P. Cole, H. Weill, R. N. Jones, and M. Ziskind, Chemical fibrosis: The model of silica. In *Symposium on the Fibrotic Process.* Edited by M. I. V. Jayson. *Ann. Rheum. Dis. (Suppl. 2),* **36**: 47–50 (1977).
139. Molina, C., *Bronchopulmonary Immunopathology.* Edinburgh, Churchill Livingstone, 1976.
140. Basten, A., Specific suppression of the immune response by T cells. In *Immunological Tolerance: Mechanisms and Potential Therapeutic Applications.* Edited by D. H. Katz and B. Benacerraf. New York, Academic, 1974, pp. 107.
141. Gaumer, H. R., J. Kaimal, M. Schuyler, and J. E. Salvaggio, Suppressor cell function in patients with asbestosis, *Am. Rev. Respir. Dis.,* **119**: Suppl. 216 (1979).

142. Bader, M. E., R. A. Bader, A. S. Tierstein, A. Miller, and I. J. Selikoff, Pulmonary function and radiographic changes in 598 workers with varying duration of exposure to asbestos, *J. Mt. Sinai Hosp.*, **37**:492–500 (1970).
143. Rossiter, C. E., L. J. Bristol, P. H. Cartier, J. G. Gilson, T. R. Grainger, G. K. Sluis-Cremer, and J. C. McDonald, Radiographic changes in chrysotile asbestos mine and mill workers of Quebec, *Arch. Environ. Health*, **24**: 388–400 (1972).
144. Ashcroft, T., and A. G. Heppleston, The optical and EM determination of pulmonary asbestos fibre concentration and its relation to human pathological reaction, *J. Clin. Pathol.*, **26**:224–234 (1973).
145. Wagner, J. C., G. Berry, J. W. Skidmore, and V. Timbrell, The effects of the inhalation of asbestos in rats, *Br. J. Cancer*, **29**:252–269 (1974).
146. Turner-Warwick, M., HLA phenotypes in asbestos workers, *Br. J. Dis. Chest*, **73**:243–244 (1979).
147. Kang, K-Y, Y. Sera, T. Okuchi, and Y. Yamamura, T-lymphocytes in asbestosis, *N. Engl. J. Med.*, **291**:735–737 (1974).
148. Kagan, E., A. Solomon, J. C. Cochrane, E. I. Beissner, and J. Gluckman, Immunological studies of patients with asbestosis. I. Studies of cell mediated immunity, *Clin. Exp. Immunol.*, **28**:261–267 (1977).
149. Kagan, E., A. Solomon, J. C. Cochrane, P. Kuba, P. Rocks, and I. Webster, Immunological studies of patients with asbestosis. II. Studies of circulating lymphoid cell numbers and humoral immunity, *Clin. Exp. Immunol.*, **28**:268–275 (1977).
150. Haslam, P., A. Lukoszek, J. A. Merchant, and M. Turner-Warwick, Lymphocyte responses to phytohaemagglutinin in patients with asbestosis and pleural mesothelioma, *Clin. Exp. Immunol.*, **31**:178–188 (1978).
151. Turner-Warwick, M., Immunology and asbestosis, *Proc. R. Soc. Med.*, **66**: 927–930 (1973).
152. Turner-Warwick, M., and P. Haslam, Antibodies in some chronic fibrosing lung diseases. I. Non-organ-specific autoantibodies, *Clin. Allergy*, **1**:83–95 (1971).
153. Turner-Warwick, M., and W. R. Parkes, Circulating rheumatoid and antinuclear factors in asbestos workers, *Br. Med. J.*, **3**:492–495 (1970).
154. Haslam, P., Immune responses to nuclear antigens in lung disease, PhD thesis, London University, 1976.
155. Haslam, P., M. Turner-Warwick, and A. Lukoszek, Antinuclear antibody and lymphocyte responses to nuclear antigens in patients with lung disease, *Clin. Exp. Immunol.*, **20**:379–395 (1975).
156. Miller, K., and E. Kagan, The in vivo effects of asbestos on macrophage membrane structure and population characteristics of macrophages: A scanning electron microscopic study, *J. Reticuloendothel. Soc.*, **20**: 159–171 (1976).
157. Miller, K., and E. Kagan, Immune adherence reactivity of rat alveolar macrophages following inhalation of crocidolite asbestos, *Clin. Exp. Immunol.*, **29**:152–158 (1977).

158. Miller, K., Z. Weintraub, and E. Kagan, The effect of asbestos on macrophages. In *The In Vitro Effects of Mineral Dusts.* Edited by R. C. Brown, M. Chamberlain, R. Davies, and I. P. Gormley. London, Academic, 1980, pp. 305–312.
159. Becklake, M. R., Asbestos-related diseases of the lung and other organs: Their epidemiology and implications for clinical practice, *Am. Rev. Respir. Dis.,* **114**:187–227 (1976).
160. Fondimare, A., and J. Desbordes, Asbestos bodies and fibres in lung tissues, *Environ. Health Perspect.,* **9**:147–156 (1974).
161. Fay, J. W. J., and J. R. Ashford, A survey of the methods developed in the National Coal Board's Pneumoconiosis Field Research for correlating environmental exposure with medical condition, *Br. J. Ind. Med.,* **18**: 175–196 (1961).
162. Rossiter, C. E., Evidence of dose-response relation in pneumoconiosis, *Trans. Soc. Occup. Med.,* **22**:83–97 (1972).
163. Schlipköter, H. W., W. Hilscher, F. Pott, and E. G. Beck, Investigations into the aetiology of coal workers' pneumoconiosis, with the use of PVN-oxide. In *Inhaled Particles,* Vol. 3. Edited by W. H. Walton. Woking, Unwin, 1971, pp. 379–389.
164. Seemayer, N. H., and N. Manojlovic, Biological effects of coal mine dusts on alveolar macrophages. In *The In Vitro Effects of Mineral Dusts.* Edited by R. C. Brown, M. Chamberlain, R. Davies, and I. P. Gormley. London, Academic, 1980, pp. 5–12.
165. Gormley, I. P., G. M. Brown, P. L. Collings, J. M. G. Davies, and J. Otlery, The cytotoxicity of respirable dusts from collieries. In *The In Vitro Effects of Mineral Dusts.* Edited by R. C. Brown, M. Chamberlain, R. Davies, and I. P. Gormley. London, Academic, 1980, pp. 19–24.
166. Lainhart, W. S., and W. K. C. Morgan, Extent and development of respiratory effects. In *Pulmonary Reactions to Coal Dust.* Edited by M. M. Key, L. E. Kerr, and M. Bundy. New York, Academic, 1971, pp. 25–56.
167. Heppleston, A. G., G. W. Civil, and A. Critchlow, The effects of duration and intermittency of exposure on the elimination of high and low rank coal dusts. In *Inhaled Particles,* Vol. 3. Edited by W. H. Walton. Woking, Unwin, 1971, pp. 261–270.
168. Lippmann, M., H. L. Eckert, H. L. Mahon, and W. K. C. Morgan, Circulating antinuclear and rheumatoid factors in coal miners, *Ann. Intern. Med.,* **79**:807–811 (1973).
169. Soutar, C. A., M. Turner-Warwick, and W. R. Parkes, Circulating antinuclear antibody and rheumatoid factor in coal pneumoconiosis, *Br. Med. J.,* **3**:145–147 (1974).
170. Wagner, J. C., and J. N. McCormick, Immunological investigations of coal workers' disease, *J. R. Soc. Med.,* **2**:49 (1967).
171. Caplan, A., R. B. Payne, and J. L. Withey, A broader concept of Caplan's syndrome related to rheumatoid factors, *Thorax,* **17**:205–212 (1962).

172. Lindars, D. C., and D. Davis, Rheumatoid pneumoconiosis, *Thorax*, 22: 525–532 (1967).
173. *The In Vitro Effects of Mineral Dusts.* Edited by R. C. Brown, M. Chamberlain, R. Davies, and J. P. Gormley. London, Academic, 1980.
174. Timár, M., Z. Adamis, E. Tatray, and G. Ungváry, In vivo and in vitro investigations on different dusts. In *The In Vitro Effects of Mineral Dusts.* Edited by R. C. Brown, M. Chamberlain, R. Davies, and I. P. Gormley. London, Academic, 1980, pp. 319–322.

12

Environmental Characterization

YAHIA HAMMAD
VENKATRAM DHARMARAJAN

Tulane University School of Medicine
New Orleans, Louisiana

MORTON CORN

The Johns Hopkins University School
of Hygiene and Public Health
Baltimore, Maryland

I. Introduction

A. Purposes of Sampling and Description of Airborne Pollutant Variations in Space and Time

The production of pollutants in the form of gases or dispersions, i.e., solid or liquid particles in air, is associated with industrial processing of materials in particular, and with human activity, in general. Thus, employed persons handle bulk materials, solvents, finished products—all of which disperse some dusts or emit gases or vapors. In the outdoor environment, the forces of nature, such as wind, disperse dusts from the surface of the earth; aerosols are emitted by vegetation, as are gases; precipitation phenomena cause fog and rainfall. Also, it is now known that gases in the atmosphere react to form a disperse state of matter such as the submicrometer aerosol in the Los Angeles smog.

There are various reasons for sampling contaminant gases and aerosols in the air. In the field of public health it is necessary to obtain estimates of the exposure of individuals to these pollutants. There are guidelines for exposure to many pollutants which have the potential to cause harmful effects after inhalation, ingestion, or dermal contact. By sampling and analyzing the air in the breathing zones of exposed individuals, we can arrive at conclusions concerning the acceptability of the individual exposure to the particular pollutant.

The determination of individual exposures to airborne contaminants can be performed for the purpose of epidemiological investigations, where excesses in morbidity or mortality are determined and related to the exposure concentrations, thus deriving a dose-response curve for the particular population exposed. Alternately, it is necessary to sample airborne contaminants to determine if workplaces or outdoor environments meet statutory requirements. Regulations which demand adherence to airborne concentrations of contaminants include the Occupational Safety and Health Act of 1970, the Clean Air Act and its Amendments of 1977, and the Mine Safety and Health Act of 1977. In the last two cases it is not only necessary to perform such sampling and to arrive at a conclusion of compliance or lack of compliance with the particular standard, but it is also necessary to document the sampling method and analytical result and to maintain the exposure record for future reference.

In research studies the investigator must often create an artificial atmosphere for the purpose of exposing animals or human subjects in the laboratory. Bottled contaminant gases and particle and aerosol generation systems are available to create artificial atmospheres. The atmospheres usually generated in laboratory studies are differentiated from those occurring in occupational environments or outdoors by their tendency to be associated with relatively constant concentrations of contaminants, while the latter environments fluctuate widely in time and space. In addition to creating environments for exposure of test species in the laboratory, there are needs for sampling that are not related to estimates of individual exposures.

There is often need to simulate an atmosphere or process stream for testing instrumentation or contaminant control equipment. Examples are the determination of the sampling efficiency of probes to sample particulate matter, or laboratory calibration of direct reading contaminant gas instrumentation in an atmosphere simulated to reproduce the condition anticipated in the field.

A host of other purposes exist for creating and sampling contaminant atmospheres. Fundamental work on particle gas interactions and particle behavior, and corrosion studies on materials, all require the development of test atmospheres and the determination of pollutant concentrations in those

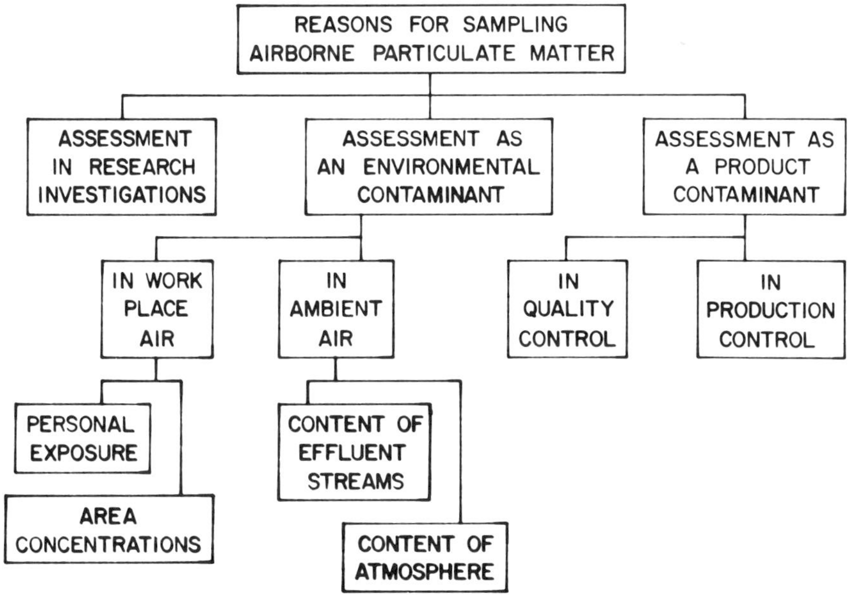

Figure 1 Diagramatic presentation of reasons for sampling airborne particulate matter.

atmospheres. Figure 1 is a diagrammatic summary of reasons for sampling airborne pollutants.

B. Expertise Associated with Sampling

The characterization of contaminant atmospheres is required in the pursuit of a variety of professions. In general, those who perform such evaluations are industrial hygienists, air pollution specialists, and perhaps chemists. The characterization of contaminant concentrations in air is not a discipline; it is a skill associated with many disciplines.

A host of general references exist to direct the professional to accepted and proven methodologies to characterize gaseous and particulate pollutants in air. They are noted here as further sources of information for the reader in this chapter.

II. Classification of Airborne Contaminants

An airborne contaminant may be defined as a substance or substances (viable or nonviable) which is suspended in air and is potentially harmful or

Table 1 General Classification of Organic Gases

HYDROCARBONS

ALIPHATIC		ALICYCLIC		AROMATIC	POLYNUCLEAR
SATURATED	UNSATURATED	SATURATED	UNSATURATED		
Ethane	Ethylene	Cyclohexane	Cyclohexene	Benzene	Indene
Methane	Acetylene	Substituted cyclohexane	Cyclopentadiene	Toluene	Naphthalene
etc.	etc.		etc.	Xylene	Terphenyl
				Styrene	Biphenyl

OXYGENATED HYDROCARBONS

KETONES	EPOXY COMPOUNDS	ETHERS	ESTERS	ALCOHOLS	ACIDS AND ACID ANHYDRIDES	ALDEHYDES
Acetone	Ethylene oxide	Ethyl ether	Methyl formate		Acetic acid	Formaldehyde
Methyl isobutyl ketone	Glycidol	Dioxane	Vinyl acetate		Phthalic anhydride	Acrolein
Cyclohexanone	Propylene oxide	Tetrahydrofuran	Phteralates			
			Isocyanates			

ALCOHOLS

PHENOLS	SATURATED ALIPHATIC	UNSATURATED ALIPHATIC	ALICYCLIC	ETHER ALCOHOLS	POLYOLS
Cresol	Ethanol	Allyl alcohol	Cyclohexanol	Methyl	Glycols
Catechol	Propanol	1-Propynol-3	Furfuryl alcohol	Ethyl	
				Butyl	
				Cellosolve	

HALOGENATED HYDROCARBONS

- SATURATED ALIPHATIC
  - Chloroform
  - Hexachloroethane
  - Tetrabromoethane
  - Iodoform
- UNSATURATED ALIPHATIC
  - Vinyl chloride
  - Allyl chloride
  - Dichloroacetylene
  - Vinyl bromide
- AROMATIC
  - Monochlorobenzene
  - O-Chlorostyrene

HYDROCARBONS WITH NITROGEN

- NITRO ALIPHATIC
  - Tetranitromethane
  - 2-Nitropropane
- NITRO AROMATIC
  - Nitrobenzene
  - Nitrotoluene
- CYANO COMPOUNDS
  - Acetonitrite
  - Methacylonitrite
- AMINES
  - Aliphatic
  - Methyl
  - Amine
  - Butyl amine
- AROMATIC AMINES
  - Aniline
  - O-Toluidine
  - Pyridine
  - Benzidine
- OTHER NON-AROMATIC AMINE AND AMIDES
  - Hydrazine
  - Ethanolamine
  - Morpholine
  - Ethyleneimine
  - Formamide

MISCELLANEOUS COMPOUNDS

- ORGANOSULFUR
  - Mercaptans
  - Disulfide
- ORGANOMETALLICS
  - Nickel carbonyl
  - Iron pentacarbonyl
- COMPOUNDS WITH O and HALOGENS
  - Phosgene
  - Epichlorohydrin
  - Methoxychlor
  - Hexafluoroacetone
- HALOGEN WITH N or S
  - Chloropicrin
  - Chloronitropropane
  - MOCA

toxic to humans, animals, vegetation, or materials. Clean, dry air contains 78.09% nitrogen and 20.94% oxygen, by volume. The remaining 0.97% of the gaseous constituents of dry air include small amounts of other inorganic and organic gases whose concentrations may differ with time and place. Water vapor is normally present in concentrations ranging from 1 to 3%. The air also contains aerosols (dispersed solid or liquid particles). They range in size from clusters of a few molecules to diameters of tens of micrometers.

In this chapter, we discuss the characterization of contaminated air for the purpose of evaluating the hazardous potential of liquid, solid, or gaseous constituents which could be inhaled by humans. At the outset it is advantageous to broadly classify the contaminants present in air into the gas phase and the disperse phase. These broad categories of contaminants present in air assist us in generalizing the entry, deposition, and effects on the respiratory system of inhaled airborne contaminants. It is not our purpose to elaborately detail any one technique or methodology, but rather to stress task approaches to provide a conceptual basis for the subject. The reader is referred to references already cited or those which will be cited in the text for completing his or her detailed understanding of specific topics.

A. Gas Phase

The airborne contaminants in the gas phase are generally referred to by industrial hygienists as being a gas or vapor; the differentiation between a gas and a vapor is that the latter is readily condensible at ambient temperatures, while a gas has a boiling point far removed from normal room temperatures, e.g., chlorine, oxides of sulfur and nitrogen, carbon monoxide, etc.

The gas phase contaminants could further be subdivided as being organic, inorganic, or organometallic. There are several hundred organic gases and vapors. They dominate the tables established by the American Conference of Governmental Industrial Hygienists and the Occupational Safety and Health Administration (OSHA) for standards of worker exposure to airborne contaminants in industry. Of the 254 gases and vapors for which there are OSHA exposure standards, 220 (86.6%) of them are organic chemicals. Of the remaining 34, 33 (or 13.0%) are inorganic gases, and one (0.4%) is an organometallic gas (i.e., nickel carbonyl). Of the organic gases, about 22% are aromatic in nature; the rest are nonaromatic.

Classification of organic gases and vapors is complicated because of their enormous number, and the variety and complexities of their structures. Table 1 is one approach to classification; it illustrates the complexities involved in categorizing organic compounds. The toxicological potential of individual organic substances are not related to this classification.

Inorganic gases can be classified according to their structures. One method of classification is presented in Table 2.

Table 2 Classification of Inorganic Gases

Category	Inorganic gases
Monoatomic	Helium, neon, argon, krypton, mercury, etc.
Diatomic	Hydrogen, fluorine, chlorine, bromine, iodine, nitrogen, oxygen
Polyatomic	
Hydrides	B_nH_x, NH_3, N_2H_4, PH_3, A_sH_3, H_2S, H_2Se, HF, HCI, HB_2, HI
Halogenides	BCI_3, BF_3, PCI_3, CIO_2, CIF_3, NF_3, OF_2, SeF_6, SF_6, SCI, SF_5, TeF_6
Oxides	O_3, H_2O_2, NO_x, SO_x, CO, CO_2, CIO_2, D_2O, etc.
Miscellaneous	HCN, $(CN)_2$, CS_2, COS

B. Disperse Phase

The disperse phase may include liquid and/or solid contaminants. In general, it is easier to sample the gaseous phase when particulate matter is not present. The presence of particulate matter as a disperse phase complicates not only the characterization of the disperse phase, but that of the gaseous phase as well. The reasons for introduction of complexity into sampling and characterization when both phases are present is that separation of the disperse phase on a filter paper, for instance, requires that the gas phase be drawn through the collected disperse phase, thus providing an opportunity for absorption of gaseous contaminants on the collected particulate phase, or vaporization of absorbed contaminants from the particulate phase to the gas. When it is known that significant quantities of particulate and gaseous contaminants are present in a contaminated atmosphere, those characterizing the atmosphere must be alert to the possible impact on results of both contaminant phases.

The most important parameter characterizing the particulate phase is its particle size. If the particles are "small" (designated here as 1 μm or less) they have very little inertia and can be sampled and evaluated without considering distortions of the sample created by inertial properties of the particles. At the other extreme, very large particles (used here to designate those greater than approximately 25 μm) tend to settle to the ground rapidly, presenting a rapidly changing component of the dispersion. If the particles are very small (here used to designate those less than approximately 0.1 μm diameter) they are associated with high coefficients of diffusion in air; they coagulate to form larger particles, thus also presenting a dynamic, rapidly changing component of the dispersion.

Figure 2 indicates sampling methods available to those preparing to sample a disperse phase. It indicates that certain decisions must be made early in the approach to characterizing a dispersion in air. The requirements

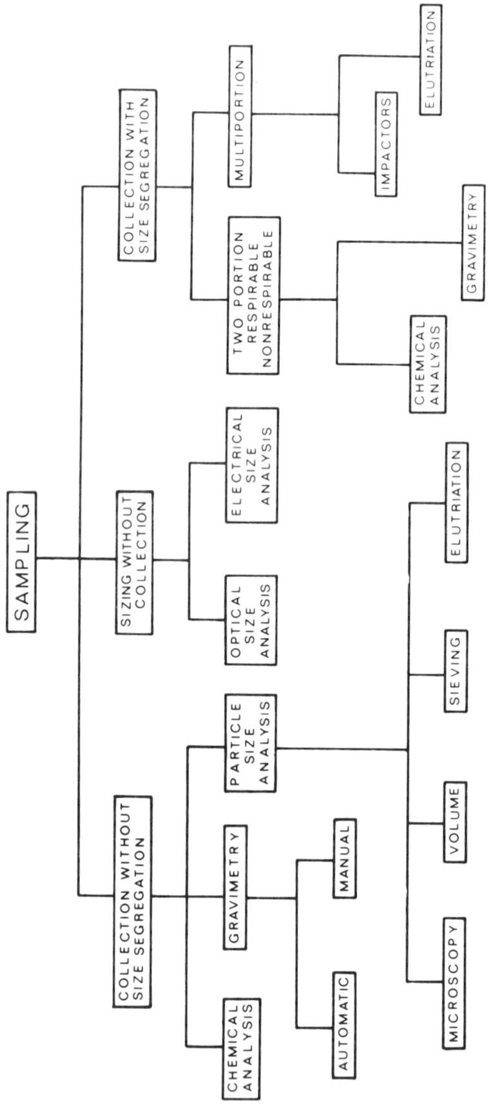

Figure 2 Diagramatic presentation of sampling methods for disperse phase of airborne pollutants.

for selection of one or the other of these methods will be treated later in this chapter. The sampling decisions are all related to the need for characterizing the dispersion with respect to particle size.

C. Properties of Aerosols Relevant to Their Generation, Sampling, and Deposition in the Respiratory System

The term *aerosol* was coined by F. G. Donnan toward the end of World War I to cover fine aerial suspensions [1]. An aerosol was to be the counterpart of the liquid colloidal suspension, the hydrosol, although it has since been realized that the analogy breaks down because of the inherent instability of the aerosol as compared with the hydrosol. Throughout this work we have applied it to systems in which particle size is sufficiently small to confer some degree of stability. Most of the airborne particles of toxicologic significance can be considered under the generic term aerosols. This category includes particulate material in either solid or liquid form and may also include gases and vapors absorbed on airborne particles. Airborne particles may be grouped into several broad categories.

Viable Particles

Airborne viable particles are primarily of two broad types: pollen and microorganisms. Although the airborne pollen grains are a vital link in the life cycle of many plants, they are associated with an unwelcomed side effect on humans, i.e., pollinosis (hay fever), a disease that severely affects 5–10% of the population of the United States [2]. The microorganisms in the air include viruses, bacteria, spores, rusts, molds, yeasts, fungi, protozoa, and algae. Many of these have purposes in the ecological cycle useful to humans; others are associated with disease in humans, animals and plants.

While most viable particulates are of natural origin, humans provide artificial sources such as sewage treatment plants and rendering plants. Direct dissemination of bacteria and viruses from people is of particular importance in indoor air. They arise from activities involving the respiratory tract such as sneezing and coughing and from the skin or wounds. They also arise from the redissemination and reentrainment of organism-bearing particulates which have accumulated in the dust of rooms, streets, sidewalks, etc. Table 3 shows the size range of airborne viable particulates [3].

Nonviable Particles

Nonviable airborne particles can be grouped into dispersion aerosols, condensation aerosols, and condensation and dispersion aerosols. *Dispersion aerosols* are formed by the transfer of powders into a state of suspension, the grinding

Table 3 Size Range of Viable Particulates

Particulate	Stoke's diameter (μm)
Viruses	0.015–0.45
Bacteria	0.3–15
Fungi	3–100
Algae	0–5
Protoza	2–10,000
Moss spores	6–30
Fern spores	20–60
Pollen grains (windborne)	10–100
Plant fragments, seeds, insects, other microfauna	100+

of solids, or atomization of liquids. Dispersion of solids requires the input of energy. Dispersion aerosols with solid particles are called dusts. Usually dusts are heterogeneous in composition and contain a wide range of particle sizes.

A *condensation aerosol* is formed when saturated vapors are condensed or when gases react chemically to form a volatile or nonvolatile product. Examples of these types of aerosols are fog and metal fumes.

Condensation and dispersion aerosols with liquid particles are called mists. On the other hand, condensation aerosols with solid disperse phase or a solid and liquid disperse phase are called "smokes." Traditionally, the term smoke has been used to describe products from incomplete combustion of fuel and other combustible material. Other nomenclature is used in the air pollution field. They include "haze," which is used in association with decreased visibility and denotes the presence of dust, mist, and pollutant gases; "smog" (smoke and fog); and "smaze" (smoke and haze).

Shapes of Airborne Particles

Aerosols present in nature or in industrial operations are associated with a variety of shapes. These shapes affect to some extent their aerodynamic behavior and consequently their site of deposition in the respiratory tract [4–6]. Also, in some cases, such as mineral fibers, the shape is directly connected to their toxic effect [7,8]. Airborne particles can be classified according to their shape into spherical, cubical, irregular, flaky, fibrous, and condensation flocs [9]. Spherical particles include atomized liquids, condensation solids (fly ash), and pollen. Various geometric shapes are formed due to formation of crystals such as sodium chloride crystals. Grinding or various processes of attrition of minerals usually produce irregular shapes. Examples of these types of particles are silica and coal dust. Mica, vermiculate, and perlite particles have unique flakes, platelets, or hollow spheroid shapes. Fibrous materials like asbestos, glass, mineral wool, cotton, wool, and a variety of synthetic materials can also be airborne. Agglomerates can result from particles combining while they are airborne or can be formed during condensation processes. They are characterized by chainlike appearance and are usually called flocs. These particles can also be formed during incomplete combustion of fuels; they can then contain a large amount of carbon. Particle shapes and physical data for particle identification can be found in the particle atlas by McCrone and Delly [10].

Particle Sizes

Perhaps no other category of toxic substances exhibits the degree of interdependence of physical characteristics and toxicity as does aerosols. One of the most important of these physical properties is the particle size. There are many direct ways of measuring the size of a particle. They include measurement of a linear dimension of the particle silhouette, the particle perimeter, or the projected area of the particle. Because these types of measurements are performed using optical or electron microscopy they cannot account for variation in particle density or in particle shape. On the other hand, there are indirect methods that measure some of the properties of the particles that can be related to the particle size. Among these properties are light scattering, electric charges on the particles, their settling velocity, diffusion, surface area, and finally the determination of the particle volume by measuring the change in electrolytic resistivity of a fluid volume containing the particle.

Because particle deposition depends primarily on particle aerodynamic properties, and because most of the particles encountered in occupational exposures are irregular in shape and of variable densities, it is necessary to define the particle size in relation to its aerodynamic behavior. The Stokes diameter (d_s) is defined as the diameter of a sphere having the same settling velocity as the particle, and a density equal to that of the bulk material from which the particle was formed. By definition, estimation of the Stokes diameter requires that we know the particle density. This parameter is not always known or in some cases, particles are formed from materials of many densities. To overcome this difficulty a new concept has been introduced; that is, describing the particle size in terms of its aerodynamic equivalent diameter (AED), d_e. It is defined as the diameter of a sphere having the same settling velocity as the particle and a density equal to 1 g/cm^3. The concept of particle aerodynamic diameter to describe particle behavior in air has been widely accepted by aerosol physicists [11] as well as by the medical profession [12–14].

The prime consideration in characterizing the potential toxic effects of airborne particulate matter is the description of the chemical composition and

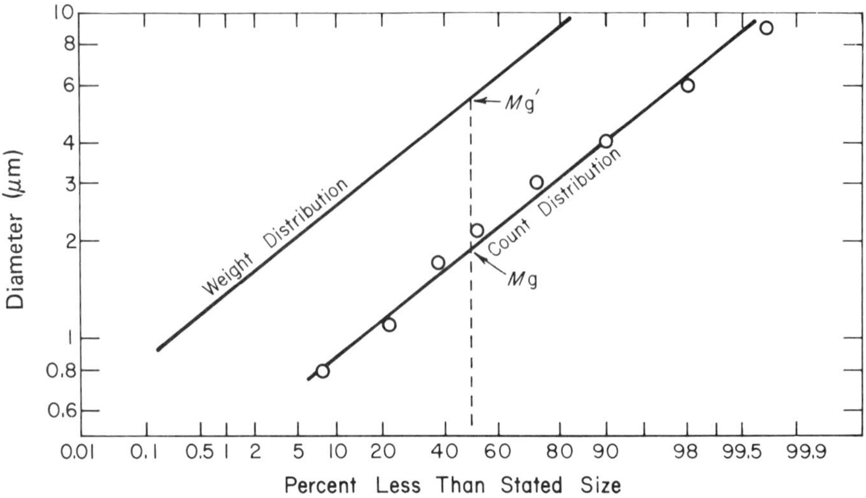

Figure 3 Typical presentation of particle size data on logarithmic probability graph paper.

the state of subdivision of the material present in a given volume of air. It should be noted that except under experimental conditions, the airborne particles constitute a distribution of sizes that differ from one population to another. Thus, the means of particle size may be the same, yet each population contains different numbers of particles or different mass concentration. Several mathematical distribution functions have been used to describe the size distribution of airborne particles. The most widely used is the logarithmic normal distribution. It is applied to the count, area as well as the weight distributions. The log-normal particle count distribution is:

$$Y = \frac{1}{\ln \sigma g \sqrt{2\pi}} \exp- \left[\frac{(\ln d - \ln Mg)^2}{2 \ln^2 \sigma g} \right] \tag{1}$$

where Y is the probability density, d the diameter of particle, σg geometric standard deviation, and Mg the geometric mean diameter. Half the number of particles in the distribution is larger that Mg and the other half is smaller than this size. In practice, a log-probability paper may be used to plot the percentage of particles less than stated size versus the logarithms of the stated size (Fig. 3). From the plot, Mg is taken at the 50% value of particle diameter d and

$$\sigma g = \frac{50\% \text{ value of d}}{16\% \text{ value of d}} = \frac{84\% \text{ value of d}}{50\% \text{ value of d}} \tag{2}$$

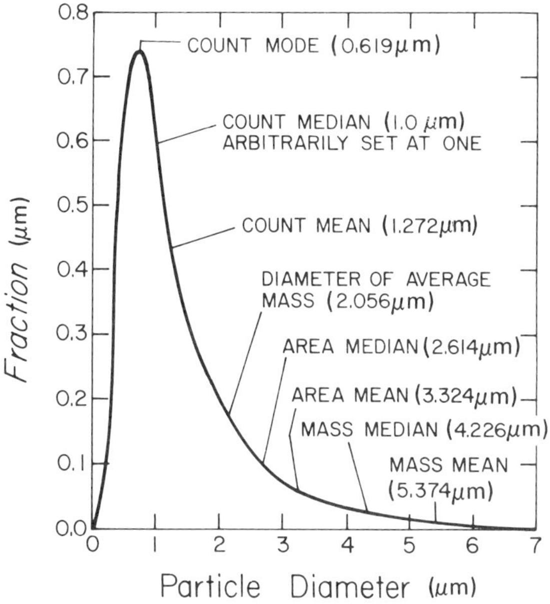

Figure 4 An example of a log normal distribution for mg = 1.0 μm and σg = 2.0 showing various average diameters.

One of the interesting properties of the log-normal distribution is that σg is the same for moments about the count, area, and weight mean geometric diameters. Also, the area median diameter Ma and mass median diameter Mg′ can be calculated from Mg and σg as follows:

$$\log_{10} \text{Ma} = \log_{10} \text{Mg} + 4.6 \log_{10}{}^2 \sigma g \qquad (3)$$

$$\log_{10} \text{Mg}' = \log_{10} \text{Mg} + 6.9 \log^2 \sigma g \qquad (4)$$

Figure 4 shows the locations of several characterizing statistical parameters of a particle size distribution curve adhering to the log normal distribution.

Surface Characteristics and Interfacial Phenomena

The properties of airborne particles related to their surface characteristics are specific area, rate of evaporation and condensation, electrostatic charge, adsorption, adhesion, and light scattering.

Surface Area and Adsorption The total surface area per unit mass of particulate matter increases rapidly with the decrease in their size. For example, a cube of 1 cm of any material has a total surface area of 6 cm^2. If it is divided into 1 mm cubes, the total surface area will be increased to 60 cm^2; further, if it is divided into 1 μm cubes the surface area will increase dramatically to 6 m^2. The subdivision of some granular materials increases their toxicity [15]. In addition, increase in surface area leads to increased chemical reaction rate and adsorption or absorption of gases on the particle surfaces. The toxicological significance of particle surface area is demonstrated by the Pylev study in which the same amounts of benzo[a]pyrene (5 mg) in a suspension with particulate matter were administered intratracheally into the lungs of rats [16]. The particles used were carbon black (3047°A in diameter and 10.6 m^2/g) and channel black (128°A in diameter and 250 m^2/g). Pylev found that elimination of the benzo[a]pyrene was inhibited by the suspension with the largest surface area. Pylev and Shabad also investigated the adsorption of benzo[a]pyrene by chrysotile asbestos. They showed that no pulmonary tumors were developed in animals treated with pure (benzene extracted) asbestos, while pulmonary tumors were found in 28.6% of the animals that received asbestos with adsorbed benzo[a]pyrene treatment [17].

Unfortunately, the specific surface area of airborne particulate matter has received little attention. Few investigations are reported, notably those by Corn et al., for suspended particulate matter for Pittsburgh [18] and its seasonal variation [19]. They also reported on the surface area of ground coal [20] and respirable dust samples from three coal mines [21]. In all of these investigations, the total particle surface area was determined by the BET method using incremental adsorption of krypton gas [22].

Evaporation and Condensation Evaporation or condensation is a diffusional mass transfer process which proceeds in proportion to the surface area exposed [23,24]. These properties are important for the stability of an aerosol if it is composed of liquid droplets or hygroscopic particles. The factors that affect the evaporation of a single droplet in still air are the droplet diameter, density, temperature, molecular weight, the diffusion coefficient of vapor from the particle, and the difference between the partial pressure at drop surface and in the surrounding air. However, for an aerosol cloud, the rate of evaporation from any given droplet is affected by the presence of other similar droplets in its vicinity. For droplets of aqueous solutions, the rate of evaporation is reduced because of the presence of the solute. For example, by addition of materials that suppress evaporation, the evaporation time of a 40 μm diameter droplet can be increased 100 fold [1].

The hygroscopic nature of a particle is an important factor in the deposition of particles in the lung. In the humid atmosphere of the lung soluble particles become droplets of solution and grow rapidly. A 4 μm sodium chloride particle in transit from the nose to the alveolar sacs would grow to about 10 μm [25]. On the other hand, a hygroscopic crystal is considerably more dense than water, and the increase in its diameter as it takes up water is less significant to lung deposition than the ratios of the diameter would suggest. That is because a dense substance has to undergo a considerable increase in diameter before there is any significant increase in its aerodynamic diameter [11]. Evaporation and condensation properties of aerosols are of vital importance in inhalation therapy. These properties as well as others have been reviewed by Morrow [12] and more recently by Newhouse and Ruffin [13].

Electrostatic Charge Aerosol particles acquire electrostatic charges either during their generation process or from collisions with atmospheric ions. The number of charges acquired by particles is limited by the breakdown strength of the surrounding medium. In the case of dry air this is about 8 esu/cm^2 or 1.6×10^{10} electrons per cm^2. It is possible to create charges which exceed this value under certain conditions; however, the usual levels observed are considerably less [1,26,27].

Charges of both signs may appear about equally after dispersion of small particles into a cloud, and the net charge of the aerosol cloud may be quite small even when individual particles in the cloud are highly charged [27]. The acquisition of opposite charges on particles affects their stability and may lead to false size data due to collision and agglomeration. The presence of electrostatic charges also causes severe problems during production of aerosols, especially those of hygienic significance, i.e., less than 10 μm. Deposition of particles in the respiratory tract is enhanced when the aerosol is charged [28,29].

Undesirable charge effects may be counteracted by exposing the aerosol to a very high bipolar concentration of ions to bring about a rapid equilibration of particle charge. This can be achieved with radioactive sources [30] or with a corona discharge in a suitably designed jet orifice [31]. Theories of electrical behavior of aerosols have been reviewed by White [26] and Whitby and Liu (see Ref. 32).

Adhesion The factors that affect the phenomenon of particle adhesion are van der Waals forces, electrostatic charges, contact points, roughness of the surface, and finally the surface tension of any liquid adsorbed on the surfaces of contact. In the case of particles present in ambient air, water vapor is adsorbed owing to the hydrogen bonding. As a result, the forces of adhesion in these cases are related to humidity. Therefore, reduction of moisture content of dust is required before dispersing it into the air. Because electrostatic charges tend to accumulate at reduced humidity, a careful balance must be sought for best dispersal results, this being a matter of experiment for a given sample. Extensive reviews of the practical and theoretical factors affecting particle adhesion were reported by Corn (see Ref. 32) and Zimon [33].

Specific Gravity

The specific gravity of a particle formed by a grinding or attrition process from a solid will be the same as that of the parent material. The same is true also for liquid droplets formed by atomization. However, because particles are subject to evaporation, condensation, surface oxidation, or agglomeration, their density will change.

When particles agglomerate the resulting particle has a different geometric form and includes void spaces. Therefore, the density of the particle cluster will be less than that of the inidvidual component particles. Thus, the density of an agglomerate may be less than one-tenth the density of the parent material [34].

In the case of porous material, there is a general tendency for the particle density to rise as the particles become finer [21,35].

It is difficult to determine individual particle densities in aerosols formed by atomization of liquid solutions. This is due to the differential drying of the liquid droplet containing a solute after initial generation [36–38].

There are few measurements of the density of suspended particulate matter in ambient air. It is estimated that the density of individual particles vary from 0.5 to 6.5 g/cm^3 [39]. The density of aerosols have been reported by Whitby et al. [40], Corn et al. [18], and Durham et al. [41].

Shape Factors

The various methods of particle size measurements should theoretically yield the same result for a perfect sphere. However, the variation between the diameters obtained by different methods increases as the particle increasingly diverges from spherical shape. Hence, the shape becomes an important factor in the correlation of results of particle sizing by different procedures. Particle shape factors are utilized to compare the particle sizes determined by microscopic measurement to those determined by an aerodynamic method, for example. Shape factors are statistical quantities and are not intended to be applied to individual particles. For nonspherical particles, the shape factors must be determined empirically. Consequently, any shape factor is valid only for a specific method of measurement of the size, specific material, and, perhaps, a specific method of preparation. Shape factors serve three main functions:

1. They are the factors of proportionality between particle size determination results by different methods.

2. They are conversion factors for expressing determination results in terms of an "equivalent" sphere.
3. They permit one to transform particle diameter into the particle surface and particle volume, respectively.

The derivation of shape factors are described in detail by Herdan [42], Hodkinson [43], and Mercer [11]. Shape factors for various materials have been extensively reported in the literature. See, for example, Kotrappa [44] for quartz; Shrag and Corn [45] for silica, mica, and fly ash; Stein and Corn [21] for respirable coal mine dust; Mercer et al. [46] for fibers, cluster, and chain aggregates; and Stein et al. [39,47] for atmospheric particles.

Aerodynamic Properties

The evaluation and control of airborne particulate hazards frequently depend on the knowledge of particle motion with respect to fluid motion. For example, the deposition of particles in the human respiratory tract, the design of sampling instruments, and the design of industrial ventilation systems for dust control are governed by the kinetic behavior of particles. The motion of particles in a fluid can result from one or more of the following processes:

1. Field forces: gravitational, electrical, magnetic
2. Particle and fluid mechanics: drag forces, inertial forces, centrifugal forces or vortex flow
3. Other processes: diffusion, thermal gradient (thermophoresis), photophoresis (photon flux), acoustic phenomena (alternating pressure field)

In this section a brief review of particle dynamics will be presented. Comprehensive treatment of this subject can be found in handbooks on aerosol physics and mechanics [1,11,32,48–51].

Sedimentation Small spherical particles falling in air rapidly attain a terminal settling velocity, closely approximated by Stokes law [1].

$$U_t = \frac{(\rho_p - \rho_f)d_s^2\ g}{18\mu_f} C_c \tag{5}$$

where C_c is the Cunningham slip correction factor:

$$C_c = 1 + \frac{A2\lambda}{d_s} + \frac{B2\lambda}{d_s} \exp - \frac{bd_s}{2\lambda} \tag{6}$$

where A = 1.234, B = 0.413, b = 0.904, and λ is the mean free path of gas molecules = 9.322×10^{-6} μm [50], for air at 20°C and 760 mmHg.

The slip correction factor modifies the basic Stokes law for particles sizes approaching the mean free of gas molecules. These particles are suspended in a noncontinuous medium and as a result their mobility increases. Generally, the slip correction factor should be applied for particles less than 2 μm in diameter.

For particles moving in air, the basic Stokes law can be modified because the density of air ρ_f (1.2×10^{-3} g/cm^3) is very small compared to the density of particles ρ_p (1.4 g/cm^3 for coal dust).

$$U_t = \frac{\rho_p d_s^2 g}{18\mu_f} C_c \tag{7}$$

from Equation 7, and from the definitions of Stokes diameter d_s and the aerodynamic diameter d_e, it can be shown that

$$d_e = d_s \sqrt{\rho_p} \tag{8}$$

Impaction When an obstacle is introduced into flowing, dust-laden air, the smaller particles are able to follow the air flow lines around the obstacle, whereas the larger particles, because of their greater inertia, are unable to change their direction with the air and are thus impacted on the obstacle. This impaction process is one of the main mechanisms for particle deposition in the respiratory tract. It is also used for aerosol sampling and sizing instruments. In Equation 7, the quantity

$$\frac{\rho_p d_s^2}{18\mu_f} C_c$$

has a dimension of time. It is called the particle relaxation time τ, the time a particle needs to adapt itself, or relax, to an applied force. If a particle is projected in still air with a velocity V, it will travel a certain distance S during time τ, before it comes to rest. This distance is called the particle stop distance and it is a characteristic of its inertial properties.

The Stokes number or impaction parameter I is a dimensionless ratio of the particle stop distance to the characteristic dimension D of the obstacle (e.g., diameter of the obstacle such as a sphere, disk, cylinder, or width of the ribbon on which particles impact):

$$I = \frac{S}{D} = \frac{V\tau}{D} = \frac{V}{D}\frac{\tau_p d_s^2}{18\mu_f} C_c = \frac{V}{D}\frac{U_t}{g} \tag{9}$$

Interception The model considered for impaction assumed particles had mass, and hence inertia, but no size except when calculating the resistance of air for cross-stream movement. By allowing for the actual particle size, an interception mechanism is considered where the particle has size, but no mass, and so follow the stream lines of air around the collector. If the streamline on which the particle center lies approaches to closer than d/2 to the collector, the particle will touch the collector and be intercepted. Interception is characterized by a parameter R, which is the ratio of the diameters of particle d and the intercepting body D:

$$R = \frac{d}{D} \tag{10}$$

Brownian Movement (Diffusion) Brownian movement was first described in 1828 by the botanist, Robert Brown. While investigating the pollen of several plants, he observed that the pollen dispersed in water had an irregular swarming motion. Half a century later, scientists found that this erratic, zigzag movement of particles is caused by their continued bombardment by the molecules of the fluid.

Particle diffusivity was investigated by Einstein in 1905 [52]. He showed that particle diffusivity can be found from:

$$D_c = C_c \frac{KT}{3\pi\mu_f d} \tag{11}$$

where D_c is the particle diffusion coefficient (cm^2/sec), K is the Boltzman constant (1.37×10^{-16} erg/°C), and, T is the absolute temperature.

The above equation shows that the diffusivity increases with the decrease in particle size and becomes significant for particles less than 0.5 μm in diameter where the root mean square Brownian displacement per second is larger than the falling distance due to gravity in the same time period.

Coagulation Coagulation of aerosols is the process of adhesion of aerosol particles upon contact with one other forming larger particles. This process causes an aerosol to become more and more coarsely dispersed. The forces and mechanisms causing coagulation are thermal, electrical, magnetic, molecular, gravitational, inertial, etc. The most important of these mechanisms is thermal coagulation where aerosols undergo numerous collisions with each other because of their random Brownian movements. The rate of coagulation depends primarily on the number concentration of the particles, available at any point in time. Thus, it can be shown that:

$$\frac{1}{N} - \frac{1}{N_o} = Kt \tag{12}$$

where N_o is the initial number of particles, N is the number of particles at time t, and K is the coefficient of coagulation.

The classic work on this subject was done by Whytlaw-Gray and Patterson [34], and more recent reviews are presented by Green and Lane [1] and Zebel (see Ref. 32).

It should be noted that, unlike gases, an aerosol cloud in a confined space is continuously changing its size distribution and mass concentration owing to:

1. Loss of particles to the floor by sedimentation
2. Loss of particles to the walls and floor by diffusion
3. Loss of particles by coagulation

III. Effects and Sites of Action of Airborne Contaminants on Respiratory System

Henderson and Haggard [53] indicated that the classification of physiologic effects of air contaminants are not entirely satisfactory because with many gases and vapors the type of physiological action depends on concentration. A vapor at one concentration may exert its principal action as an anesthetic, whereas at lower concentration, with no anesthetic effect, it may injure the nervous system. Henderson and Haggard, however, presented a broad physiological classification for gases and vapors that was widely accepted by toxicologists in the occupational health field. In this section, we will attempt to expand that classification to include airborne particulates.

A. Asphyxiants

This category of gases consists of those that have the capacity to deprive tissues of oxygen through some means other than interference with the mechanics of respiration. They can be separated into two distinct groups, simple asphyxiants and chemical asphyxiants.

Simple axphyxiants are physiologically inert gases that when present in sufficient quantity in the inspired air prevent body tissues from receiving an adequate oxygen supply. Nitrogen, hydrogen, and helium are examples of this type of gas.

Chemical asphyxiants prevent the body from utilizing an adequate oxygen supply. Two classic examples of this category are carbon monoxide and cyanides. Carbon monoxide (CO) toxicity is based on its affinity for hemoglobin, which is over 200 times that of oxygen for the hemoglobin molecule. CO combines with hemoglobin to form carboxyhemoglobin, reducing the total oxygen-carrying capacity of circulating blood. In contrast to CO, cyanide interferes with a great many enzymes, the most significant of which is cytochrome oxidase. Thus, it prevents the utilization of O_2 by the tissues.

B. Irritants

Irritants are corrosive materials that inflame moist and mucous surfaces. Usually the concentration factor is of greater significance than the duration of exposure.

The inflammatory process is essentially the same regardless of the site of action of the compound, but the symptoms differ. The differences in the sites of action mainly reflect differences in solubility, boiling points, and volatility of the irritant materials. Inflammation of the upper respiratory tract leads to rhinitis, pharyngitis, and laryngitis; inflammation of the bronchi results in bronchitis and bronchopneumonia; inflammation of the lungs leads to pulmonary edema and pneumonia.

The solubility of an irritant is the most important factor in determining its site of action within the respiratory tract. Highly soluble materials primarily affect the upper respiratory tract. Examples in this category include ammonia, alkaline dusts, hydrogen chloride, and sulfur dioxide. Compounds of intermediate solubility affect both upper respiratory tract and pulmonary tissue. Halogens, ozone, and toluene diisocyanate (TDI) are examples of compounds with intermediate solubility. Insoluble materials like nitrogen dioxide and phosgene affect the terminal respiratory passages and air sacs. It should be noted that there are some exceptions; for example, bromobenzyl cyanide, an upper respiratory tract irritant, is a relatively insoluble vapor [54].

Irritants are also subdivided into primary and secondary categories. A primary irritant causes no systemic toxic effect because the products formed on the respiratory tract tissues are nontoxic. Examples of this category are hydrochloric acid and sulfuric acid. Secondary irritants not only irritate the mucous membranes of the respiratory tract but also a significant systemic effect results from the absorption of the compound. Hydrogen sulfide and many aromatic hydrocarbons are examples of this type.

Because irritants constitute the majority of airborne contaminants affecting the respiratory system, it is interesting to note that they can be further classified in terms of their effects on the mechanics of respiration. One group of irritants increases the flow resistance, decreases compliance, and at high concentrations decreases breathing frequency. Irritants in this group include sulfur dioxide, sulfuric acid, formaldehyde, and acrolein. The other group has slight effects on the resistance but decreases compliance and increases respiratory rate. Irritants in this group include oxides of nitrogen and ozone.

C. Anesthetics and Narcotics

This group includes a large number of volatile hydrocarbons of wide industrial use. While these gases and vapors have little or no effect on the lungs, they act as simple anesthesia after they have been absorbed into the blood. For some, the action is limited to functional disturbances; others may injure other organs of the body. Examples of the first category are nitrous oxide, ethers, and aldehydes. Anesthetic vapors may injure the visceral organs (chlorinated hydrocarbons), the hematopoietic system (benzene), or the nervous system (methyl alcohol, carbon disulfide, and esters or organic acids).

D. Systemic Poisons

The airborne contaminants that can be classified as systemic poisons include materials that cause organic injury to visceral organs, hematopoietic system, and the nervous systems as mentioned in the previous sections. They also include toxic metals: lead, mercury, cadmium, manganese, beryllium, etc., as well as toxic nonmetallic inorganic materials such as arsenic, phosphorus, and sulfur.

E. Sensitizers

Sensitizers are those materials that produce an antigen-antibody complex resulting in an allergic-type reaction in the body. The end results of this reaction in the body may be the release of histamine, the formation of reagin antibody, or complement-fixing complexes of antigen and precipitating antibody. These reactions can be immediate or delayed for up to 12 hr. Recently, it was found that other pathways may be activated, with similar end results. Thus, chemicals that are not protein in nature, e.g., isocyanates or sulfur dioxide, may precipitate reactions similar to those caused by antigen-antibody reactions. These reactions result in complex biochemical alterations of the tracheobronchial airway smooth muscle tone, causing bronchoconstriction and consequently an increase in airway resistance.

Examples of proteinaceous sensitizing materials are castor oil, pollen, and other ill-defined agents causing farmer's lungs, byssinosis, and bagassosis. Nonproteinaceous materials may precipitate disorders similar to allergic reactions and include TDI, diphenyl methane diisocyanate (MDI), and sulfur dioxide.

F. Fibrosis

Since fibroblasts are present in the interstitium of the lungs, these cells can be stimulated to form excessive amounts of reticulin or collagen. Excessive collagen formation is likely to accompany prolonged or chronic pulmonary inflammation. The pathogenesis of pulmonary fibrosis caused by deposition of some types of dust is not entirely clear, and various theories explaining this process have been suggested [55]. The accepted theory at the present time is that based on destruction of lung macrophage. It is postulated that since the macrophage contains small vesicles holding potent enzymes, these substances may be released by certain ingested particles, but not all particles, thus altering the cell milieu and causing premature death of the macrophage. The products released by the macrophage stimulate the fibroblast to lay down adequate amounts of collagen that promote tissue fibrosis [56]. Free crystalline silica is a typical example of airborne particulates causing such reaction. It has been also suggested that long asbestos fibers not completely engulfed within the macrophage permit leakage of macrophage content, and this material might also stimulate the increased activity of fibroblasts [57].

It should be noted that exposure to sublethal doses of the oxides of nitrogen may at first cause pulmonary edema, but later bronchopneumonia and bronchiolitis obliterans develop. The later condition is usually associated with interstitial fibrosis. This type of pulmonary fibrosis is also known as silo-filler's disease [58].

G. Carcinogens

Of all the occupational health aspects of concern to professional workers in the disciplines involved with occupational medicine and industrial hygiene, the role of carcinogenic agents is the most vexing and perhaps the most poorly understood. Over 1500 chemical substances are suspected to have a potential as chemical carcinogens.

Various airborne contaminants have been shown to induce cancer in the various tissues of the respiratory tract. A correlation between radon exposure and lung cancer was reported in uranium mines in the United States [59], iron ore mines in Sweden [60], and hematile mines in England [61]. Other occupational exposure with established risks of lung cancer include nickel workers [62], asbestos workers [63], and gas workers [64].

IV. Standards and Guidelines for Airborne Concentrations of Potentially Toxic Chemicals

Prior to enactment of the Occupational Safety and Health Act of 1970, the principal guidelines for the concentrations of airborne contaminants to which workers should be exposed were those developed by the American Conference of Governmental Industrial Hygienists; they are known as threshold limit values [65]. Threshold limit values (TLV) have a time base for permissible exposure. Thus, the TLV-time weighted average (TLV-TWA) is the concentration to which nearly all workers may be repeatedly exposed, day after day, for a normal 8 hr workday or 40 hr workweek for 40 years. The TLV-short-term exposure limit (TLV-STEL) is the maximum concentration to which workers can be exposed for a period of up to 15 continuous minutes without suffering from (1) intolerable irritation, (2) chronic or irreversible tissue change, or (3) narcosis of sufficient degree to increase accident proneness, impair self-rescue, or materially reduce work efficiency. No more than four excursions per day are permitted within this limit, with at least 50 min between exposure periods, and provided the TLV-TWA also is not exceeded. The STEL is associated with a 15 min maximal concentration. A third TLV, the TLV-ceiling (TLV-C), is the concentration which is not exceeded, even instantaneously.

TLV are guidelines. The ACGIH cautions "that they are not intended as absolute boundaries between safe and dangerous conditions." The TLV are reviewed by ACGIH annually, as new information becomes available. There are now TLV for approximately 600 substances; new compounds and changes to those on the list occur annually. Supporting evidence for TLV is contained in Documentation of Threshold Limit Values [65]. It should be noted that compounds which have been associated with cancer in humans, or are suspected of being human carcinogens, are not assigned TLV; exposure to these agents should be avoided.

The 1968 TLV values were adopted by OSHA as legal standards. Table Z-1 of OSHA standard is a compendium of the 1968 TLV *but under OSHA they are applicable to a single 8 hr period of exposure and are legally enforceable.* In addition, OSHA adopts on an ongoing basis permanent standards for toxic substances in the work environment. A permanent OSHA standard includes many provisions in addition to the permissible exposure limit (PEL) for the substance in air. OSHA must adhere to the U.S. Administrative Procedures Act to adopt standards. Thus, standards must be proposed, public hearings must be held, posthearing comment periods permitted, etc. Standards can also be legally challenged in the courts. Standard setting is a slow process; OSHA has promulgated approximately 20 permanent standards for toxic substances (called "health standards") since its inception in 1970. Because of these procedural safeguards in standard setting, OSHA would have to follow the same lengthy process to revise the 1968 TLV. So we see that although ACGIH reviews TLV annually, OSHA adopted 1968 TLV early in the Agency's operation and continues to use these values as legal standards, with few exceptions, i.e., asbestos.

Only a small fraction of the many thousands of chemicals used in industry and commerce are listed by ACGIH as TLV or are covered by OSHA as standards. The medical or environmental professional should utilize TLV and OSHA standards as the basis for judging the adequacy of breathing air in the work environment. Where a TLV or OSHA standard is not relevant, the existing toxicological literature must be consulted to establish an unofficial guideline for good practice.

V. Sampling Strategies for Epidemiologic Survey

A. Types of Surveys

The predominant purpose of occupational epidemiology is the search for causal associations between diseases and environmental exposure. Ideally, an epidemiological hypothesis should specify:

1. The characteristics of the persons to whom the hypothesis applies, i.e., the population
2. The cause being investigated, i.e., environmental exposure
3. The expected effect or disease

Thus, a dose-response relationship is derived that specifies the amount of the cause needed to lead to a stated incidence of the effect. Another relationship is also sought, that is, a time-response relationship. It specifies the time period that will elapse between exposure to the cause and observation of the effect.

Epidemiological studies can be characterized by whether the ascertainment of cause and effect relate to a single point (cross-sectional) or to two different points in time (longitudinal).

One of the difficulties associated with a longitudinal study is the waiting time that elapses between the selection of the population and the development of disease (prospective study). This difficulty can be eliminated if the cause and effect under investigation are such that they can both be ascertained from existing records (retrospective study).

The contribution of the industrial hygienist in these investigations is to evaluate the environmental exposure, e.g., to determine the dose received by every individual of the population under investigation. Environmental surveys conducted in conjunction with cross-sectional and prospective studies are relatively easy to design and perform, since all the pertinent information about industrial processes, raw materials, final products and by-products, and their toxic potential can be gathered at the time of the survey. Also, environmental and health measurements are obtained simultaneously.

The present state of the art in knowledge and technology can be also applied in planning and executing the environmental survey. Another important aspect is the standardization of sampling methods throughout all the phases of the prospective study.

Retrospective investigations suffer from serious limitations because of lack or uncertainty of information about previous exposure. For example, sampling for free silica, asbestos, synthetic mineral fibers such as fibrous glass and mineral wool, and cotton dust at the present time is performed according to standard methods recommended by NIOSH that differ from the sampling methods utilized in the past. As a result, a whole range of investigations have been carried out to determine if there is any correlation between the current and obsolete methods. Some of these have met with success, but most often poor correlations are obtained [66–68]. Due to technological progress, some drastic changes in industrial operations may have occurred in the past, which lead to alterations in physical and chemical properties as well as concentration of airborne contaminants. A typical case is the exposure to free silica in the Vermont granite sheds. The advent of pneumatic tools and new cutting and polishing machines caused dust concentrations to increase by factors of 10 to 100 as compared with manual operations. On the other hand, the quartz content of the respirable fraction diminished from 13–17% to about 9% [66]. Comparison between present and past exposure was obtained by reconstructing earlier working conditions using contemporary tools and work practice of the 1920s [69].

B. Approach to Occupational Environmental Survey

In a study of the health status of the workers in any industry, work environment must be defined in some meaningful way. Many variables affecting the host, agent, and environment should be taken into consideration and the possible confounding variables should be eliminated or at least controlled.

Selection of Plants

The identification of plants to be included in an epidemiological study should represent a profile of the whole industry. Theoretically, random or stratified random sampling can be utilized to identify the plants. However, for practical and logistic reasons other important factors may influence the selection process. For example, the selected plants should cover a wide spectrum of exposure to provide meaningful qualitative environmental distinctions. Inclusion of modern and old plants can serve that purpose, since modern plants usually utilize automated enclosed systems and to some extent efficient ventilation, while older plants are most likely to use batch processes. They can also provide more distinct categories for studies of time-response relationships. Due to technological progress and change of processes in some plants, past exposure of workers can be better estimated if older industrial processes are still utilized in the old plants. Sometimes, unique processes not usually present in all plants of any given industry may provide insight about the toxic properties of the agent under investigation. In an epidemiological study on the etiologic factor of byssinosis, El-Batawi and Shash [70] found that workers carding medical cotton have neither byssinosis nor significant changes in ventilatory capacity during the day. They concluded that the active agent is water soluble and that byssinosis did not result from the cellulose fraction of cotton dust. This significant contribution to the understanding of that disease could have been missed entirely if the investigators included only carding operations from textile industry in their study.

As much as there are valid reasons for selection and inclusion of certain plants in a health survey, there are valid reasons to eliminate others. In an epidemiological study of the health status of workers engaged in the production of synthetic mineral fibers carried out by Tulane Medical Center (H. Weill, personal communication, 1979), plants processing, or were known to have used, asbestos in their insulation products were not included in the study. Similarly, plants producing textile-type glass fibers (usually larger than 6 μm in diameter) were not included because these fibers are not in the respirable range.

It should be noted that the abovementioned process of selection and elimination should be performed after a thorough understanding of the industry's raw materials, products, by-products, and processing operations. The team, usually industrial hygienists, epidemiologists, and statisticians engaged in the selection process, should visit some representative plants of the industry.

Exposure Classification

Effective exposure classification schemes should satisfy the following criteria: (1) identify the exposure of every worker in the population; (2) reduce the number of potential toxic materials to a minimum; (3) each exposure group in the scheme should be homogeneous and cover a range adequate for meaningful distinctions between groups; and (4) the number of workers in each group should be large enough for statistical analysis.

Various exposure classification schemes have been reported in the literature. The classifications were based on concentration of the airborne contaminant, work area, job titles, duration of employment, or a combination of two or more factors such as the concept of dust years, where the dust concentration multiplied by the years of employment is utilized for ranking of exposure.

Concentration of Airborne Contaminant Classification of exposure according to concentration of the contaminant has been successful only in the situations where a single etiologic agent is encountered, such as silica [66] or cotton dust [71]. It is a simplistic approach that does not take into consideration the time factor (duration of exposure). Its use has been abandoned and more sophisticated classifications have been developed.

Work Areas and Job Titles In the chemicals industries (paints and coatings, plastics, rubber, etc.), where the workers are simultaneously exposed to many types of airborne contaminants, development of classification schemes becomes very difficult. The toxic agents may have different effects that manifest themselves over variable time periods from the onset of exposure. This is further complicated by the possible unknown chemical reactions taking place during the industrial processes, and the synergistic or antagonistic toxic effects in humans. Also, because of the nature of the industrial processes, various components are used that vary from one day to another depending on the production schedule. Workers may be transferred from one job to another because of promotion or other reasons. Under these circumstances, the determination of the dose becomes virtually impossible. Under these circunstances exposure classification on a qualitative basis and to some extent quantitatively can be achieved by dividing the workers into groups according to production departments, work areas, or job titles performing similar operations and/or exposed to similar agents.

Mancuso et al., in their mortality study in the rubber industry [72], could not develop a scheme for exposure classifications. They divided the workers into four groups according to the production departments of the manufacturering company. However, they concluded that the total duration of work by category is necessary and that classification by department is probably inadequate because of the many causes of mortality and multiple exposures within and between departments.

In a mortality study of steel workers, Lloyd and Ciocco [73] and Lloyd et al. [74] were able to classify the workers in 54 work areas. They showed that cause-specific mortality was associated with work areas, without recording the specific environmental toxic substances. McMichael et al. [75, 76] and Gamble and Spirtas [77] in another study of the health experience of rubber industry workers used a different classification scheme. They indicated that many jobs in the rubber industry cannot be objectively classified according to exposure. Also, because of the variety of jobs involved with different processes in a department, classification by department is not adequate. Consequently, the investigators developed what they called occupational titles. These categories comprise a number of jobs grouped together on the basis of operation (types of machine and/or process), stock (calendar, tread, beads), and product (tubes, tires, flaps). For example, different jobs of building industrial, passenger, truck, and tractor tires were combined into one occupational title called tire building, which in any one plant might comprise four to five different departments. In this way, about 70 occupational titles were developed. The investigators stated that this classification scheme reduces the dilution effect which occurs when workers at low risk are combined with workers at high risk, and thereby pinpoint the areas of greater risk. Their scheme showed that lymphatic leukemia cases spent more times in jobs that have higher exposure to solvents than did the nonleukemia controls. It also showed that particular adhesive systems cause temporary losses in lung functions in two of the seven tested occupational titles.

Indices of Exposure The two classification schemes mentioned above are associated with major defects. They classify individuals according to concentration of airborne contaminant or their job duties at the time of the survey and do not take into consideration the variation of exposure or job changes during the period of employment. What is needed is an "index of exposure" that allows for total work history, inclusive of various exposures, and the corresponding times of that exposure. The closest common model that integrates the life time exposure or dose is:

$$D = \sum_{i=1}^{i} (C_j T_j) \tag{13}$$

where n is the number of times an individual has changed workplaces during his or her employment, T is the time spent in the same workplace, C_j is concentration of airborne contaminant, and J is the workplace. It should be noted that inherent in the above definition is the assumption that exposure to say 1.0 mg/m^3 of silica dust for 1 year is equivalent to 0.1 mg/m^3 for 10 years, an assumption that is not always valid especially for a chronic disease with a long latent period (asbestosis, silicosis) where the jobs of significance are those early in the work history.

Jahr [78] proposed an exposure index that would attach more importance to exposure a long time ago relative to more recent exposure, and would continue to increase after exposure had ended. He used time to weight exposure as follows:

$$D_W = \sum_{j=1}^{N} (Y - Y_j \div 1)C_j \tag{14}$$

where D_W is the weighted dose, Y is year of examination of individual, Y_j is year with mean exposure C_j, and N is the total number of years, starting with the first year of exposure.

One of the drawbacks of Jahr's model is that it ignores lung elimination. Thus, the two models would represent the extremes in construction of cumulative exposure indices. The first model takes no account of when exposure took place and the second takes no account of elimination. The British Thoracic and Tuberculosis Association (BTTA) [79] proposed a third model where elimination is taken into account. It is based on the assumption that over a long period dust is eliminated from the lungs at a rate proportional to the amount retained, and that risk is measured as cumulative dose weighted by residence time of each contribution. Hence, a family of measures of risk is produced. This family is characterized by the rate of exponential decay, or half-life time. The extremes being the cumulative dose (first model) with a half-life of zero and the cumulative dose weighted by time since exposure (second model) with a half-time of infinity.

The first model has been used extensively in the past for studies of dust exposure in the cotton textile industry [80], asbestos-cement industry [81], granite sheds [82], and gold mines in South Africa [83], as well as others. It has also been used in nondusty exposures such as vinyl chloride [84].

Berry et al. [85] were the first to correlate the health experience of workers and their asbestos dust exposure utilizing the three models. As expected, their data showed striking differences between the first and second models. They encountered some difficulties in utilizing the third model because half-life times could not be determined with adequate precision.

Duration and Number of Samples Usually, the duration of sampling is determined by the time necessary to obtain sufficient amounts of the airborne contaminant for accurate analysis. Hence, the duration will be based on the sensitivity of the analytical procedure, the concentration of the particular contaminant in air, and the sampling flow rate.

In the cases of contaminants whose toxicological properties warrant short-term and ceiling limit values, short-term (10–20 min) samples are utilized to define peak concentrations and estimate peak excursion durations. For standards based on time-weighted average concentrations, the samples are obtained over a full shift, or the time-weighted average exposure can be calculated from consecutive short-term samples.

The above mentioned instrumental/analytical and legal restrictions should not prevent the industrial hygienist from taking other influencing factors into consideration. The sampling period, for example, should represent some indentifiable period of time of the worker's exposure, usually a minimum of one complete cycle of his or her activity. This is particularly important in studying nonroutine or batch-type activities, which are characteristic of many industrial operations. Other examples are highly automated and enclosed operations, where processing is done automatically and the operator's exposure is relatively uniform. However, the worker can be exposed to an entirely different pattern during maintenance or trouble-shooting operations.

Roach [86] suggested that for substances that produce an acute response and for which peak concentrations may be of real significance, the sampling time should be related to the biological half-life of the contaminant in the body. Assuming that the body burden (x) of a given contaminant builds up in an exponential fashion, he was able to show that the maximum value of the coefficient of variation for the body burden during a sampling time t is:

$$CV(x) = 0.59 \frac{t^{1/2}}{T} CV(C) \tag{15}$$

where T is the biological half life of the substance in the bocy and CV(C) is the coefficient of variation of the concentration of the contaminant in air. On the basis of the above equation, Roach recommended that sampling time should be one-tenth of the biological half-life of the contaminant in the body. For this period, CV(x) is less than 19% of CV(C) and the average body burden would equal that attained in exposure to a constant concentration at the average level of that period.

In an ideal situation, each potentially exposed worker should be individually sampled. In most cases, however, we have to resort to a sampling strategy that produces the most efficient use of sampling resources. For compliance purposes, the industrial hygienist attempts to identify the employee(s) with maximum possible risk. For example, in a grinding operation, the worker operating the grinder would most likely be the employee at maximum risk from exposure to toxic particulates. The further the person is located from the source of generation the lower the possibility of significant exposure. However, this simple example is usually the exception rather than the rule. Workers' exposures are further complicated by their mobility, work practices, air movement within a work room, and the location of ventilation and exhaust systems. If the maximum-risk worker cannot be selected with reasonable certainty, then it is necessary to resort to random sampling from the group of workers (N). The objective of the procedure is to select a subgroup of adequate size (n) so that there is a high probability $(1 - \alpha)$ that the random sample contains at least one worker out of the high-risk workers (No). Hence, the following probability equation can be solved for n:

$$1 - \frac{(N - No)!}{(N - No - n)!} \frac{(N - n)!}{N} \leqslant 1 - \alpha \qquad (16)$$

Table 4 gives the required sample size n of a random sample drawn from a group of size N = 1 to 50 which ensures with 90% confidence that at least one individual from the highest 10% exposure group is contained in the sample.

It can readily be seen that this selection method depends solely on the total number of workers and, regardless of the environmental conditions, (n) will always be the same.

Afterward, the compliance officer or industrial hygienist obtains breathing zone samples for the selected group of workers and determines whether their exposure exceeds the standards set forth by OSHA. The NIOSH statistical procedures [87–90] for calculating the 95% lower confidence limit (LCL) should be utilized to make one of the following three decisions regarding the worker's exposure level:

1. Noncompliance

Table 4 Size of Partial Sample[a]

Size of group N	Number of required samples
8	7
9	8
10	9
11–12	10
13–14	11
15–17	12
18–20	13
21–24	14
25–29	15
30–37	16
38–49	17
50	18

[a]For top 10% and confidence 0.90.

2. No action
3. No decision

By "noncompliance" (during the sampling period) it is meant that the decision has been reached with a given probability that the worker's exposure level exceeds the Federal standard. By "no action" (during the sampling period) it is meant that the decision has been reached with a given probability that the worker's exposure level does not exceed the standard. Finally, by the "no decision" choice, it is meant that neither of the above choices can be asserted with a sufficiently high probability.

For environmental surveys geared to be utilized in conjunction with an epidemiological study, we are not interested in a high-risk individual as such. What we are trying to estimate is the exposure of the workers so that the dose can be related to the health experinece of the worker. In statistical terms we are trying to estimate a measure of central tendency (mean, median, etc.) and measure of dispersion (range, standard deviation, etc.) of the worker's exposure. If the true exposure of a group of workers is μ mg/m^3, (population mean) and a sample of size n yields a mean exposure $\bar{x}$ mg/m^3, then the error E in estimating the population mean is

$$E = \bar{x} - \mu \tag{17}$$

If the population standard deviation is σ mg/m^3, the quantity

$$\frac{\bar{x} - \mu}{\frac{\sigma}{\sqrt{n}}} \quad \text{or} \quad \frac{E}{\frac{\sigma}{\sqrt{n}}}$$

is a value of a random variable having or approximating a standard normal distribution. We can assert with a probability of $1 - \alpha$ that

$$-Z\frac{\alpha}{2} < \frac{E/\sigma}{\sqrt{n}} < Z\frac{\alpha}{2} \tag{18}$$

Where $Z(\alpha/2)$ is such that the normal curve area to its right equals $\alpha/2$, then

$$E < Z\frac{\alpha}{2}\frac{\sigma}{\sqrt{n}} \tag{19}$$

or

$$n < \left[\frac{Z(\alpha/2)\,\sigma}{E}\right]^2 \tag{20}$$

If we select the sample size n so that

$$n = \left[\frac{Z(\alpha/2)\,\sigma}{E}\right]^2 \tag{21}$$

then we can say that with a probability of $1 - \alpha$ the error in estimating N by means of $\bar{x}$ will be less than E.

The limitation of this procedure is that it requires previous knowledge of σ. A good estimate of the population standard deviation can be obtained from previous surveys carried out in similar industries or from a pilot study. It should also be noted that various investigations have shown that environmental data are usually better described by fitting a log normal distribution to the measurements [91]. The estimation procedure of the number of samples may be adjusted accordingly if the geometric standard deviation is larger than 1.4 [87].

Industrial Hygiene Records Record keeping has been one of the essential tools for industrial hygienists in managing, monitoring, and documenting their efforts in the evaluation and control of employee exposure. At the present time, regulatory standards require that certain records be kept regarding the exposure of employees as well as their health status. Industry, governmental agencies, and research institutions are also utilizing the exposure records as the primary source for statistical and epidemiological investigations. Physicians may need the employee's exposure data if a causal relationship is suspected between exposure and illness. In addition, corporate legal and employee relations staff consider the industrial hygiene records essential for health-related grievances and arbitration cases and for compensation claims.

Because industrial hygiene studies produce a large amount of data of various types, the records cannot be easily presented in a universal form. Generally, they should include field notes that describe the type of contaminant(s), type of sample (personal or area), method of collection, site and/or job description, and department. Where chemicals are used, an inventory of all materials and their health and safety material data sheets should be kept. Industrial hygiene records may also include a description of industrial processes, any changes in the operations, and the dates of such changes together with the availability and performance of personal protective equipment as well as industrial ventilation and exhaust systems.

Recognizing the necessity and importance of records and faced with a growing accumulation of data, there have been numerous efforts to apply recent computer technology to the retention and efficient utilization of industrial hygiene records. These efforts have usually been made in conjunction with, or as part of a larger effort to computerize the data generated by the combined functions of the industrial hygiene (environmental monitoring), medical (biological monitoring), and personnel (work history) departments [92–97].

For a detailed description of industrial hygiene records, reports, and data automation, the reader may consult handbooks on industrial hygiene [98,99]. The reader should also be acquainted with the federal and state regulations and requirements pertinent to the situation in question.

VI. Sampling Methods for Gas Phase Pollutants

There are several distinct and different methods available for sampling gas phase pollutants. They depend upon the chemical and physical nature of the gas or vapor. The sampling method chosen for detecting a leak or peak concentration during a spill or accident will be different from those used for the determination of average exposure to employees in an epidemiological study. In many instances, the sampling and the analysis steps occur in situ simultaneously, and the two steps are often indistinguishable. These methods are referred to as "direct reading" techniques or instruments. In contrast, an indirect sampling method is one in which the sample is collected, for example on a substrate, and then sent to a laboratory for subsequent analysis. Direct and indirect sampling tecyniques will now be discussed separately.

A. Direct Reading Methods for Gases

The technological revolution in solid state electronics has vastly contributed to the development of scores of new, portable, sensitive, reliable, and rapidly responding instruments for the direct measurement of gas phase pollutants. The wide array of instruments available to the modern industrial hygienist ranges from simple, manually operated gas detector tubes for detecting leaks or instantaneous concentrations to completely automatic continuous measurement computer-controlled instruments with digital readouts. The latter can be installed at remote locations; they yield statistical summaries by the hour, shift, day, or week, activate audio and visual alarm signals, and trigger shutdown operations in accidents or emergencies.

Direct reading methods and instruments for gases will now be described; they are based on the measurement of a specific chemical or physical property of the gaseous species.

B. Direct Reading Colorimetric Indicator Tubes

Colorimetric indicator tubes or detector tubes depend on formation of a colored stain formed on a substrate coated with a chemical in a glass tube. The chemical specifically reacts with the desired gas or vapor to form a colored reaction product.

Detector tubes are glass tubes containing support materials such as silica gel, alumina, ground glass, pumice, or resin of uniform grain size, coated with specific chemical(s) for each gaseous species to be detected. The tube is sealed at both the ends. In operation, the seals at both ends are broken and a known volume of air at a specific flow rate is drawn through the detector tube. Depending upon the concentration of the desired gas, the chemical reaction, and the kinetics of the reaction, a colored stain of a certain length is produced in the detector tube. The concentration of the gas in the sample is proportional to the length of the stain. A calibration curve of stain length versus pollutant concentration is provided by the manufacturer.

Some detector tubes have more than one substrate or column. The first column may filter out the other interfering gases, or may oxidize or reduce the gas and render it suitable for reaction with materials in the second part of the tube. More than a hundred different detector tubes are commercially available. It is difficult to classify these tubes into any general scheme because of the variety of gases measured and the many chemical reactions utilized to obtain visual indicators of the reaction [100–102].

The accuracy, reliability, and sensitivity of the detector tube is different for each gas. Factors influencing tube characteristics are: the specificity, sensitivity and the speed of reaction; intensity and the contrast of the colored stain compared to the color of the impregnated substrate; packing of the

Table 5 Properties of Selected Detector Tubes for Gases and Vapors[a]

Gas	TLV (ppm)	Measurable concentration (ppm)	Indicating color change	Shelf life	Useful temperature range (°C)	Useful humidity range	Interferences
Acetone	1000	500–5000	Yellow-dark orange brown	Unlimited	–	–	–
Acroylonitrile	20	10–500	Orange-brown	Unlimited	–	–	Several non-halogenetic organic vapors
Ammonia	25	25–250	Pink-Pale yellow	1 year	0–40	0–100% RM	Amines
		1–25%	Pink-purple blue	Unlimited	–	–	Hydrogen sulfide
Arsine	0.05	5–160	White-brown black	3 years	–	–	Hydrogen sulfide Phosphine
Benzene	10 (1.0 ?)	5–50	White-reddish brown	–	0–40	5–80	–
Butadiene	1000	30–600	Pale yellow-blue	3 years	–	–	Unsaturated hydrocarbons
Carbon dioxide	5000	2500–25,000	Blue purple-pale pink	3 years	–10–40	0–100	Acid gases at high concentration
Carbon monoxide	50	25–250	Pale yellow-green and blue	1 year	0–40	0–100	–

Carbon tetrachloride	10	5–50	Yellow-blue	6 months	5–30	0–100	Phosgene
Chlorine	1	0.5–5	White to yellow	1 year	0–40	10–90	Bromine, chlorine dioxide, ozone, nitrogen dioxide
Chloroform	50(10)	75–600	Grayish white-reddish orange	6 months	–	–	Halogens and halides
Ethyl mercaptan	0.5	1–26	White-yellow	1 year	–	–	Methyl sulfide, chlorine, methyl mercaptan, NO_2, CO, etc.
Ethylene dichloride	100	10–400	White-orange	1 year	10–38	0–80	Chlorine, bromine, trichloroethylene
Furan	5	500–16,000	Yellow orange-dark brown	Unlimited	–	–	Organic vapors (nonhalogenated)
Hydrogen cyanide	10	5–50	Yellow-red	1 year	0–30	0–100	–
Hydrogen sulfide	10	5–60	White-pale brown	1 year	0–40	0–100	Sulfur dioxide

Table 5 (Continued)

Gas	TLV (ppm)	Measurable concentration (ppm)	Indicating color change	Shelf life	Useful temperature range (°C)	Useful humidity range	Interferences
Methyl bromide	20	5–50	White-brown	1 year	0–40	20–200	Halogens, hydrogen halides and halogenated hydrocarbons
Methyl isobutyl ketone	100	50–10,000	Orange-blue green	Unlimited	–	–	Organic vapors (nonhalogenated)
Nickel carbonyl	0.001	20–700	Pale yellow-blackish purple	6 months	–	–	Hydrogen sulfide, sulfur dioxide
Nitrogen dioxide	5	2.5–25	Yellow to dark gray	–	0–40	0–100	Ozone, chlorine, chlorine dioxide, bromine, iodine
Phosgene	0.1	0.5–50	White-reddish brown	1 year	–	–	Chlorine, nitrogen dioxide, hydrogen chloride
Phosphine	0.3	5–90	Pale blue-yellow brown	Unlimited	–	–	Hydrogen sulfide

Sulfur dioxide	5	2.5–25	Blue purple-white	1 year	0–40	0–100	Hydrogen sulfide, nitrogen dioxide
Tetrahydrofuran	200	0.1%–5.0%	Yellow orange-blue green	Unlimited	–	–	Organic vapors
Toluene	100	50–500	White-brown	–	10–30	0–100	Benzene, xylene, toluene, hexane
Trichloroethylene	100	50–500	White-orange	–	0–40	20–100	Chlorine, bromine, iodine, hydrogen halides, halogenated hydrocarbons

[a]The information about specific tubes was derived from several sources. The properties of detector tubes for the same compound may be different for different manufacturers.

The names and addresses of some vendors are given below:

1. Bacharach Instrument Co., 625 Alpha Dr., Pittsburgh, Pennsylvania.
2. National Environmental Instruments Co., (Bendix) 1865 Post Road, P.O. Box 590, Pilgrim Station, Warwick, Rhode Island.
3. National Draeger, Inc., Parkway View Drive, Pittsburgh, Pennsylvania.
4. Matheson Gas Products, P.O. Box 85, 932 Paterson Plank Rd., East Rutherford, New Jersey.
5. Mine Safety Appliances Co., 400 Penn Center Bldg., Pittsburgh, Pennsylvania.

support material; shelf life of the reagent; and quality control during tube manufacture and calibration. Most of the currently available detector tubes are short-term detector tubes. This, combined with its limited sensitivity, makes detector tubes useful only for measurements of peak concentration, episodic excursions, leaks, etc. Detector tubes are not well suited for estimating the time-weighted average exposures of workers to pollutant gases. Table 5 gives a list of selected detector tubes along with other pertinent information.

C. Direct Reading Physical Instruments for Analyzing Gases and Vapors

Many of the direct reading commercially available instruments are designed for measuring specific gases and vapors; some have universal application (in a limited sense). All the instruments are based on measurement of some physical or physicochemical property of the gas or gases. The various steps of classic analysis, i.e., sample collection, sample preparation, or conditioning, analysis, and the calculation of concentration are all accomplished almost instantaneously and automatically. Because many of the instruments are deceptively simple to operate and the responses are so rapid, the user may have a false sense of security with regard to the result. These instruments should only be used by one familiar with their scope and limitation.

Two kinds of direct reading monitors for gases are available: (1) continuous, in which the air is continuously sampled and a response or measurement of the concentration of the desired gas is either continuously recorded on chart paper or is displayed on a meter (the response time of such instruments may vary from milliseconds to a few minutes); and (2) grab sampling, in which an appropriate volume of air is obtained during a fixed period of time and the amount of a given gas in that volume is determined. The grab sampling instruments measure peak or instantaneous concentrations only.

The various physical properties on which these instruments are designed are listed below:

1. Electrochemical properties
   - Electrical conductivity in liquid phase
   - Potentiometry
   - Coulometry
2. Spectroscopic or spectrophotometric properties
   - Infrared absorption
   - Ultraviolet and visible light absorption
   - Spectral emission
   - Chemiluminescence
   - Photometric measurements of surface deposit

3. Thermal methods
   Thermal conductivity
   Heat of combustion
   Flame ionization

4. Miscellaneous
   Radioactivity
   Paramagnetism
   Quadrupole mass spectrometry
   Electron capture
   Electrom impact spectrometry

The theory and operating principles of instruments based on some of the analytical techniques listed above are discussed in Section VIII. An in-depth discussion of these instruments is beyond the scope of this book. However, Table 6 summarizes the various direct reading instruments commercially available, their potential, sensitivity, range, specificity, portability, and so on.

D. Indirect Reading Methods

In spite of the tremendous progress made with direct reading instrumentation technology, one often must depend upon the classic methods of sampling and analysis. These consist of the following steps:

1. Collection of representative air samples, either as is or on some solid or liquid substrate where the desired species is stabilized physically or chemically
2. Storage and transportation to a laboratory
3. Recovery and separation of the desired species and conditioning of the sample
4. Quantitative analytical determination of the species
5. Expression of the results

In this section we discuss the sampling, storage, and transportation steps. The recovery, separation, and analytical measurement steps will be discussed in Section VIII.

E. Collection Devices for Gases and Vapors

The various collection devices used for sampling gases are of four types: air displacement, condensation, absorption, and adsorption techniques. The ultimate choice of the collection method will depend upon several factors,

Table 6 Selected Physical Methods Employed in Air Analysis

No.	Method	Principle of operation	Type of sampling	Range: Lower (ppm)	Range: Upper (ppm)	Application and remarks
A	Absorption (volumetric, gasometric, or manometric)	Measured volume of gas-air mixture is absorbed by reagent and volume shrinkage determined. Pressure reduction may also be measured	Grab	300	100%	Selective; oxygen deficiency determinator; high concentration of gases; special forms will detect lower concentrations; U.S. Bureau of Mines describes a portable form for field use, and several compact models are available
B	Absorption (gravimetric)	Gas-air or vapor-air mixture is trapped on equilibrated absorbent such as activated charcoal or silica gel. Change in weight represents weight of contaminant in known air volume	Continuous	<1	Depends on amount sampled	Nonselective; used primarily for total solvents when a mixture of solvents is encountered; absorbed material when eluted can be measured by gas chromatography
C	Electrical conductivity	Gas-air mixture is absorbed in a solution whose electrical conductivity is measured before and after absorption	Grab or continuous	0.01	1%	Selective and can be applied to all acid or alkaline gases and also to vapors which can be burned to CO_2, SO_2, or HCl; field instrument is available

D	Heat of combustion					
	(1) combustible gas indicator	Gas-air or vapor mixture is passed over a heated (above gas combustion temperature) platinum wire which is part of a balanced electrical resistance bridge. The combustion of the gas on the wire unbalances the bridge	Grab	20	1000	Selective; field instrument was designed primarily for benzol but can be applied to other combustible gases not removed by water vapor absorbent which is provided and necessary to the proper operation of the instrument
	(2) Explosimeter	Explosimeter is a less sensitive form of the above instrument for explosive concentrations of combustible gases	Grab	10% of lower inflammable limit 1% in most sensitive inst.	5%	Water vapor absorbent not necessary because of lower sensitivity; instrument is used for explosive and flammability determinations; single meter calibrations for all gases the product of whose molecular heat of combination and the lower explosive limit is a constant
	(3) CO indicator (Hopcalite)	Gas is passed over a catalyst (Hopcalite) which converts CO to CO_2 and the heat of combustion is mea-	Continuous	10	10000	Used in the field (portable apparatus) and tunnels for CO determination; water vapor and oil fumes can poison catalyst

Table 6 (Continued)

No.	Method	Principle of operation	Type of sampling	Range: Lower (ppm)	Range: Upper (ppm)	Application and remarks
		sured by a thermopile which is connected to a galvanometer				and are removed before passing over catalyst
E	Interferometer	Refractivity of gas-air or vapor-air mixture as compared to dry air is measured by comparison of interference fringes or Fraunhofer lines when light is passed through gas-air mixture	Grab	12 to 127	10–100%	Nonselective; sensitivity depends on refractivity of gas or vapor; CO_2 and moisture interfere and must be removed; apparatus made in both portable and laboratory types
F	Spectrum absorption					
	(1) Ultraviolet	Gas-air or vapor-air mixture is passed through a tube with an ultraviolet light source at one end and a photoelectric cell at the other; gases or vapors which have absorption bands in the ultraviolet or near ultra-	Grab or continuous	1	0.01–1	Sensitive to several gases and vapors; maximum sensitivity for mercury vapor; water vapor and CO_2 do not interfere; field instruments for mercury, trichloroethylene, and perchloroethylene have been developed. By using mercurioxide

	violet absorb light and diminish cell response which is registered by a calibrated meter				at controlled temperatures mercury vapor detectors of the spectrum absorption type can be used with gases such as carbon monoxide and ethylene, and can be used to detect vapors such as benzene, ethanol, and others
(2) Infrared	Gas-air or vapor-air mixture is passed through a tube with a source of infrared (heated filament) at one end and a thermopile for recording absorption of infrared at the other end; gases or vapors having absorption bands in infrared absorb the infrared rays and diminish amount of heat reaching the thermopile; this is registered by a calibrated galvanometer or ammeter; differential pressure unit is also used	Grab or continuous	1	10%	Sensitive to all heteroatomic gases and vapors; bands for absorption in infrared vary with gases just as in ultraviolet bands; thus the methods may be made selective by the development of screening filters; field infrared unit is available for CO and CO_2; British manufacturer can supply instrument for any heteroatomic gas specified

Table 6 (Continued)

No.	Method	Principle of operation	Type of sampling	Range		Application and remarks
				Lower (ppm)	Upper (ppm)	
	(3) Mass spectrum	Separates according to mass gaseous ions formed in an evacuated system; abundance of each ionic species is measured electrically by electrometer tube and amplifier	Grab or continuous	1	5000	Applicable to all gases and vapors but requires expensive and elaborate equipment; only adapted for laboratory handling of samples collected on silica gel and revaporized or grab samples
G	Thermal conductivity	Gas or vapor mixture is passed over a heated wire (below ignition temperature); change in heat loss of wire to surrounding gas mixture is registered by change in wire resistance measured on a balanced Wheatstone bridge	Grab or continuous	25	10%	Nonselective; water vapor and carbon dioxide interfere and must be removed; greatest application in field is to high concentrations such as in flue gas analyzers
H	Vapor pressure	Gas or vapor-air mixture is passed over a cooled condensing surface in a confined chamber;	Grab	10	1%	Selective; only high concentrations, 1000 ppm or greater, can be obtained by grab samples; appli-

		the chamber is then evacuated and the condensed gas allowed to evaporate and its pressure measured. Icewater, dry ice-acetone, or liquid air mixtures may be used depending upon contaminant sampled				cable in field only to vapors or gases for which icewater or dry ice-acetone mixtures can be used since liquid air is difficult to obtain and handle; contaminants must be immiscible with water; sensitivity depends on contaminant sample and amount of air sampled in continuous method
I	Gas chromatograph	Absorbs gas or liquid injected into a carrier gas stream of helium, hydrogen, nitrogen, or argon on a temperature-controlled absorbent column	Grab or liquid	1	1%	Selective; can be used to identify solvents and separate gas mixtures by selective elution; many types of detectors including several of those above
J	Electrochemical cell	The gas sample is catalytically oxidized (or reduced) at an electrode which is maintained at a fixed potential; the current flow is proportional to the partial pressure of the gas in the sample	Grab or continuous	0.01	1000	Commercially available instruments for CO, SO_2, H_2S, and NO_x

Table 6 (Continued)

No.	Method	Principle of operation	Type of sampling	Range: Lower (ppm)	Range: Upper (ppm)	Application and remarks
K	Photoionization	Gas or vapor sample is ionized by ultra-violet radiation. Electrodes collect the ions and the resultant current flow is proportional to the concentration	Grab or continuous	0.1	1000	The commercially available device is partially selective in that major components of air are not photoionized; organics can be measured by this method
L	Solid state electrolytic sensor	Metal and non-metal oxides act to convert the gas sample into ions or complexes which are collected as an electrical signal. The signal is proportional to the concentration	Grab or continuous	1	1000	Relatively nonselective; commercially available; depending on application can be very useful

Source: From Ref. 101.

such as the objective of the analysis, the chemical characteristics of the gas analyzed, the sensitivity of the subsequent analytical method, the convenience of collection, and storage and transportation of samples. The individual collection techniques are discussed below:

Air Displacement Techniques

In these techniques an unaltered sample of the air is collected during a short or a long time interval. One of the simplest methods is to evacuate a flask or container using a vacuum pump, seal the flask (with a stopcock or heat seal), and then open the flask at the sampling site to obtain a known volume sample of the air. The flask is closed and sent to the laboratory for analysis of the sample. An aspirator bottle filled with water and then drained at the sampling site can also be used. The volume of the sample conveniently collected by these methods is restricted to about 1–5 liters. Samples can also be collected by using small portable pumps to displace air into bags made of synthetic materials (Teflon, mylar, polyvinyl chloride, Saran, Tedlar, etc.). The reactivity, permeability, and absorbability of the desired species with the plastic bag used for collection must be known. Long-term samples can be collected by slowly filling the bag over a long period of time. These methods can be used for grab or for short-term and long-term (8 hr) sampling. They yield integrated time-weighted average concentrations, and not concentration fluctuations with time. The analytical methods for these samples must be very sensitive, because relatively small volumes of air are collected. Both area and personal samples can be collected using plastic bags. A new gas collection method utilizes a 100 ml stainless steel tank with two ports [103]. A critical orifice is attached to one of the ports; the other port has arrangements to evacuate and seal the tank. The method of collection is based on the pressure difference inside and outside the tank being greater than the critical pressure needed to maintain critical air flow in the orifice. The unit can be used for sample collection for as long as 8–10 hr, without a pump or another energy source (passive collection). The volume of air collected can be determined by measuring the initial and final pressures of air in the tank. It is important in these methods to determine the stability and integrity of the desired species during the lag time between collection and analysis.

Condensation Techniques

In this method, the air sample is passed through a condenser, cold finger, or U tube cooled below the boiling or freezing point of the sampled gas or vapor. The gas or vapor species to be collected liquefies or solidifies, and the remaining air, such as oxygen or nitrogen, passes through. The sample is concentrated; further separation and recovery are usually simple. Transportation of these samples over long distances can present problems.

Water in the air must be removed by dessication before sample collection to prevent formation of ice. The dessicant material must not absorb the material being sampled.

Absorption Techniques

The term absorption is used here to mean dissolution of a gas in a suitable solvent, or reaction with a suitable chemical dissolved in a solvent. Gas bubblers, scrubbers, washers, or impingers are other terms used to denote absorption apparatus. Gas absorbers of different sizes and shapes, mostly made of glass, are available commercially.

A gas absorber promotes intimate contact between the gas and the liquid phases. Because of the high solubility or reactivity of the material being sampled, it is absorbed in the liquid phase.

The efficiency of absorption is affected by the time, surface area, and intimacy of contact between the two phases. Absorption is promoted by drawing air through beaded or spiral columns of liquid or through a sintered or fritted glass tube immersed in the liquid. A drop or two of a foaming agent can be added to promote contact through foaming.

The gases either dissolve in the solvent or react; in the latter case the product is fixed in the absorbing medium. Although not ideal, this method of sampling can be adapted for personal monitoring. In recent years, some spill-proof impingers have been designed which should make this sampling technique more amenable for personal monitoring (spill-proof Mini-impinger, supplied in United States by Daco Products, Co., Inc., Montclair, N.J.). Depending upon the collection medium, efficiency, sensitivity of the analytical method, etc., both long- and short-term samples are possible with absorption techniques.

Adsorption Techniques

In adsorption techniques, the gas molecules are attached to the active sites on the surface of a solid or liquid. The gas molecules do not react with the surface; they are held by physical forces. Hundreds of organic solvents and vapors and many inorganic gases can be readily adsorbed on suitable media and subsequently desorbed in the laboratory for analysis. Perhaps the most widely used adsorbing medium is activated charcoal. Silica gels, alumina, molecular sieves, zeolites, etc., are all finding application for sampling of specific gases.

The adsorption devices consist of a glass tube, 5–10 mm in diameter and 50–130 mm in length, containing a few milligrams to grams of an adsorbing medium. The adsorbing medium is generally granulated (4–40 mesh size) to provide a large surface area for adsorption.

In operation, air is drawn through the tube at suitable flow rates from a few milliliters per minute to liters per minute. The gases to be analyzed are adsorbed in the medium and stabilized. The tubes are then capped; they can be transported readily, if necessary. For analysis the adsorbed gases are then desorbed, either thermally or chemically, separated, and analyzed using a suitable analytical method, usually gas or liquid chromatography. Infrared, ultraviolet, visible, and mass spectrometry can also be used for the final determination.

The choice of the adsorbing medium, flow rates to use, and the final method of determination will depend upon a number of factors, such as the chemical structure of the gas or vapor, its polarity, adsorbability, desorbability, retention or breakthrough period, and expected concentration.

A recent development in collection of gases based on adsorption is passive sampling. As the name denotes, these samplers do not need the conventional air movers (electrically or manually operated pumps or bellows) for collection. The adsorbent or absorbent (usually charcoal) is kept in small badgelike containers, which have a window covered with certain synthetic membranes. The membranes allow either the diffusion [104–106] or the permeation [107,108] of selected gases through the membrane to the adsorbent. The diffusion or permeation is dependent only on the ambient concentration of the analyte gas (the other variables such as the surface area, thickness of membrane, etc., being constant). At the end of the sampling period, the gases are desorbed from the adsorbent and analyzed by conventional methods. The amount of the analyte on the adsorbent can be correlated to a time-weighted average concentration by laboratory calibration. Several studies [106,108] have shown good correlation between the concentrations measured by this technique and by conventional methods.

F. Calibration and Standardization of Instruments

In all analytical techniques, whether direct or indirect, calibration and standardization of the instrument is of paramount importance. Preferably, the calibration should always be performed against a primary standard. For example, the measurement or adjustment of air flows should be calibrated against a spirometer or a soap bubble meter. It should be recognized that dry and wet test meters, rotameters, etc., are secondary standards for flow measurements. They are less accurate devices because they have been calibrated against a primary standard.

Most of the new or not well established techniques should be thoroughly and critically evaluated before adoption in a survey. For these purposes, it is often necessary to generate standard atmospheres, samples, solutions, or conditions against which the new method is tested. The standard conditions should simulate actual measurement conditions as closely as possible in terms of concentrations, humidities, pressures, temperatures, and impurities or interferences. In circumstances where this is not possible, the new method should be compared with an established and generally accepted method.

VII. Sampling Methods for Disperse Phase Pollutants

Sampling of airborne particulate matter is carried out for a variety of reasons. One of the most important purposes of dust sampling is to relate the dust concentration to the health experience of the population at risk. The environmentalist measures one or more of the properties of dust expected to be related to the disease caused by that particular type dust. These properties include the concentration of dust expressed by number, surface area, and mass of the total dust cloud or a certain size fraction of it. In designing the dust sampling instruments, some forces are utilized to measure that property under investigation. Generally, these forces are gravitational, inertial, thermal, or electrical. These forces have been discussed in more detail in Section II.C.

The objectives of aerosol sampling are:

1. To detect working places with unsatisfactory conditions and determine the causes of these conditions
2. To determine the effectiveness of control methods and equipment
3. To provide records of dust conditions and to assess trends of dust concentrations
4. To correlate dust exposure with the health experience of the exposed population
5. To create and control dust exposure in research and experimental investigations
6. To ascertain the delivery of predetermined doses in inhalation therapy
7. To comply with standards and regulations

A. Selection of Sampling Methods

The selection of sampling method depends primarily on the airborne contaminant, the purposes of the survey, and the subsequent sample analysis. In the evaluation of an environmental contaminant, sampling may be performed to assess occupational exposures. In this case, sampling procedures are utilized which determine either the exposure of selected individual workers, i.e., personal samples, or the concentration and/or properties of airborne particulates at selected work sites, i.e., area samples. Sampling may also be performed outside the workplaces to determine the properties and concentrations of particulate matter emitted to the atmosphere in an effluent stream or as a pollutant in community air.

Before undertaking any sampling program, one has to ascertain if the particular situation is covered by statutory requirements promulgated in detail by a federal, state, or local regulatory agency. If the situation is regulated, then the decision by an investigator to diverge from the official regulatory agency procedures is a major one, for the individual then carries the burden of proof to prove the equivalency of the selected unofficial method [109].

It is important to note that several biological parameters may influence the choice of sampling and analytical methods. For the assessment of a potential health hazard, the masured property of particulate matter should be related to action of the hazardous causative agent at the critical site in the body. For example, for particulate matter containing a highly soluble chemical component that can act as a cumulative systemic poison, the route of entry to the human body is of secondary importance. The total amount of the component that enters the body is of primary importance, because the agent will dissolve in body fluids and subsequently enter the blood circulation when inhaled and/or cleared from the lungs and swallowed. Consequently, the quantification of the total amount of the chemical present in airborne form is sought. Conversely, some highly insoluble dusts, such as crystalline free silica, which act in the pulmonary compartment of the respiratory tract to cause silicosis, would not constitute a hazard unless the free silica is present within a particle size that deposits in the pulmonary compartment. In this case, the method of quantification should reflect that portion of airborne dust that will deposit in the human respiratory tract distal to the ciliated epithelium [110].

In the following classification, the methods of sampling are presented according to the purpose of sampling, the property of the sample to be measured, and the method of analysis to be used.

Collection without Size Separation

This mode of collection represents the capture of what is commonly known as total suspended particulate matter (TSPM). Collection of TSPM may be accomplished with filters, electrostatic precipitators, thermal precipitators, or impactors.

Gravimetric and chemical analysis of TSPM require the collection of adequate quantities of particulate matter, usually more than 1 mg. This usually requires sampling at high flow rates and/or for long periods of time.

One of the most important properties of a dust sampler is its collection efficiency. This efficiency will depend on the collection mechanism, particle size, and dust loading. Electrostatic precipitators may significantly reduce collection efficiency for smaller particle sizes [11,111]. The collection efficiency of filters will vary according to filtering medium and nominal pore size. Generally, membrane filters and fiber glass filters are very efficient. The efficiencies of most filtering materials used in industrial hygiene are discussed in detail by Lippman (see Ref. 100). Thermal precipitation is one of the most efficient mechanisms of collection of particles. It collects virtually all particles down to 0.01 μm in diameter [11]. However, because of the limited flow rates required and consequently small collection quantities of particulate matter, it is used only as a research instrument for aerosol physics.

Gravimetric determination of the collected TSPM may be automatically obtained by methods such as β attenuation [100], light extinction [112], frequency shift of a vibrating crystal [113], or by conventional weighing methods.

Particle Size Determination of Collected Dust

The significance of particle size in relation to dust properties and its potential health effects have been discussed in previous sections. In this part, the various methods of particle sizing will be presented.

The particle size analysis of TSPM can be accomplished by microscopy, sieving, elutriation, or other specific methods [111]. Microscopy requires small samples ($< 10\ \mu$g); the sample size requirements for the remainder of the methods is usually equal to or larger than the amounts required for chemical and gravimetric analyses.

Optical microscopy is one of the oldest methods of particle size determination and it is still one of the preferred methods because of its simplicity. The collected particles are viewed under a microscope and the individual particles are measured with a calibrated eyepiece graticule. If the sample was collected on a transparent medium, for example when an impactor or thermal precipitator was used, or if the sample was collected on a membrane filter that can be made transparent by means of immersion oil, the sample may be directly observed. In other cases, it is necessary to transfer the sample onto a microscope slide.

The determination of particle size by microscopy is limited by the resolution of the microscope ($> 0.2\ \mu$m). The reliability of the sizing data depends primarily on the number of particles counted. Also, the errors arising from subsequent mathematical conversion of projected area sizes to aerodynamic or weight sizes can be very large [113,114].

The determination of particle size by electron microscopy has advantages and disadvantages when compared to optical microscopy. Although the same collection methods are used, particles to be examined by transmission and scanning electron microscopy are usually transferred to a special substrate. Sample transfer and preparation require experience and skill; it is also a very tedious process, a major drawback of the method. Although the lower limit of size resolution is on the order of 10–100 Å, the presence of particles larger than 5 μm and/or volatile particles may cause significant errors; the latter will evaporate in the microscope vacuum. The errors associated with conversion of projected area size to aerodynamic and weight size are similar to those encountered in optical microscopy.

Particle size determination by sieving is usually performed on particles larger than 37–40 μm. Recently, the introduction of electrodeposited micromesh sieves has extended the particle size down to about 5 μm. Sieve analysis requires 2–5 g of sample for reliable analysis. The particle size range and the relatively large amount of dust needed for analysis limit the applications of sieve analysis. The differential particle sedimentation in a fluid is dependent on the particle size. This principle has been used extensively for particle size analysis. The fluid can be a gas (air, helium) or liquid that does not dissolve the particles (water, alcohol). The force field can be gravity or centrifugal force. Gravitational forces can be used to classify particles down to 1 μm [115]. Centrifugal sedimentation devices are used to shorten the time involved in analysis and further extend the minimum particle size to 0.01 μm [116].

Particle size distributions based on particle volume can be determined by the electric resistivity method. The size limits of this method are about 1–200 μm. The Coulter Counter is a size classifier utilizing the electric resistivity principle. It was originally developed to count blood cells. It is used extensively at the present time for particle size analysis [11] and the determination of particle shape factors [45].

Collection with Size Segregation

Various instruments that segregate particulate matter into size classes are available. They have the advantage of providing the particle size distribution directly, as well as particles in fractions suitable for determination of total weight or weight of individual chemical components, thus eliminating the need for one or more transfer steps.

Cascade or multistage impactors have been in use since 1945, when May [117] first described the device. There are a number of commercially available impactors with size separation down to 0.2 μm and air flow rates up to 1200 liters/min. Sampling and sizing problems with impactors include sample losses of entry, bounce and blow off of particles from collection stages, and losses of particles to the wall. Impactors may be used in a reliable and reproducible manner with proper impactor selection and care in usage [118].

Aerosol spectrometers using gravitational [47,119,120] or centrifugal [121,122] forces have been used as size classifiers. The use of these devices in field instruments has been limited because of the complexity of backup apparatus, the very small amount of dust samples, or the relatively high cost of the instrument.

Size Determination without Collection

In this type of sampling, the particle size distribution is determined while it is in its airborne state. Instruments of this type utilize either the electrostatic or light-scattering properties of particles. The particle size determined by light scattering is influenced by the refractive index of the particles as well as their shape. The uncertainty in measuring the size of a dust of unknown chemical composition varies from about 30 to 200% [112]. For this reason, these instruments should be calibrated prior to sampling with particles representative of the dust to be sized. The lower limit of particle diameters determined by optical spectrometers is about 0.1–0.4 μm.

Particle size determination based on the motion of charged particles in an electrical field is one of the few available techniques for particle less than 1.0 μm [11,100]. The applications of this type of instruments are limited by the upper size, i.e., 1.0 μm, that can be analyzed. A complete size distribution can be obtained by the coupling of this instrument with another size-selective instrument such as an optical spectrometer. However, the conversion between several methods of particle sizing introduces ambiguities that should be avoided specially in cases of statutory requirements.

Size-Selective Samplers

Size-selective samplers have been utilized to collect the "respirable fraction" of airborne dust cloud. Two conventions define collection characteristics of respirable dust:

1. The British Medical Research Council (MRC)
2. The U.S. Department of Energy (formerly the AEC) and the American Conference of Governmental Industrial Hygienists (DOE/ACGIH)

A comparison between these two conventions and median in vivo data for particle deposition in the pulmonary compartment of the human respiratory tract has been reported by Lippman (see Ref. 100). The MRC convention is satisfied by horizontal elutriators, while the DOE/ACGIH convention is closely adhered to by cyclone dust collectors [100] and more recently by a single-stage impactor [123]. Theoretical and experimental studies show that the elutriator/cyclone and elutriator/impactor ratios are about 1.2 [124-127] and 0.52 [123], respectively. Although results for respirable dust collected using elutriators and cyclones are comparable, a major difficulty with the elutriator is the requirement that the sampler be operated in a horizontal oreintation. This constraint limits the applicability of elutriators to area-type sampling.

A promising new technique of size-selective dust sampling has been reported by Cahill et al. [128], where two Nucleopore filters of different sizes (8.0 and 0.4 μm) are operated in series. The investigators have shown that under specific operating conditions, particles collected on the 8.0 μm filter represent the fraction that would deposit in the upper respiratory tract. Particles passing the 8.0 μm filter and collecting on the 0.4 μm filter satisfy the DOE/ACGIH convention.

Another size-selective sampler utilized at the present time for cotton dust sampling is the vertical elutriator [129]. It was developed by Lynch [130] in 1970 to obtain lint-free cotton dust. It is operated as a stationary "area sampler." The theoretical penetration of particles through the elutriator is [131]:

$$P = 1 - \frac{de^2}{225}$$

which corresponds to a cutoff aerodynamic diameter equal to 15 μm. Although this instrument has been used extensively in epidemiological surveys in the cotton textile industry [71], cotton ginning [132], and the cotton seed industry [133], few studies of its performance have been reported in the literature [134,135].

VIII. Analysis of Samples

The term *analysis of samples* may refer to methods for either qualitative or quantitative analysis of samples. Qualitative analysis answers the question, What is in the sample? Quantitative analysis answers the question, How much?

A. Qualitative Analysis

A commonly held but erroneous view is that small quantities of hazardous chemicals in bulk materials can be directly translated into small nonhazardous quantities of airborne material. "Trace" quantities of a bulk material can become a large proportion of the airborne contaminant in either the gaseous or the particulate state. This concentrating effect occurs because trace ingredients may be more volatile than other ingredients, or solids may contain smaller particle sizes which are more easily made airborne. Whatever the mechanisms involved, this phenomenon necessitates that initial determinations of airborne contaminants be performed. Conclusions cannot be reached on the basis of bulk material composition. The latter merely serve to identify chemicals to be determined in the sample. In many instances the tradename of a substance makes it difficult to identify components, but usually if the manufacturer of the product is queried, the composition of the substance is made available, at least in qualitative terms, which is sufficient for directing the initial determination.

In many cases, depending upon the manufacturing process or the nature of application, unknown by-products can be produced from side reactions, reactions with other pollutants in air, thermal degradation, or photochemical reactions. In some industries, the raw materials themselves are so complex it is difficult to identify the chemicals that become airborne during their cracking, refining, processing, etc. Under these circumstances, before they can be quantitated, it is essential to identify the chemicals present by qualitative analysis. In the case of inorganic components, qualitative chemical tests are made to confirm the identity of the various possible structures from which the correct structure will emerge.

The organic contaminants can be in either gaseous or particulate form. For mixtures, large samples have to be collected and separated using appropriate techniques for gases and/or particulates. Details of separation are discussed elsewhere in this section. After separation, physical properties, i.e., melting point, boiling point, and elemental composition, are determined; also, the ultraviolet, infrared, mass, and nuclear magnetic resonance spectra of the compounds are noted. Usually with these data the chemical structure of the organic compound can be predicted. Confirmatory tests such as those for functional groups, derivation, and tests on derivatives, etc., are performed to confirm the predicted structure. In recent years, the combination of gas chromatography and mass spectrometric techniques (GC-MS) has been routinely used for the separation and identification of complex organic mixtures.

Books are available which deal with the subjects of systematic identification of organic compounds [136–138] and contributions to GC-MS interfacing for separation and analysis of organic compounds [139–142].

B. Quantitative Analysis

Quantitative analysis consists of four basic steps:

1. Sampling
2. Separation and/or sample preparation

3. Analytical determination
4. Expression of results

The sampling methods for gaseous and particulate contaminants were presented in Sections VI and VII. In this section, we discuss the different methods used in separation and/or preparation of samples prior to chemical analysis.

Separation and/or Preparation of Samples for Analysis

Sample preparation is dependent upon the final analytical procedures to be used, as well as the nature of the sample in hand. In many instances, sample separation or preparation is not required because the sampling process itself is specific and selective for the analysis of the desired pollutant. The interfering species were either not collected or were suitably masked using chelating agents or chemical complexes. For example, in the determination of chlorine in air using the methyl organge method, chlorine bleaches the red-colored methyl orange dye when air is sampled through a solution containing methyl orange at a pH of less than 2.0. The solution is returned to the laboratory and the optical density of the solution is directly measured [143]. However, in many instances elaborate chemical separations are required before one can proceed with the analysis.

The particulate sample which requires separation and chemical analysis usually arrives at the laboratory after collection on a filter. The gaseous samples arrive in plastic bags, adsorbed on charcoal or some other substrate, or in an absorbing solution. In most instances (except for x-ray diffraction and the fluorescence or neutron activation techniques), the particulate samples are stripped from the filter and dissolved before separations. For microscopic measurements, the filter material itself is sometimes rendered transparent by adding immersion oil, or dissolved with organic solvents (membrane filters). The particulates can be stripped from filters using ultrasonic devices or by selectively destroying the filter. (For example, a glass filter is destroyed with hydrofluoric acid.) Inorganic particulates such as the oxides and sulfides of the metals are leached off the filters using hydrochloric and nitric acids. For organic particulates, the species are normally dissolved in a suitable organic solvent.

The gases (from flasks, bags, etc.) are sometimes used as is for analysis. The adsorbed samples are desorbed by extraction into some suitable solvent before analysis. Absorbing solutions are sometimes used as is, evaporated to dryness, and the residue dissolved with some other solvent, or extracted directly with other solvents. All these operations yield a complex mixture of dissolved analytes which have to be separated before they can be analyzed.

The following physical and chemical methods of separation are used:

Distillation

Solvent extraction

Chromatography (column, gas, liquid, thin-layer, and ion exchange chromatography)

Ion exchange and exclusion

Dialysis

Precipitation, coprecipitation, and adsorption

Flotation

Zone melting

Biological methods

Only solvent extraction and chromatographic separation techniques are extensively utilized for the analysis of pollutants in air. Sequestering or masking the interfering ion or ions with suitable mono- or polydentate chelating agent is another technique used, especially in inorganic analysis.

Solvent extraction is a process in which the analyte of interest is transferred from one solvent phase to a second solvent which is immiscible with the first. Most of the solvent extractions are from an aqueous phase to an organic phase. Solvent extraction is limited with organic analyses because it is difficult to obtain clean separations. Solvent extraction is used extensively for metal analyses [144], especially with colorimetric or spectrophotometric analysis. It has also been used with atomic absorption techniques for metals, for eliminating matrix interferences, and for enhancing the sensitivities [145, 146].

Chromatographic methods of separation include column, liquid, gas, thin-layer, and ion exchange chromatographic techniques. In column or adsorption chromatography, a solution containing a mixture of solutes (the mobile phase) is passed through a column containing a stationary and inert material (stationary phase) such as alumina, cellulose, starch, calcium carbonate, celite, silicid acid, and charcoal. The solutes are separated as the mixture moves through the column. The separation and resolution is dependent upon a number of factors of both the columns and solute. The structure, polarity, the solvent used, and the affinity of solute for the adsorbent are also significant factors.

In gas chromatography the mobile phase is a mixture of gases swept over the stationary phase by an inert carrier gas such as nitrogen, helium, or argon. The stationary phase can be either a solid material or a liquid coated on a solid, packed in a small-bore stainless steel, nickel, copper, aluminum, or glass tube. Table 7 lists a few of the many substrates used as the stationary materials and their application in separation. The development of capillary

Table 7 Substrates Used in Gas Chromatography and the Kinds of Separations

Substrate materials	Separations
n-Dodecane	C_6 Hydrocarbons
n-Octadecane	C_7 to C_9 Hydrocarbons
Aircraft engine oil (Bright stock)	High-boiling hydrocarbons
Silicone (550)	General hydrocarbons and organo-metallics
Diethylene glycol monoethyl ether	Paraffins, olefins, and acetylenes
Paraffin wax	Amines
Dioctylphthalate	General purpose, including ketones, esters, fluorinated hydrocarbons
Di-2-ethylhexylsebacate	General hydrocarbons, chlorinated hydrocarbons

Source: Adapted from Ref. 149.

column chromatography [148,149] has increased the speed and efficiency of separations. Extremely complex organic mixtures (even isomers) can be resolved using this technique.

For organic substances having boiling points above 400°C the separations with gas chromatography become difficult. In such cases they can be separated in liquid form using column chromatography. In column chromatography, where the driving force is normally gravity, unusually large columns and extremely long times would be required for separation of complex mixtures. To overcome this problem, a new technique referred to as High-pressure or performance liquid chromatography (HPLC) has been developed. In this technique, small diameter columns are used and the solutes are forced through the columns under very high pressure (4000–6000 psi). Recent developments in HPLC [150] technology have made this technique an invaluable tool for many separations and it has become a common instrument in most well-equipped laboratories.

In paper and thin-layer chromatography (TLC) the stationary phase is the filter paper itself or a thin layer of a substrate coated on a glass plate. The mixture of solutes is spotted at the end of the filter paper or the TLC plate and is eluted with a solvent either rising by capillary action or descending by gravity. With the elution of solvent, the solutes migrate differentially and are separated. This technique is used primarily as a qualitative technique. It is valuable when a sample contains a number of unknown substances and a quick method is needed to determine their number. In many instances identification is also possible.

Table 8 Classification of Analytical Methods According to the Frequency of Their Application in the NIOSH Manual of Analytical Methods

Description of the method	Number of applications	% Use
Gas chromatography	202	60
Atomic absorption spectroscopy	41	12
UV-Visible spectrophotometry	40	12
Anodic stripping voltammetry	16	5
Ion-specific electrode	9	3
High-pressure liquid chromatography	7	2
X-ray diffraction	4	1
Gravimetry, catalytic Rx, titration, fluorescence, turbidimetry, infrared, microscopy, differential thermal analysis	18	5% (Every technique <1% individually)
TOTAL	337	

GC, HPLC, and TLC techniques are generally used for organic compounds. Ion exchange chromatography [151] is relevant to inorganic compounds because, as the name indicates, ions are needed for this separation. The separation is based on exchange of cations or anions with the stationary phase. The stationary phase in ion exchange consists of polymeric resins with specific functional exchange groups. With the advent of atomic absorption spectroscopy ion exchange chromatographic separation for the analysis of inorganic cations has decreased.

The above brief description of chromatographic methods of separation highlights their versatility and usefulness in separations. Since its inception in 1951 more than 40,000 publications have appeared in the field of chromatography.

Sample preparation involves processes required to bring the analytes in the sample to a special state, as demanded by the particular analytical method employed for determination. The preparation steps depend upon a number of factors, such as the nature of the sample, the concentration of analytes, and the specific analytical method to be used. In many instances after sample separation, a few steps such as back extraction, adjustment of pH, addition of chelating agents, dilutions or concentrations by evaporation, and making other derivatives of the desired species, are required before final analysis. It is preferable to minimize the number of separation and preparation steps to avoid sample losses.

Table 8 gives a frequency distribution of all the analytical methods in the three volumes of the 1977 edition of the NIOSH Manual of Analytical

Methods [143]. This current and comprehensive manual not only includes determination of pollutants in air, but also many biological analytical methods of importance in occupational disease, such as determinations of metal in blood, urine, and tissue.

C. Gas Chromatography

Gas chromatography is mainly used for the separation and determination of mixtures of organic gases, vapors, volatile organic solvents, and some inorganic gases. A schematic flow diagram of a typical gas chromatographic instrument is given in Figure 5. It consists of a carrier gas source, a sample injection port, a column, a detector, and a recorder. The injection port, the column (containing either solid, or a liquid coated on a solid, substrate), and the detector are kept hot (as high as 400°C) using thermostats. A plug of sample, either as a gas mixture or solution, is introduced at the sample injection point. The carrier gas (usually helium, nitrogen, or argon) sweeps the sample (all gases now) to the column. As the sample migrates through the column it is separated and individual components enter the detector. The total amount of each individual component is detected and recorded to yield a "chromatogram." The entire sequence of events normally takes minutes. From the chromatogram, the number of components, the identity of components, and the concentration of each component of the mixture can be readily determined. In modern gas chromatographs, microprocessors and computers are used to analyze the chromatogram and print out results.

The column, the heart of any chromatographic method, consists of a tube packed with a solid material or solid coated with a thin layer of an appropriate solvent. The column may be straight, bent, or coiled and made of glass, stainless steel, aluminum, and copper tubing; they are usually 5–8 mm in internal diameter and 10–100 m long. Columns are packed with firebrick or chromosorb of 30–60 mesh size, and coated with the appropriate solvent. The right selection of column material is based mainly on experience and/or trial and error. Column technology has been reported in the literature [152, 153].

Three different kinds of gas chromatograph detectors are commonly used; thermal conductivity, flame ionization, and electron capture. The thermal conductivity detector (TCD) is based on the principle that a hot body will lose heat at a rate which depends upon the composition of the surrounding gas. TCD can be used universally for all compounds. Its sensitivity is limited and good flow control is needed to achieve acceptable reproducibility.

In the flame ionization detector (FID), the effluent gas from the column is mixed with hydrogen and burned in air or oxygen. Ions and electrons formed in the flame enter an electrode gap and decrease the gap

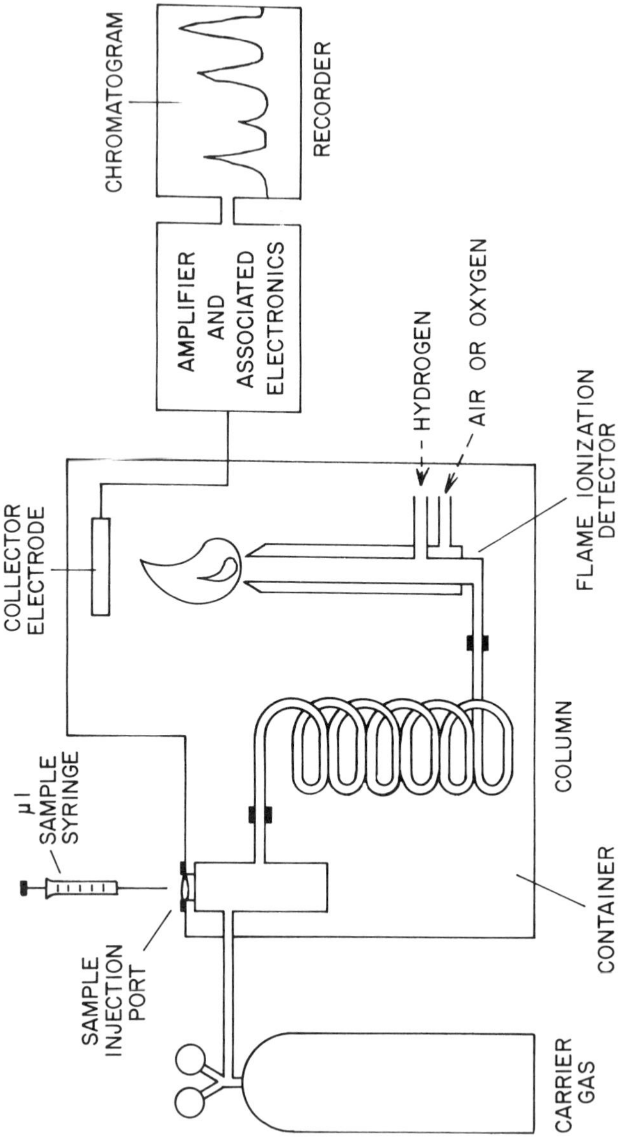

Figure 5 A gas chromatograph with flame ionization detector.

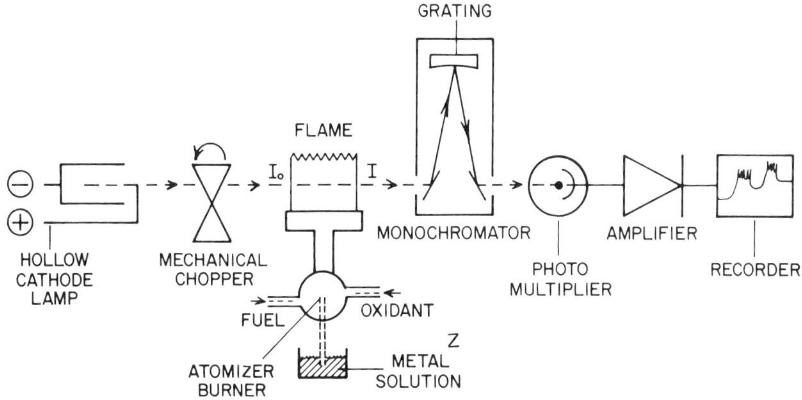

Figure 6 Atomic absorption spectroscopy.

resistance, permitting increased current flow, which is measured. FID detectors are extensively used in environmental analysis of organic compounds because they do not respond to common air pollutants, inert gases, water, nitrogen, and oxygen. FID also does not respond to carbon disulfide, a common solvent used for desorption and dissolution of organic compounds.

Electron capture detectors (ECD) measure the loss of signal rather than a positively produced electrical current, as in FID. As the carrier gas flows through the detector, a tritium or nickel-63 source ionizes the nitrogen molecules and slow electrons are formed. The slow electrons produce a steady current in a voltage field. If the sample contains molecules which absorb electrons, then this current will be reduced in proportion to the concentration of the sample. The loss of current is a measure of the concentration of the desired species. ECD is extremely sensitive to certain molecules such as alkyl halides, conjugated carbonyls, nitrites, nitrates, and organometallics. This selectively has made this detector especially valuable for analysis of pesticides. Selected recent application of GC methods for environmental characterization are reported elsewhere [154–158].

D. Atomic Absorption Spectroscopy

When a solution containing metal ions is atomized either by aspiration into a flame or injection into a heated zone, the bulk of the atoms in the atom cloud so formed will be in their ground state. These ground state atoms can absorb radiation at discrete wavelengths characteristic of an element and can get into an excited state. The excited atoms in turn emit radiation on returning to the ground state. The amount of energy absorbed or emitted is a function of the number of atoms present and hence may serve as a measure of the concentration of the respective elements in the sample.

The atomic absorption (AA) spectrometer consists of a source, some means of atomization, a monochromator, a detector, and a chopper for modulating the source. Figure 6 is schematic diagram of a typical atomic absorption spectrometer. The source is a hollow cathode lamp. The cathode of the lamp is made out of the element to be determined. The sample to be analyzed is generally atomized in a flame using conventional atomizers and burners. Other methods of atomization include cathode sputtering, heated graphite tubes, graphite rods, or tantalum boats. Radiation from the source traverses the atomic population representing the sample. The resonance radiation frequencies will be absorbed by the atoms in the flame, and the absorption is measured using a monochromator for resolution and a conventional photomultiplier tube system. The emissions from the flame and the background radiation are rejected by the chopper modulation of the source and by synchronizing the photomultiplier system to the same frequency.

Atomic absorption spectroscopic methods are applicable exclusively to metal determinations. A unique hollow cathode lamp, emitting a unique resonant line, is used for each individual metal. Because this unique frequency radiation can be absorbed only by that metal, interferences are excluded. However, there are some interferences under certain conditions due to formation of refractory compounds in the flame, and some specific and nonspecific molecular absorptions. Atomic absorption methods have become the most widely used technique for the determination of metals in all kinds of matrices such as air, water, biological samples, oil, and coal [143,145,146, 159,160].

E. Ultraviolet-Visible Spectrophotometry

Ultraviolet-visible spectrophotometry is an absorption spectroscopic method. The extent of absorption (or transmittance) of radiant energy (UV-visible region) at a characteristic wavelength by a solution of the analyte is compared to a series of analyte standard solutions. The absorption of UV and visible radiations caused electronic transitions in molecules. The amount and wavelength of absorption are dependent on the structure of the molecule. Organic compounds containing nitrogen, oxygen, sulfur, halogens, and conjugated and benzenoid structures strongly absorb in the UV-visible region. In dilute solutions, to a limited extent, absorption is proportional to the concentration, which is the basis for all spectrophotometric analytical methods.

Spectrophotometers consist of a source of UV and visible light, a monochromator and associated optics, a sample cell or cuvette, and the photomultiplier tube system for the measurement of radiant energy. A schematic

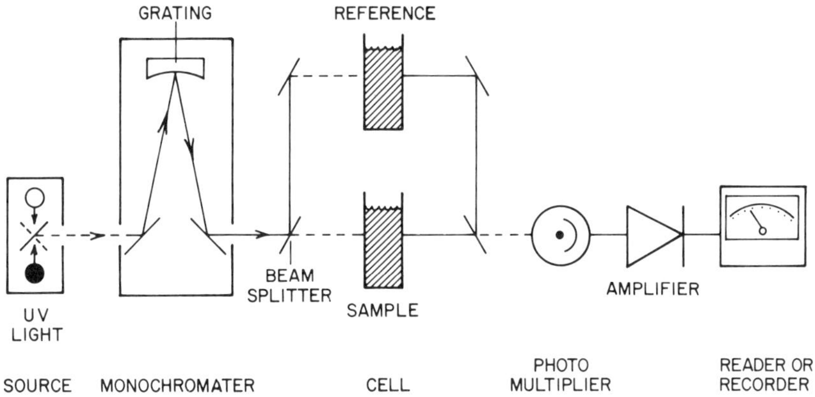

Figure 7 Ultraviolet visible spectrophotometer.

diagram of a spectrophotometer is given in Figure 7. The spectrophotometric absorption measurements are usually performed in solutions (aqueous or organic). Separations and sample preparations are of major importance in these methods. The prepared sample solution must be uniquely colored or be absorbing at a wavelength where other species in the sample do not absorb. The absorbances of the sample and the standards prepared identically are measured at specific wavelengths in matched cells. The concentration of the analyte can then be measured from the standard calibration curve.

Organic, inorganic, and organometallics can all be determined spectrophotometrically [161,162]. Because all gases and particulates can be dissolved in one form or the other, to form an absorbing species, they can theoretically be determined by spectrophotometric methods. The sensitivity, specificity, reliability, etc., are all different for each procedure, and are dependent on the structure of the particular analyte and the sample preparation procedures.

F. Miscellaneous Methods

Anodic Stripping Voltammetry [163-165]

This is an electrochemical technique especially suited for analysis of metals. It is based on electrolytically depositing (or reducing) all the metals onto a solid electrode or amalgamating on a mercury cathode. After all the metals are coated on the electrode, the polarity of the electrodes are reversed. The potential impressed on the anode is swept. When the specific oxidation potential of the desired metal is exceeded, all the metal on the electrode is oxidized (stripped from the electrode), causing a jump in the current. The current is proportional to the concentration or total amount of the metal present on the electrode. This method has very high sensitivity and is inherently free of interferences.

Ion-Specific Electrodes [166–168]

Ion-specific glass membrane electrodes are primarily used for the measurement of inorganic anions and some cations, primarily chloride, bromide, fluoride, cyanide, thiocyanide, and iodide in air and biological samples. The principle of operation is very similar to a pH electrode, which is selective for hydrogen ions. These electrodes are simple to use and have good sensitivity combined with rapid responses.

High-Pressure Liquid Chromatography [150,151]

This method is essentially similar to the gas chromatographic method except that the mobile phase is also a liquid containing the solutes. Because it is more difficult to pass a liquid through a packed column, high pressures are employed. The separated solute, as it comes out of the column, is measured using UV-absorption techniques. Sophisticated data display and analysis, as in GC techniques, have become standard features of this method. HPLC methods are used wherever GC methods cannot be employed (high boiling solutes).

X-ray Diffraction [169]

This technique is primarily used for the measurement of crystalline materials. X-rays are diffracted at specific angles depending on the crystal structure. The angle provides the specificity, and the intensity of the diffracted beam provides for quantitative measurements. The method has good sensitivity and is rapid. The equipment is expensive, and trained professionals are needed to perform the analysis.

G. Expression of the Results

The gaseous contaminant concentration is usually expressed in parts per million (ppm; volume/volume) or the equivalent, milligrams per cubic meter. The concentration of particulate contaminants is usually expressed as the latter, but in the case of certain fibrous (asbestos, glass) material, they are also expressed as number per unit volume. The ppm is related to the mg/m^3 of a gas by the following formula (using ideal gas laws).

$$\text{ppm} = \text{mg/m}^3 \times \frac{22.4 \text{ (liters)}}{\text{MW (g)}}$$

for 0°C and 760 mmHg pressure. A mg/m^3 unit is recommended for universal use.

IX. Applications of Environmental Characterization in Occupational Lung Disease Research

Environmental characterization in occupational lung disease research is primarily concerned with the estimation of the dose of airborne contaminant that enters and adversely affects the lungs. To achieve that objective, we must understand (1) how the exposure occurs, (2) the location of the respiratory system where deposition or adsorption occurs, and (3) to some extent, the identity of the mechanism or toxic property of air contaminant that causes the effect. In this section we will consider some examples of airborne contaminants and how investigators were able to relate the dose to the effects on the lungs.

A. Gas Phase

A 5 year longitudinal investigation of workers engaged in the manufacture of TDI in a new plant, with baseline clinical, immunologic and physiological data obtained prior to the beginning of operation and exposure to TDI vapor has recently been completed [170]. At the inception of the study, workers' exposure was estimated by continuous readout area monitors (Model 7000 TDI Area Monitor, MDA Scientific, Inc., Park Ridge, Illinois) installed at strategic positions in the plant. Careful examination of the concentration profiles obtained over a period of 2 years showed that area monitors did not provide adequate description of the individual work exposure because environmental conditions in the various industrial operations were markedly different and workers were quite mobile. For example, the physical structure of the TDI manufacturing plant is open and unprotected. As a result, windspeed and direction, humidity, temperature, precipitation, and movement of the workers will cause a completely different pattern of exposures in comparison to the drumming operations. The drumming building is physically enclosed, and consequently workers' movement is restricted. In 1975, a new personal sampler became available (MCM Model 4000). This sampler is capable of providing a continuous profile of the workers' exposure over an 8 hr working shift. The sampling and supporting apparatus also electronically integrates and records the total dose for the 8 hr in ppm-hr units. Using personal sampling instruments, the investigators generated a complete description of the exposure of the working population (143 workers). Information from over 2000 personal samples covering 42 job titles were utilized to correlate the respiratory health experience of the workers to their exposure. Spirometric measurements, respiratory symptoms, and atopic status of the workers were related to the cumulative exposure as well as to peak exposures, i.e., length of time above each of the levels 0.005, 0.01, 0.02, 0.04, 0.06, and 0.08 ppm.

B. Disperse Phase

Most particulate toxic substances encountered in the workplace are clearly defined chemical compounds that can be measured with a high degree of specificity. Hence, for any given compound, the route of entry, site of deposition, and mode of action depend in some measure on the size of the particle. However, in some cases we are faced with the problem of differentiating between several classes of compounds in a mixed atmosphere which adds complexity to sampling method selection. Also, it is sometimes necessary to make, and clearly state alongside the results, either certain simplifying assumptions or certain qualifications for the application of results. Workers in the asbestos cement industry are exposed to cement, free silica, and chrysotile and crocidolite asbestos in a particulate form [81]. The complexity of the problem is further complicated because, for asbestos, the parameter of greatest biological relevance is difficult to define but is probably associated with fiber dimension [7,8]. In early epidemiological studies, health effects were correlated with dust concentration measurements made with the impinger. Since very few fibers were seen, a count of all particles present was used as an index of overall dustiness. More recently, the TLV has been based on counts of fibers longer than 5 μm as determined by light microscopy. Thus it became highly desirable to develop information that may lead to conversion of particulate concentration to fiber concentration in the asbestos cement industry. Hammad et al. [68] were able to show that if average concentrations of particle counts or fiber counts are used to rank exposure of workers into broad categories, similar conclusions concerning relative level of exposure could be reached by either method, which explains the high correlation between the health experience of asbestos cement workers and particle counts in these studies. Since the length of asbestos fibers is related to their toxic effects, Hammad et al. also reported on correlation between particle concentration and fiber concentration for selected fiber lengths. Correlation coefficients obtained for longer fibers are better than those for shorter fibers, which is probably due to counting errors associated with the detection of small fibers by light microscopy. Obviously, one may suggest using electron microscopy for better precision of small fiber counts. However, though it can be scientifically satisfying, it is so tedious that very few samples can be evaluated, and because of larger variability of workers' exposure, the true accuracy of the exposure estimate is lower than it would have been if many samples had been taken by the less precise method, i.e., light microscopy.

Other challenging situations are encountered in evaluation of workers' exposure to organic particulate matter, such as enzyme detergents and cotton dust. Weill and co-workers investigated the respiratory reaction of workers exposed to enzyme detergent dusts [171]. The detergents contain amylase, nonenzyme protein, nutrients, inorganic salts, and between 0.1 and 1% proteolytic enzyme. The concentration of airborne dust was determined by high-volume sampling pumps and the proteolytic enzyme content of the collected dust was further determined by the N-dimethyl casein method [172]. It was therefore possible to relate the clinical and physiological features of the affected workers to the concentration of the enzyme itself rather than to the total dust concentration. They were also able to show that below certain enzyme dust levels, sensitization to the enzyme was not demonstrated in new workers and respiratory symptoms in previously sensitized workers were abated.

Although cotton dust is accepted as the cause of byssinosis among exposed workers, the causative agent(s) is not yet known. Numerous studies have been performed to correlate dust concentration and medical findings, but with such a heterogeneous generic dust, different and sometimes confusing results were obtained. Cases of byssinosis have been diagnosed in practically all stages of textile processing—ginning, pressing, carding, spinning, and weaving. The prevalence rates are usually higher in the early stages of the industrial processes. Jones et al. [173] in their investigation of 486 workers in three cotton textile mills also found what they called the "mill effect," i.e., workers with byssinosis (5.7%) were unequally distributed with respect to job category and mill, and these variables, rather than the current dust exposure levels, accounted for the observed distribution of byssinosis prevalence rates. They attributed this mill effect to the variation in biological potency of the different types of cotton utilized by the mills. In a study of cottonseed mills, these same authors found that for exposed workers, a significant mean functional decline over the working shift was present on Monday but absent on Friday, indicating an acute bronchoconstrictor response [133]. However, the prevalence of byssinosis was only 2.3%. It is interesting to note that, in the report published by Hammad et al. [174] on dust concentrations in these studies, the elutriated dust concentrations in the textile mills (0.1–9.2 mg/m^3) are less than those in the cottonseed mills (0.20–14 mg/m^3), supporting the hypothesis of the variability of the biological potency of raw cotton dust. Also, because of the narrow range of dust concentration and wide variability of particle sizes in textile operations, the vertical elutriator provides a good estimate of the dose received by the workers. Conversely, because of the wide range of dust concentrations and narrow range of particle sizes in cottonseed mills, personal sampling provides a better estimate of the dose.

References

1. Green, H. L., and W. R. Lane, *Particulate Clouds: Dusts, Smokes and Mists,* 2nd Ed. London, E. & F. N. Spon Ltd., 1964.
2. Jacobson, A. R., and S. C. Morris, *Air Pollution,* Vol. 1. Edited by A. C. Sterm. New York, Academic, 1976, pp. 169–170.
3. Edmonds, R. L., *Ecological Systems Approaches to Aerobiology.* Edited by W. S. Benninghoff and R. L. Edmonds. Ann Arbor, Michigan, University of Michigan, 1972, pp. 6–11.
4. McNown, J. A., and J. Malaika, Effects of particle shape on settling velocity at low Reynolds Number, *Trans. Am. Geophys. Un.,* **31**:74–82 (1950).
5. Kunkel, W. B., Magnitude and character of errors produced by shape factors in Stokes' Law estimates of particle radius, *J. Appl. Phys.,* **19**:1056–1058 (1948).
6. Timbrell, V., The inhalation of fibrous dusts, *Ann. N.Y. Acad. Sci.,* **132**: 255–273 (1965).
7. Stanton, M. F., and C. Wrench, Mechanisms of mesothelioma induction with asbestos and fibrous glass, *J. Natl. Cancer Inst.,* **48**:797–821 (1972).
8. Stanton, M. F., M. Lagard, A. Tegeris, E. Miller, M. May, and E. Kent, Carcinogenicity of fibrous glass: Pleural response in the rat in relation to fiber dimension, *J. Natl. Cancer Inst.,* **58**:587–603 (1977).
9. Whitby, K. T., A. B. Algren, R. C. Jordan, and J. C. Annis, The ASHAE air-borne dust survey, *Heating, Piping, Air Cond.,* **29**:185–192 (1957).
10. McCrone, W. C., and J. G. Delly, *The Particle Atlas,* 3rd Ed. Ann Arbor, Michigan, Ann Arbor Sci. Publ., 1978.
11. Mercer, T. T., *Aerosol Technology in Hazard Evaluation.* New York, Academic, 1973.
12. Morrow, P. E., Aerosol characterization and deposition. *Am. Rev. Respir. Dis.,* **110**:(Part 2)88–99 (1974).
13. Newhouse, M. T., and R. E. Ruffin, Deposition and fate of aerosolized drugs, *Chest,* **73**:935–943 (1978).
14. Hiller, C., M. Mazumder, D. Wilson, and R. Bone, Aerodynamic size distribution of metered-dose bronchodilator aerosol, *Am. Rev. Respir. Dis.,* **118**:311–317 (1978).
15. Hatch, T. F., and P. Gross, *Pulmonary Deposition and Retention of Inhaled Aerosol.* New York, Academic, 1964, pp. 121–122.
16. Pylev, L. N., Effect of the dispersion of soot in deposition of 3,4-Benzopyrene in lung tissue of rats. *Gig. Sanit.,* **32**:19–23 (1967).
17. Pylev, L. N., and L. M. Shabad, *Biologic Effects of Asbestos.* Lyon, IARC, 1973, pp. 99–105.
18. Corn, M. L., T. L. Montgomery, and R. J. Reitzer, Atmospheric particulates: Specific surface areas and densities, *Science,* **159**:1350–1351 (1968).
19. Corn, M., T. L. Montgomery, and N. A. Esemn, Suspended particulate matter: Seasonal variation in specific surface areas and densities, *Environ. Sci. Technol.,* **5**:155–158 (1971).

20. Corn, M., F. Stein, Y. Hammad, S. Manekshaw, W. Bell, S. J. Penkalaand, and R. Freedman, Physical and chemical characteristics of "respirable" coal mine dust, *Ann. N.Y. Acad. Sci.*, **200**:17–30 (1972).
21. Stein, F., and M. Corn, Shape factors of narrow size range samples of respirable coal mine dust, *Powder Technol.*, **13**:133–141 (1976).
22. Branauer, S., P. H. Emmett, and E. Teller, Adsorption of gases in multimolecular layers, *J. Am. Chem. Soc.*, **60**:309–319 (1938).
23. Fuchs, N. A., *Evaporation and Droplet Growth in Gaseous Media.* London, Pergamon, 1959.
24. Mason, B. J., *The Physics of Clouds.* Oxford, Clarendon, 1959.
25. Milburn, R. H., W. L. Crider, and S. D. Morton, The retention of hygroscopic dusts in the human lungs, *Arch. Ind. Health*, **15**:59–62 (1957).
26. White, H. J., *Industrial Electrostatic Precipitation.* Reading, Massachusetts, Addison-Wesley, 1963.
27. Dellavalle, J. M., C. Orr, and B. L. Hinkle, The aggregation of aerosols, *Br. J. Appl. Phys. (Suppl.)*, **3**:189–206 (1954).
28. Fry, F. A., and A. Black, Regional deposition and clearance of particles in the human nose, *Aerosol Sci.*, **4**:113–124 (1973).
29. Fraser, D. A., The deposition of unipolar charged particles in the lungs of animals, *Arch. Environ. Health*, **13**:152–157 (1966).
30. Mercer, T. T., Aerosol production and characterization: Some consideration for improving correlation on field and laboratory derived data, *Health Phys.*, **10**:873–887 (1964).
31. Whitby, K., Homogeneous aerosol generators. Tech. No. 13, Minneapolis, Univ. of Minnesota, NP-10020, 1961.
32. Davies, C. N. (Ed.), *Aerosol Science.* New York, Academic, 1966.
33. Zimon, A. D., *Adhesion of Dusts and Powders.* New York, Plenum, 1969.
34. Whytlaw-Gray, R., and H. S. Patterson, *Smoke.* London, Edward Arnold, 1932.
35. Bairne, T., and J. M. Hutcheon, The shape of ground petroleum coke particles, *Br. J. Appl. Phys. (Suppl.)*, **3**:S76–S81 (1954).
36. Stein, F., N. Esmen, and M. Corn, The density of uranine aerosol particles, *Am. Ind. Hyg. Assoc. J.*, **27**:428–430 (1966).
37. Sehmel, G. A., The density of uranine particles produced by a spinning disc aerosol generator, *Am. Ind. Hyg. Assoc. J.*, **28**:491–492 (1967).
38. McKnight, M. E., and M. I. Tillery, On the density of uranine, *Am. Ind. Hyg. Assoc. J.*, **28**:498–499 (1967).
39. Stein, F., N. A. Esmen, and M. Corn, The shape of atmospheric particles in Pittsburgh air, *Atmos. Environ.*, **3**:443–453 (1969).
40. Whitby, K. T., A. B. Algren, and R. C. Jordan, Size distribution and concentration of air-borne dust, *Heat P.A.C.*, **27**(Part II):121–128 (1900).
41. Durham, J. L., W. E. Wilson, T. G. Ellestad, K. Willeke, and K. T. Whitby, Comparison of volume and mass distribution for Denver aerosols, *Atmos. Environ.*, **9**:717–722 (1975).
42. Herdan, G., *Small Particle Statistics*, 2nd Ed. London, Butterworths, 1960.

43. Hodkinson, J. R., The effect of particle shape on measures for the size and concentration of suspended and settled particles, *Am. Ind. Hyg. Assoc. J.,* **26**:64–71 (1965).
44. Kotrappa, P., Shape factors for quartz aerosol in respirable size range, *Aerosol Sci.,* **2**:353–359 (1971).
45. Schrag, K. R., and M. Corn, Comparison of particle size determined with the Coulter counter and optical microscopy, *Am. Ind. Hyg. Assoc. J.,* **31**:446–453 (1970).
46. Mercer, T. T., P. E. Morrow, and W. Stober (Eds.), *Assessment of Airborne Particles.* Springfield, Illinois, Charles C. Thomas, 1972.
47. Stein, F., R. Quinlan, and M. Corn, The ratio between projected area diameter and equivalent diameter of particulates in Pittsburgh air, *Am. Ind. Hyg. Assoc. J.,* **27**:39–46 (1966).
48. Richardson, E. G. (Ed.), *Aerodynamic Capture of Particles.* London, Pergamon, 1960.
49. Fuchs, N. A., *The Mechanics of Aerosols.* New York, Pergamon, 1964.
50. Dennis, R. (Ed.), *Handbook on Aerosols.* Technical Information Center, Energy Research and Development Administration, Springfield, Virginia, 1976.
51. Friedlander, S. K., *Smoke, Dust and Haze.* New York, John Wiley, 1977.
52. Einstein, A., *Investigations of the Theory of the Brownian Movement.* New York, Dover, 1956, p. 75.
53. Henderson, Y., and H. W. Haggard, *Noxious Gases,* 2nd Ed. New York, Reinhold, 1943.
54. Casarett, L. J., Toxicology of the respiratory system in toxicology: The basic science of poisons. Edited by L. J. Casarett and J. Doull. New York, Macmillian, 1975, pp. 201–224.
55. Parkes, W. R., *Occupational Lung Disorders.* London, Butterworths, 1974, pp. 85–95.
56. Heppleston, A. G., The fibrogenic action of silica, *Br. Med. Bull.,* **25**(3): 282–287 (1969).
57. Bruch, J., Response of cell cultures to asbestos fibers, *Environ. Health Perspect.,* **9**:253–254 (1976).
58. Spencer, H., *Pathology of the Lung: Excluding Pulmonary Tuberculosis,* 2nd Ed. Oxford, Pergamon, 1976, p. 677.
59. Lundin, F. E., J. Wagoner, and V. E. Archer, Radon daughter exposure and respiratory cancer, quantitative and temporal aspect. NIOSH and NIEHS Joint Monograph, No. 1, 1971.
60. Jorgensen, H. S., A study of mortality from lung cancer among miners in Kiruna, 1950–1970, *Work Environ. Health,* **10**:126–133 (1973).
61. Boyd, J. T., R. Doll, J. S. Faulds, and J. Leiper, Cancer of the lung in iron ore (haematite) miners, *Br. J. Ind. Med.,* **27**:97–105 (1970).
62. Doll, R., Cancer of the lung and nose in nickel miners, *Br. J. Ind. Med.,* **15**:217–223 (1958).
63. Selikoff, I. J., J. Churg, and E. C. Hammond, Asbestos exposure and neoplasia, *JAMA,* **188**:22–26 (1964).

64. Doll, R., R. E. W. Fisher, E. J. Gammon, W. Gunn, G. O. Hughes, F. H. Tyrer, and W. Wilson, Mortality of gas workers with special reference to cancers of the lung and bladder, chronic bronchitis, and pneumoconiosis, *Br. J. Ind. Med.,* **22**:1–12 (1965).
65. 1977 Threshold limit values for chemical substances and physical agents in workroom environment with intended changes. American Conference of Governmental Industrial Hygienists, P.O. Box 1937, Cincinnati, Ohio, 45201.
66. Theriault, G. P., W. A. Burgess, L. DiBerardinis, and J. M. Peters, Dust exposure in the Vermont granite sheds, *Arch. Environ. Health,* **28**:12–17 (1974 .)
67. Lynch, J. R., H. E. Ayer, and D. L. Johnson, The interrelationships of selected asbestos exposure indices, *Am. Ind. Hyg. Assoc. J.,* **31**:598–604 (1970).
68. Hammad, Y. Y., J. E. Diem, and H. Weill, Evaluation of dust exposure in asbestos cement manufacturing operations, *Am. Ind. Hyg. Assoc. J.,* **40**:490–495 (1979).
69. Ayer, H. E., J. M. Dement, K. A. Busch, H. B. Ashe, B. T. H. Leradie, W. A. Burgess, and L. DiBerardinis, A monumental study: Reconstruction of a 1920 granite shed, *Am. Ind. Hyg. Assoc. J.,* **34**:206–211 (1973).
70. El-Batawi, M. A., and S. E. Shash, An epidemiological study on aeriological factors in byssinosis, *Arch. Gewerb. Pathol. Gewerbhyg.,* **19**:393–402 (1962).
71. Merchant, J. A., J. C. Lumsden, K. H. Kilburn, W. M. O'Fallon, J. R. Ujda, V. H. Germino, and J. D. Hamilton, Dose response studies in cotton textile workers, *J. Occup. Med.,* **15**:222–230 (1973).
72. Mancuso, T. F., A. Ciocco, and A. A. El-Attar, An epidemiologic approach to the rubber industry, *J. Occup. Med.,* **10**:213–232 (1968).
73. Lloyd, W., and A. Ciocco, Long term mortality study of steelworkers. I. Methodology, *J. Occup. Med.,* **11**:299–310 (1969).
74. Lloyd, J. W., F. E. Lundin, Jr., C. K. Redmond, and P. B. Greiser, Long term mortality study of steel workers. IV. Mortality by work area, *J. Occup. Med.,* **12**:151–157 (1970).
75. McMichael, A. J., R. Spirtas, and L. L. Kupper, An epidemiologic study of mortality within a cohort of rubber workers, *J. Occup. Med.,* **16**:458–464 (1974).
76. McMichael, A. J., R. Spirtas, L. L. Kupper, and J. F. Gamble, Solvent exposure and leukemia among rubber workers: An epidemiologic study, *J. Occup. Med.,* **17**:234–246 (1975).
77. Gamble, J. F., and R. Spirtas, Job classification and utilization of complete work histories in occupational epidemiology, *J. Occup. Med.,* **18**:399–404 (1976).
78. Jahr, J., Dose-response basis for setting a quartz threshold limit value, *Arch. Environ. Health,* **29**:338–340 (1974).
79. British Thoracic and Tuberculosis Association Report from the Research Committee: Opportunist mycobacterial pulmonary infection and occupational dust exposure: An investigation in England and Wales, *Tubercle,* **56**:295–310 (1975).

80. Berry, G., M. K. B. Molyneux, and J. B. L. Tombleson, Relationships between dust level and byssinosis and bronchitis in Lancashire cotton mills, *Br. J. Ind. Med.*, **31**:18–27 (1974).
81. Weill, H., M. M. Ziskind, C. Waggenspack, and C. E. Rossiter, Lung function consequences of dust exposure in asbestos cement manufacturing plants, *Arch. Environ. Health,* **30**:88–97 (1975).
82. Theriault, G. P., J. M. Peters, and W. M. Johnson, Pulmonary function and roentgenographic changes in granite dust exposure, *Arch. Environ. Health,* **28**:23–27 (1974).
83. Beedle, D. G., E. Harris, and G. K. Sluis-Cremer, The relationship between the amount of dust breathed and incidence of silicosis in pneumoconiosis. In *Proceedings of the International Conference.* Edited by H. A. Shapiro. Johanesburg, 1969, pp. 473–477.
84. Kramer, C. G., and F. E. Mutchler, The correlation of clinical and environmental measurements for workers exposed to vinyl chloride, *Am. Ind. Hyg. Assoc. J.,* **33**:19–30 (1972).
85. Berry, G., J. C. Gilson, S. Holmes, H. C. Lewinsohn, and S. A. Roach, Asbestosis: A study of dose-response relationships in an asbestos textile factory, *Br. J. Ind. Med.,* **36**:98–112 (1979).
86. Roach, S. A., A more rational basis for air sampling programs, *Am. Ind. Hyg. Assoc. J.,* **27**:1–12 (1966).
87. National Institute for Occupational Safety and Health: Occupational exposure sampling strategy manual. U.S. Department of Health, Education and Welfare Publication No. 77-173, 1977.
88. National Institute for Occupational Safety and Health: Statistical methods for the determination of noncompliance with occupational health standards. U.S. Department of Health, Education and Welfare Publication No. 75-159, 1975.
89. National Institute for Occupational Safety and Health: Handbook of statistical tests for evaluating employee exposure to air contaminants. U.S. Department of Health, Education and Welfare Publication No. 75-147, 1975.
90. Bar-Shalom, Y., A. Segall, and D. Budenaers, Decision and estimation procedures for air contaminants, *Am. Ind. Hyg. Assoc. J.,* **37**:469–473 (1976).
91. Esmen, N., and Y. Hammad, Log-normality of environmental sampling data, *J. Eiviron. Sci. Health,* **A12**:29–41 (1977).
92. Ott, M. G., H. R. Hoyle, R. R. Langer, and H. C. Scharnweber, Linking industrial hygiene and health records, *Am. Ind. Hyg. Assoc. J.,* **36**: 760–766 (1975).
93. Jennings, H., and K. L. Rohrer, A computerized industrial hygiene program, *Plant Eng.,* **30**:149–151 (1976).
94. Ott, M. G., Linking industrial hygiene and health records, *J. Occup. Med.,* **19**:388–390 (1977).
95. Berrett, C. D., and H. D. Belk, A computerized occupational medical surveillance program, *J. Occup. Med.,* **19**:732–736 (1977).

96. Kerr, P., Recording occupational health data for future analysis, *J. Occup. Med.,* **20**:197–203 (1978).
97. Snyder, P. J., Z. G. Bell, and R. J. Samelson, The computerization of industrial hygiene records, *Am. Ind. Hyg. Assoc. J.,* **40**:709–720 (1979).
98. Clayton, G. D., and F. E. Clayton (Eds.), *Patty's Industrial Hygiene and Toxicology,* Vol. I. John Wiley, New York, 1978.
99. Cralley, L. V., and L. J. Cralley (Eds.), *Patty's Industrial Hygiene and Toxicology,* Vol. III. New York, John Wiley, 1979.
100. American Conference of Governmental Industrial Hygienists, *Air Sampling Instruments,* 5th Ed., Cincinnati, Ohio, 1978.
101. Brief, R. S., *Basic Industrial Hygiene: A Training Manual.* American Industrial Hygiene Association, Akron, Ohio, 1975, pp. 51–55.
102. *Direct Reading Colorimetric Indicator Tubes Manual,* 1st Ed. American Industrial Hygiene Association, Akron, Ohio, 1976.
103. Personal atmospheric gas sampler with a critical orifice. Part I. Development and evaluation. Developed by Naval Research Laboratory, Washington, D.C., under a NIOSH Contract. Report No. 7693, 1977.
104. Tompkins, F. C., Jr., and R. L. Goldsmith, A new personal dosimeter for monitoring of industrial pollutants, *Am. Ind. Hyg. Assoc. J.,* **38**:371–377 (1977).
105. McCammon, C. S., and J. W. Woodfin, An evaluation of a passive monitor for mercury vapor, *Am. Ind. Hyg. Assoc. J.,* **38**:378–386 (1977).
106. Bamberger, R. L., G. G. Esposito, B. W. Jacobs, G. E. Podolak, and J. F. Mazur, A new personal sampler for organic vapors, *Am. Ind. Hyg. Assoc. J.,* **39**:701–708 (1978).
107. Nelms, L. H., K. D. Reisznev, and P. W. West, Personal vinyl chloride monitoring device with permeation technique for sampling, *Anal. Chem.,* **49**:994-998 (1977).
108. West, P. W., and K. D. Reiszner, Field tests of a permeation-type personal monitor for vinyl chloride, *Am. Ind. Hyg. Assoc. J.,* **39**:645–650 (1978).
109. OSHA Safety and Health Standards, 29 CRF 1904, 1900, pp. 13(f).
110. Muir, D. C. F., *Clinical Aspects of Inhaled Particles.* London, Wm. Heinemann, 1972.
111. Silverman, L., C. E. Billings, and M. W. First, *Particle Size Analysis in Industrial Hygiene.* New York, Academic, 1971.
112. Hodkinson, J. R., The optical measurement of aerosols. In *Aerosol Science.* Edited by C. N. Davies. New York, Academic, 1966, pp. 287–357.
113. Liu, B. Y. H., R. N. Berglund, and J. K. Agarwal, Experimental studies of optical particle counters, *Atmos. Environ.,* **8**:717–732 (1974).
114. Esmen, N. A., On error bounds of estimating size-weight distribution from microscopic sizing, *Iran. J. Sci. Technol.,* **3**:169–191 (1974).
115. Allen, T., *Particle Size Measurement,* 2nd Ed. London, Chapman and Hall, 1974.
116. Whitby, K. T., A rapid general purpose centrifuge sedimentation method for measurement of size distribution of small particles. I. Aparatus and method, *Heat. Pip. Air Cond.,* **61**:33–47 (1955).

117. May, K. R., The cascade impactor: An instrument for sampling coarse aerosols, *J. Sci. Instrum.*, **22**:187–195 (1945).

118. Marple, V. A., and K. Willeke. In *Proceedings of the Symposium on Fine Particles.* Edited by B. Y. H. Liu. New York, Academic, 1976, pp. 411–446.

119. Timbrell, V., The terminal velocity and size of airborne dust particles, *Br. J. Appl. Phys.*, **5**(Suppl. 3):S86–S90 (1954).

120. Timbrell, V. In *Assessment of Airborne Particles.* Edited by T. T. Mercer, P. E. Morrow, and W. Stoker. Springfield, Illinois, Charles C. Thomas, 1972, pp. 290–330.

121. Stober, W. In *Proceedings of the Symposium on Fine Particles.* Edited by B. Y. H. Liu. New York, Academic, 1976, pp. 351–397.

122. Abed-Navandi, M. A. Berner, and O. Preining. In *Proceedings of the Symposium on Fine Particles.* Edited by B. Y. H. Liu. New York, Academic, 1976, pp. 447–464.

123. Treaftis, H. N., T. F. Tomb, and C. D. Taylor, Comparison of respirable coal mine dust concentrations measured with an MRE and a newly developed two-stage impactor sampler, *Am. Ind. Hyg. Assoc. J.*, **39**:891–897 (1978).

124. Lynch, J. R., Evaluation of single-selective presamplers. I. Theoretical cyclone and elutriator relationship, *Am. Ind. Hyg. Assoc. J.*, **31**:548–551 (1970).

125. Moss, O. F., and H. Ettinger, Respirable dust characteristics of polydisperse aerosols, *Am. Ind. Hyg. Assoc. J.*, **31**:546–547 (1970).

126. Maguire, B. A., and D. Barker, A gravimetric dust sampling instrument (SIMPEDS): Preliminary underground trials, *Ann. Occup. Hyg.*, **12**:197–201 (1969).

127. Knight, G., and K. Lichti, A comparison of cyclone and horizontal elutriator size selectors, *Am. Ind. Hyg. Assoc. J.*, **31**:437–441 (1970).

128. Cahill, T. A., L. L. Ashbaugh, J. B. Barone, R. A. Eldred, P. J. Feeney, F. G. Flocchini, C. Goodart, D. J. Shadoan, and G. W. Wolfe, Analysis of respirable fractions in atmospheric particulates via sequential filtration, *J. Air Poll. Control Assoc.*, **27**:675–678 (1977).

129. National Institute for Occupational Safety and Health, U.S. Department of Health, Education and Welfare: Criteria for a recommended standard . . . occupational exposure to cotton dust. HEW Publ No. (NIOSH) 75-118, 1974.

130. Lynch, J. R., Transactions of the National Conference on Cotton Dust Health. Edited by D. A. Fraser and M. C. Battigelli, Chapel Hill, University of North Carolina, 1970, pp. 33–43.

131. Walton, W. H., Theory of size classification of airborne dust clouds by elutriation, *Br. J. Appl. Phys.*, **5**(Suppl. 3):S29–S39 (1954).

132. Palmer, A., W. Finnegan, O. Herwitt, R. Waxweiler, and J. Jones, Prevalence of byssinosis in cotton gins in lower Rio Grande Valley of Texas, and Messilu Valley of New Mexico. Cincinnati, Ohio, U.S. Dept. of Health, Education and Welfare, Public Health Service, Center for Disease Control, National Institute for Occupational Safety and Health, 1974.

133. Jones, R. N., J. Carr, H. Glindmeyer, J. E. Diem, and H. Weill, Respiratory health and dust levels in cottonseed mills, *Thorax*, **32**:281–286 (1977).

134. Classen, B. J. Sampling discrepancies of the cotton dust vertical elutriator. In *Proceedings of the 1978 Beltwide Cotton Production Research Conferences, Special Conference on Cotton Dust.* Edited by J. M. Brown, National Cotton Council of America, Memphis, Tennessee, 1978.
135. Robert, K. Q., Cotton dust sampling efficiency of the vertical elutriator, *Am. Ind. Hyg. Assoc. J.,* **40**:535–542 (1974).
136. Silverstein, M., and G. C. Bassler, *Spectrometric Identification of Organic Compounds,* 2nd Ed. New York, John Wiley, 1967.
137. Shrimer, R. L., R. C. Fuson, and D. Y. Curtin, *Systematic Identification of Organic Compounds,* 5th Ed. New York, John Wiley, 1964.
138. Dyer, J. R., *Applications of Absorption Spectroscopy of Organic Compounds.* Englewood Cliffs, New Jersey, Prentice Hall, 1965.
139. Grob, K., and G. Grob, Gas-liquid chromatographic-mass spectrometric investigation of C_6-C_{20} organic compounds in an urban atmosphere. An application of ultratrace analysis on capillary columns, *J. Chromatogr.* **62**:1–13 (1971).
140. Ryhage, R., and S. Wikstrom, Gas chromatography-mass spectrometry. In *Mass Spectrometry: Techniques and Applications.* Edited by G. W. A. Milne. New York, John Wiley, 1971, pp. 91–119.
141. Henderson, W., and G. Steel, Total-effluent gas chromatography-mass spectrometry, *Anal. Chem.,* **44**:2302–2307 (1972).
142. Schulze, P., and K. H. Kaiser, The direct coupling of high resolution glass open tubular columns to a mass spectrometer, *Chromatographia,* **4**:381–387 (1971).
143. NIOSH Manual of Analytical Methods, 2nd Ed. Department of HEW Public Health Service, National Institute for Occupational Safety and Health, Cincinnati, Ohio, 1977.
144. Morrison, G., and H. Freiser, *Solvent Extraction in Analytical Chemistry.* New York, John Wiley, 1957.
145. Sachdev, S. L., and P. W. West, Concentration of trace metals by solvent extraction and their determination by atomic absorption spectrophotometry, *Environ. Sci. Technol.,* **4**:749–751 (1970).
146. Dharmarajan, V., Development of analytical methods for the determination of airborne inorganic particulates. Ph.D. Dissertation, Louisiana State University, Baton Rouge, Louisiana, 1972.
147. Berg, E. W., *Physical and Chemical Methods of Separation,* Vol. 8. New York, McGraw-Hill, 1963, pp. 80–106.
148. Novotny, M., Contemporary capillary gas chromatography, *Anal. Chem.,* **50**:16A–32A (1978).
149. Bursey, J. T., D. Smith, J. E. Bunch, R. N. Williams, R. E. Berkley, and E. D. Pellizasi, Application of capillary GC/MS/computer techniques to identification and quantitation of organic components in environmental samples, *Am. Lab.,* **9**:35–42 (1977).
150. Majors, R. E., Recent advances in high performance liquid chromatography: Packings, columns, *J. Chromotogr. Sci.,* **15**:334–351 (1977).
151. Harold, F. W., Ion exchange and liquid column chromatography, *Anal. Chem.,* **50**:36R–50R (1978).

152. Bainlescu, G. E., *Stationary Phases in Gas Chromatography.* Rome, Pergamon, 1975.
153. Grab, R. L., *Modern practice of Gas Chromatography.* New York, Wiley Interscience, 1977.
154. Cram, S. P., and T. H. Risby, Gas chromatography, *Anal. Chem.,* **50**: 213R–243R (1977).
155. Saltzman, B. E., and W. R. Burg, Air pollution, *Anal. Chem.,* **49**:1R–16R (1977).
156. Pellizari, E. D., J. E. Bunch, R. E. Berkley, and J. McRae, Determination of trace hazardous organic vapor pollutants in ambient atmosphere by gas chromatography/mass spectrometry/computer, *Anal. Chem.,* **48**:803–807 (1976).
157. Karasek, F. W., D. W. Denney, K. W. Chan, and R. E. Clement, Analysis of complex organic mixtures on airborne particulate matter, *Anal. Chem.,* **50**:82–88 (1978).
158. Greimke, R. A., and I. C. Lewis, Development of a gas chromatographic-ultraviolet absorption spectromatric method for monitoring petroleum pitch volatiles in the environment, *Anal. Chem.,* **47**:2151–2156 (1975).
159. Hieftje, G. M., and T. R. Copeland, Falme emission, atomic absorption and atomic fluorescence spectrometry, *Anal. Chem.,* **50**:300R–327R (1978).
160. Siemer, D. D., Analysis of trace metals in air, *Sci. Technol.,* **12**:539–543 (1978).
161. Howell, J. A., and L. G. Hargis, Ultraviolet and hight absorption spectrometry, *Anal. Chem.,* **50**:243R–261R (1978).
162. Willard, H. H., L. L. Merrit, and J. A. Dean, *Instrumental Methods of Analysis.* New York, Van Nostrand, 1974.
163. Vydra, F., K. Stubic, and E. Julakova, *Electrochemical Stripping Analysis.* New York, Wiley, 1976.
164. Cahill, F. P. J., and G. W. Van Loon, Trace analysis by atomic absorption spectroscopy and anodic stripping voltammetry, *Am. Lab.,* **8**:11–15 (1976).
165. Ferren, W., Analysis of environmental samples by means of anodic stripping voltammetry, *Am. Lab.,* **10**:52–60 (1978).
166. Bailey, P. L., *Analysis with Ion Selective Electrodes.* London, Heyden, 1976.
167. Bainlescu, G. E., and V. V. Cosofret, *Applications of Ion Selective Membrane Electrodes in Organic Analysis.* New York, Halstead, 1977.
168. Buck, R. O., Ion selective electrodes, *Anal. Chem.,* **50**:17R–29R (1978).
169. Liebhafsky, H. A., G. H. Pfeiffer, E. H. Winslow, and P. D. Zemany, *X-rays, Electrons, and Analytical Chemistry-Spectrochemical Analysis with X-rays.* New York, Wiley Interscience, 1972.
170. Weill, H., Respiratory and immunologic evaluation of isocyanate exposure in a new manufacturing plant. Final Report, NIOSH Contract No. 210-75-0006, 1979.
171. Weill, H., L. C. Waddell, and M. Ziskind, A study of workers exposed to detergent enzymes, *JAMA,* **217**:425–433 (1971).

172. Yuan, L., G. E. Means, and R. E. Feeney, The action of proteolytic enzymes on N,N-dimethyl proteins, *J. Biol. Chem.,* **244**:789–793 (1969).
173. Jones, R. N., J. E. Diem, H. Glindmeyer, V. Dharmarajan, Y. Hammad, J. Carr, and H. Weill, Mill effect and dose-response relationships in byssinosis, *Br. J. Ind. Med.,* **36**:305–313 (1979).
174. Hammad, Y. Y., V. Dharmarajan, and H. Weill, Sampling of cotton dust for epidemiologic investigations, *Chest,* **79S**:108S–113S.

13

Epidemiology

J. CORBETT MC DONALD

TUC Centenary Institute of Occupational Health
Lodon School of Hygiene and Tropical Medicine
London, England

I. Introduction

The practice of medicine is based on knowledge of where and why diseases occur and on knowledge of disease processes. Epidemiology is primarily concerned with distributions of disease and its determinants, while pathological and physiological sciences focus on disease mechanisms. These two approaches are complementary, overlapping, and equally essential, both for the clinician who must diagnose and treat individual patients and, perhaps more obviously, for those who provide health care for population groups such as those employed in various occupations and industries.

All diseases, including those of the lung and respiratory tract, are caused by a multiplicity of factors, working directly and indirectly, and their outcome is also multifactorial. Underlying this general rule are evolutionary and ecological concepts of adaptation, whereby we have inherited and acquired resistance, often of a high order, to a wide range of potentially harmful agents and circumstances. Challenges to this resistance may result in subclinical changes, to acute and chronic disease when the adaptive mechanisms are overstretched, and to death when they fail.

This etiological theory implies that humans will be most vulnerable when faced by new factors to which we have had little opportunity to adapt, as in the social and industrial environments. It also follows that if the patterns of causation and of resistance are complex, disease incidence and outcome will vary correspondingly. Although it may be convenient to consider specific causal agents in the work environment, such as chlorine, crocidolite, beryllium, toluene diisocyanate, *R. burnetti,* etc., and to prescribe specific methods of treatment and control, the outcome will be largely determined by many other factors. These are age, sex, place of residence, social circumstances, health and nutritional status, and tobacco and alcohol consumption, to name only a few. Herein lies the scientific enigma of how general laws can be derived from unique events and the practitioner's quandary of how best to apply these laws in the specific circumstances of the patient or community. The principles of epidemiology and of quantitative logic (statistics) are designed to cope with these problems, and physicians who understand them are likely to have some advantage in their work.

It is in the essence of epidemiology that observed facts and occurrences are related whenever possible to an appropriate denominator. The results are expressed as a simple *proportion* or percentage, when time is of minor importance, or as rates of *prevalence* at a point in time, or of *incidence,* per unit of time. The purpose of such rates and proportions is to allow useful comparisons to be made. These will be informative only if like is compared with like, so it is necessary that the statistics should either be specific for such obvious factors as age, sex, and occupation, which might confound any comparison, or be adjusted to allow for them.

Simple statistics describing the population distribution of disease are the building blocks of epidemiology and can be used for a variety of purposes. First, they permit a balanced picture to be formed of the frequency and severity of sickness suffered by a particular community, essential for determining priorities and the planning of health services. Second, they allow etiological hypotheses to be tested by examination of the degree of correlation between indices of disease occurrence and the presence of suspected agents. Third, measures of prevention, treatment, and control can be evaluated in a similar manner.

Since some readers of this book may be more concerned with the clinical than the group approach to medical practice, the relevance of epidemiology to them is worth some comment. The sick person looks to the doctor for diagnosis and prognosis, safe and effective treatment, and advice on the way his or her life and affairs should be adjusted. Diagnosis is a matter of probability, taking into account all available evidence: personal and environmental history, symptoms, physical signs, and laboratory tests. Epidemiological descriptions of disease entities put the range of variation of these components in reasonable perspective. Choice of therapy is made after cautious interpretation of the controlled and uncontrolled findings of others, as to both benefit and risk. Each patient is part of a sequential experiment, adding to the physician's own knowledge or prejudice in proportion to his or her epidemiological insight. Finally, it is worth remembering that many discoveries in medicine concerning disease causation have come from simple epidemiological observations by clinicians. Practicing physicians have good opportunities which deserve the best methodology.

This chapter is written with the research needs of those in clinicial and occupational health practice in mind. Emphasis is on basic principles of survey design, applicable to common problems and limited resources. This is not to belittle such studies; history does not suggest that much would have been lost had the "professionals" been forced to observe similar limits. Most of the examples are taken from personal, sometimes outdated experience, because I am familiar with it and need not be reluctant in pointing to the faults.

A few comments must first be made on the most fundamental ingredient in any scientific endeavour–the objective. Under the rhetorical statement, "God is the answer," the seer wrote, "But what is the question?" Before embarking on any epidemiological study, it cannot be too strongly stated that an attainable objective or answerable question must be clearly and unambiguously defined. Such expressions as "Our aim was to investigate . . . " or "We sought to determine the causes of . . . " are far too vague. Both the general and specific aims of the work must be stated precisely and in operational and measurable terms. For the most part, epidemiology is a practical science to be used for decision making. Having clearly defined the question, it is a useful discipline to ask what we shall do with the answer. Whatever the results of the inquiry, there may only be two or three conceivable lines of possible action; it is important that the inquiry at least be capable of discriminating between these.

I have chosen to start with experimental designs used in evaluation so that the reader may better appreciate the many ways in which observational studies fall short of the "scientific" experiment, and the possible sources of error which result. This emphasis will indicate, too, the prime importance of sound study design without which precision in measurement, computer sophistication, and complex statistical analysis can achieve little.

II. Evaluation

Evaluation studies test not only the efficacy of therapeutic or preventive measures but also the validity of the concepts of causation and disease mechanism on which the control regime is based. For example, workers exposed to noxious dusts are x-rayed periodically in the hope that withdrawal of those showing early changes will reduce the subsequent incidence of pneumoconiosis and associated disease. Evaluation of such procedures, commonly used in occupational medicine for various hazards, tests both their effectiveness and the hypothesis that the disease in question will not seriously progress after cessation of exposure. This example illustrates the difficulty of interpreting inquiries to evaluate routine screening. Failure may reflect either that the method is based on an incorrect theory or that the procedure (or some part of it) is ineffective. It may be important to distinguish between these two explanations, and to do so, individual components of the screening procedure will have to be tested separately. Do the subjects all come for x-ray? Is the x-ray technique adequate? Are x-rays properly read? Given that each part appears satisfactory, there then remains the question of overall effectiveness. We can observe systematically what happens in industries where regular screening is applied, but the fundamental question is what would have happened without it. The traditional approach to this type of question is subjective, to judge the results against our past experience. But is is easy to see how readily one can be misled. Some of the main sources of error are discussed fully by Campbell and Stanley [1]; they are as follows:

1. *Changing circumstances.* Working conditions are improving everywhere so there is likely to be less disease now than in the past, anyway; on the other hand, cigarette smoking may have increased.
2. *Aging.* The working population may have reached an age when complications with long latency are becoming manifest.
3. *Ascertainment.* Lung cancer and other diseases may now be better diagnosed and so apparently more frequent than in the past.
4. *Regression.* Control measures are used when situations are bad; in general, the worst tends to improve and the best to deteriorate.
5. *Selection.* Industrial plants available for study are often the better organized and more cooperative; their workers may therefore fare better than average.
6. *Losses.* Labor turnover, which affects both the risk of dust diseases and their detection, may be higher or lower than average in the plants under study.

A. Experimental Designs

The six threats to unbiased assessment ("internal validity") just listed have led during the past 50 years to the use of randomized controlled trials (RCT), first in agriculture and education, then in the evaluation of drugs and vaccines, and more recently, in health and social services. Even the strict experimental design has its weaknesses, but first let us examine how it achieves its high level of internal validity. The assessment of influenza vaccine is a classic example, where RCT have demonstrated their value, both in studies conducted in industry by the Medical Research Council in Britain, and by the U.S. Armed Forces Epidemiological Board.

Since there is no test by which clinical susceptibility to influenza virus infection can be reliably measured, the only way of obtaining two groups of men comparable in this respect is by random allocation, using sampling numbers or some similar procedure. Except by chance, the probability of which can be calculated statistically, the two groups thus formed can be expected to experience the same subsequent influenza attack rate. One group is vaccinated, the other given a similar but inactive placebo; both are then observed in like manner for a specified period of time. Neither the volunteers nor those responsible for diagnosis and recording of illness in the follow-up period are given the identity of the experimental or control subjects. The possibility of subjective bias is thus removed, and the study is then designated "double-blind." Trials of this design (shown diagramatically in Fig. 1) [2] are now commonplace and most physicians are probably familiar with them; however, they have their problems and limitations.

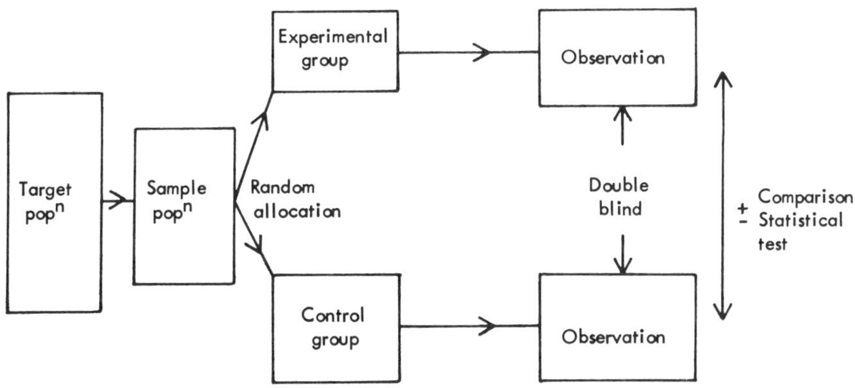

Figure 1 The experimental design. (Based on Greenberg and Mattison, 1955 [2].)

One problem is that randomization does not guarantee equality, any more than tossing coins will ensure an equal number of heads and tails. In a trial with which I was associated, vaccine and placebo injections were given, but there was no subsequent influenza outbreak—a frustratingly frequent occurrence. For idle curiosity, we analyzed sickness absence attributed to influenza in the two groups during the previous winter. The incidence in controls was more than twice that experienced by the vaccinated, a difference we would happily have attributed to immunization, had the order of events been reversed!

Clinical trials usually entail serious ethical questions, since the control subjects are deliberately deprived of some supposedly useful treatment. This can be justified only during the rather short period of time after potential value and safety have been claimed but before the public and medical profession have made up their minds. The ethical problem can sometimes be reduced by offering something of comparable value to the controls. In several MRC trials, it was the practice to give influenza virus A vaccine to one group and influenza virus B vaccine to the other. It was a reasonable gamble that both types of infection would seldom occur simultaneously. In a large trial in the British chemical industry [3], this paid off by enabling both A and B vaccines to be evaluated with some indication of the duration of protection.

Ethical questions aside, randomization and the double-blind system are easier to describe than to achieve. Thus, in the matter of routine screening just mentioned, it would be well-nigh impossible to randomize dust-exposed workers, and it is hard to imagine an acceptable placebo with which to compare the chest x-ray examination. Even in trials of drugs and vaccines, the double-blind code may be broken by unforeseen clues to identity. These breaches are seldom serious, however, and ingenuity in trial design can overcome many obstacles.

More fundamental objections to the experimental design lie elsewhere. These are discussed quite fully by Campbell and Stanley, and also by Carol Weiss in her excellent monograph on evaluation research [4]. First, everything about an RCT is so highly controlled that it becomes unreal and its results therefore difficult to generalize to the ordinary world. In the terminology of Campbell and Stanley, it lacks "external validity." Second, the RCT demands a degree of rigidity which usually prevents the application of lessons learned, until the trial has run its full course. Finally, it is very expensive in both time and effort, so its use must be reserved for questions of critical importance in which precision and internal validity are essential.

B. Nonexperimental Designs

The disenchantment with strict experimental designs which has grown among those concerned with educational and social services has still not reached medicine. The almost missionary zeal of such writers as Cochrane [5] for the wider application of RCT to health services has yet to convince many administrators that anything more than conventional experience and "evolutionary wisdom" are needed. Evaluation in the field of occupational lung disease is confined to trials of vaccines and chemotherapeutic agents for specific respiratory infections and a very few controlled studies of surgery and radiotherapy for lung cancer. It should be more widely known, therefore, that there are several quasiexperimental designs of high internal validity. Their application requires no less rigor than the RCT, but many of the latter's limitations and difficulties are avoided. The interested reader should consult Campbell and Stanley for a detailed account of these designs. Here, we shall consider only the group known collectively as time-series.

A simple nonexperimental method is the "before-and-after" study. For example, the prevalence of byssinotic symptoms among workers in a textile mill might be recorded before the introduction of a new dust-control process and then again afterward. Evidence of this kind is weak, but better than nothing. It can be strengthened considerably by making, not one but, a *series* of prevalence measurements, at intervals before and after the introduction of the new machinery. In this way, both the trend and the variability in prevalence can be assessed before and after and any interruption in pattern stands out. As shown schematically in Figure 2, this can be quite impressive. Such evidence can be virtually conclusive when similar time-series observations are made in several plants, preferably at irregular intervals and in random order. This constitutes the full multiple time-series design, illustrated in Figure 3. The virtue of this approach is that it lends itself well to the real world of hospitals, clinics, factories, and mines. In these situations it is seldom possible to make the same change simultaneously everywhere, but with sufficient planning and rigorous care, this constraint can be turned to advantage. Since the design essentially entails a series of extended before-and-after experiments, the main difficulty is to obtain data free from subject and observer bias. In some situations—in the evaluation of therapy, for example—it may be feasible to achieve double-blind standards. More commonly, however, the intervention cannot be disguised and much then depends on objective measurements by observers kept as ignorant as possible of events.

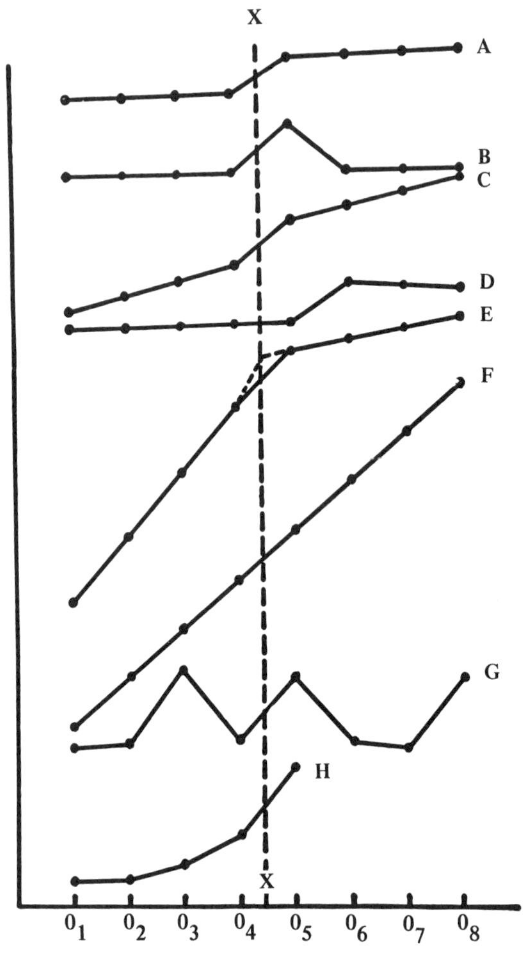

Figure 2 Some possible outcome patterns from the introduction of an experimental variable at point *X* into a time series of measurements, O_1 O_8. Except for *D*, the O_4–O_5 gain is the same for all time series, while the legitimacy of inferring an effect varies widely, being strongest in *A* and *B*, and totally unjustified in *F*, *G*, and *H*. (Reproduced with permission from Campbell, Donald T., and Stanley, Julian C. Experimental and quasiexperimental designs for research. In *Handbook of Research on Teaching*, Gage, ed., p. 38. Copyright 1963 by the American Educational Research Association, Washington, D.C.)

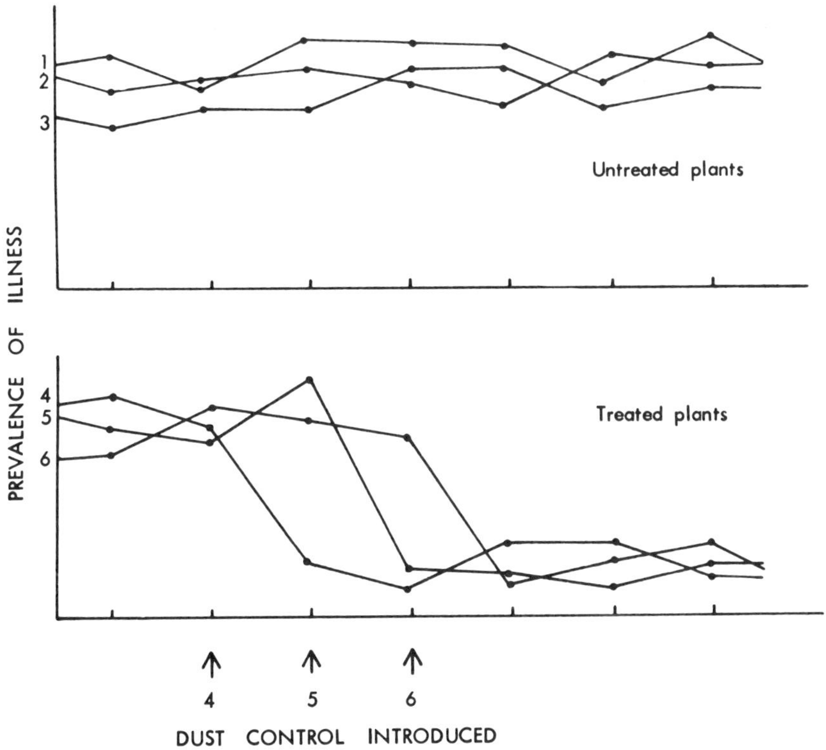

Figure 3 A multiple time-series.

III. Etiological Research

Cause and effect are difficult to distinguish from coincidental association even when both are witnessed. Chronic, insidious and malignant chest dieseases, complicated as they are by multiple facets of human susceptibility and long latent periods, highlight the complexity of the task. Philosophically speaking, causation can never be proved; it can only be considered as a working hypothesis until disproved. As stated by Hill [6], we must approach each situation with the questions, "Is there any other way of explaining the set of facts before us? Is there any other answer equally, or more, likely than cause and effect?"

In etiological research, the first question to be established is whether the time and place associations between the response (disease) and the stimuli (suspected causal factors) are greater than might be expected by chance, taking accounts of confounding variables. In assessing chance (see Chapter 15), the level of certainty we require—0.5, 0.05, or whatever—is a matter of opinion and of circumstances. Moreover, tests of statistical significance cannot be applied *after* the event; the hypothesis must first be defined, a survey conducted, and the results then tested.

We come then to the question of whether an observed association is causal or coincidental. In judging this, we have to consider two issues: the plausibility of the hypothesis; and the possibility that chance is the explanation, even though unlikely. As noted by a distinguised statistician, R. A. Fisher, "The one chance in a million will undoubtedly occur, with no less and no more than its appropriate frequency, however surprised we may be that it should occur to us."

For these reasons, we must take account of the number of confirmatory studies, the evidence of rational dose-response relationships, and whether the suspected factor is the major cause or only one of many. Thus, governments took action to discourage smoking, albeit belatedly, only after (1) many investigations had demonstrated an association with lung cancer, (2) the risk appeared directly proportional to cigarette consumption, and (3) most cases of the disease were evidently explained by this single cause. Other questions and other decision makers may require less evidence, but the same principles will hold.

Plausibility is a more subjective issue and depends on whether the hypothesis fits well with current beliefs on pathogenesis. The results of *in vitro* and animal experiments, and even quite simple anatomical considerations, will all influence our judgement. The fact that tobacco smoke is inhaled and not ingested favors a causal relationship with lung cancer; so too does the presence of known carcinogens. Curiously, even the induction of bladder cancer in rats adds weight to the evidence.

Convincing information on causality can be obtained from well-designed human experiments, but such studies are seldom feasible. The ethical problems are great and their external validity has always to be questioned; nevertheless, they have been used in studying the pathogenicity of respiratory viruses [7], live-attenuated influenza vaccine strains [8], and in provocative testing with suspected allergens [9].

A. Longitudinal Studies

Of three basic survey designs open to epidemiologists, none can achieve the internal validity of the experimental model but longitudinal (cohort) studies may have considerable strength equal indeed to that of a multiple time series. Consider several groups of workers, similar in age and health, who are exposed at different times to a specific airborne dust. If they consistently manifest the same respiratory signs and symptoms some 4 to 6 weeks later, whereas groups not exposed remain well, this clearly suggests cause and effect. The case is made stronger if both the proportion of workers attacked and the severity of their illness are directly related to the dust concentration experienced. These points illustrate the essential characteristics of a longitudinal study: defined populations, subsequent exposure, later measurements of attack rate, and an "expected" basis for comparison. However, seldom are all these features present and the absence of any one may introduce its own type of bias.

Study Population

The population to be studied should be defined *before* exposure, with sufficient information to confirm that the exposure groups were similar at the start. Some form of medical examination of each person prior to exposure is ideal, but not always possible. Cohorts are commonly defined as all persons employed in a particular plant on a given day. This is not satisfactory; such employees have survived heterogeneous selective forces operating over differing time periods. Men adversely affected by their work tend to leave and those employed longest in the cohort are the least susceptible. This problem of survivor bias is particularly important in working environments in which there are particles, gases, or vapors, to which some employees respond acutely. This was evident in a survey made some years ago among grain workers in the St. Lawrence river ports. The gangs were mainly men who had worked many years in very bad conditions without obvious ill effect; those who had been forced to move to other types of work might well have been less healthy but were not available for examination.

Exposure

Exposure has two main components, duration and concentration, and measurements of the latter are often poor or lacking. Duration is always a major factor and is sometimes the only exposure index available. Bias is created when disability or death, caused by the exposure, leads to a change in job or termination of employment. Since those who survive at work for a long time accumulate the greatest exposure and vice versa, dose-response relationships are disturbed. This source of error cannot be overcome by survey design but may be reduced by selecting an appropriate method of analysis [10].

In a large cohort study of mortality in Quebec chrysotile miners and millers, our first analysis did not deal adequately with this problem. A "dust index" was calculated for each worker, as the product of time and average dust concentration, and mortality then examined in dust-index groups. Table

1 sets out age-corrected death rates (all causes) thus obtained [11]. The falling trend in mortality below the level of 400 million particles per cubic foot is probably an artefact caused by selective survival, which is only overcome, and to an unknown extent, at high exposures. In later analyses, a sounder approach was followed. Only deaths 20 years or more after first employment were counted, and mortality was examined in four mutually exclusive groups, divided by years of service. Some data taken from a paper by McDonald and Liddell [12] illustrate the result (Table 2). The rows demonstrate much the same pattern as in Table 1, but the columns now show that mortality increased with average dust concentration in men who had worked 5 years or more. A reverse trend is seen in those with lesser service, probably due to selection of fitter men for dusty and more physically demanding jobs. Other approaches to the analysis of cohort data are discussed by Liddell et al. [10].

There are some situations in which length of exposure is independent of length of survival. For example, factory workers employed during the second World War on the manufacture of gas-mask filter pads from crocidolite asbestos in England [13] and in Canada [14] suffered a very high mortality from malignant mesothelioma some 20 to 30 years later. The longest period of exposure was 2.5 years and therefore quite unrelated to outcome. Reports on longitudinal studies of lung cancer (and of other respiratory disease), in relation to tobacco consumption, illustrate a different point in that they commonly ignore duration and classify the subjects only by intensity, e.g., by cigarettes consumed per day. This approach makes the reasonable assumption that, for practical purposes, smoking habit is an unchanging personal characteristic almost akin to sex, race, or hair color. In studies of susceptibility to acute respiratory disease in persons of different blood groups [15], the assumption becomes a certainty. In measuring the effect of cessation of cigarette smoking, survival-exposure interactions again become a problem. Exsmokers who achieve long periods of abstention certainly reduce their exposure but only to the extent that they survive to do so.

Table 1 Equivalent Average Death Rates per 1000 Men by Dust Index

Dust index (10^6 particles/ ft^3 per year)	<10	10–	100–	200–	400–	800–	All
No. of men	3006	3408	1148	1002	842	575	9981
Rate, all causes	264.1	260.4	257.6	240.6	262.9	312.5	263.1

Source: After McDonald et al. (1971)[11].

Table 2 Standardized Mortality Rates, All Causes, in Men 20 Years and More After First Employment, by Gross Service and Average Dust Concentration

Average dust concentration (10^6 particles/ft^3 per year)	Years of service			
	<1	1–5	5–20	>20
Low	1.12	1.12	1.10	0.98
Medium	1.13	1.09	1.07	0.89
High	0.95	1.12	1.22	1.07
Very high	1.03	1.04	1.26	1.50
Total	1.07	1.09	1.15	1.07

Source: After McDonald and Liddell (1979)[12].

Follow-Up

Very few long-term cohort studies maintain complete observation on all subjects. Every loss is a potential source of error, and most losses occur in persons employed for short periods and varying levels of exposure. Unfortunately, short-term employees may be those with poorest health, but more easily traced if they become sick or die. If these speculations are correct, the health effects of exposure may be obscured. Bias in the opposite direction, however, may result from diagnostic practices. Diseases suspected to be occupational in origin are, for many reasons, more carefully sought in workers with long employment and heavy exposure than in those whose health was unlikely to have been affected. In the Quebec chrysotile study, autopsy rates rose from 11% for those with minimal exposure to 22% in the highest dust-exposure category; these differences could well have affected the certification of such causes of death as lung cancer and pneumoconiosis. However, the most serious deficiency in any cohort study is that the follow-up is too short for the disease in question. It has been repeatedly stressed that occupational studies of chronic respiratory and malignant diseases must focus on workers at least 20 years after first employment, and preferably much longer. In respiratory cancer, at least, evidence of an increased risk within 20 years points to selective factors rather than to the job. But failure to demonstrate risk in cohorts, where few subjects were followed sufficiently long, is even more serious.

Basis for Comparison

As already explained, longitudinal studies copy the logic of the experimental model; internal comparison is thus the first method of analysis to be considered. A cohort must be expected to differ from the general population by virtue of the selective criteria by which it was defined. It is then assumed that division of the cohort into subcohorts, differing in their degree of exposure, will approximate random allocation and so result in groups comparable in their subsequent experience. Although this is a useful working assumption, there may well be problems, for example,

1. Even in large surveys, the number of subjects in each exposure group, after allowance for differences in age, sex, era, and other variables, may not be sufficient for stable comparisons.
2. Without evidence from some external standard, there is no assurance that the group with minimal exposure adequately estimates the effect of no exposure. Exposures in the past may have been higher than supposed or the effects of even minimal exposure may be quite significant.
3. Information on exposure may be too poor to allow reliable internal comparisons, and dilution may obscure real effects.

For one or other of these reasons, an appropriate external standard population must often be sought. However, for reasons given below, this too presents serious difficulties and perfect comparisons can seldom be made. Indeed, in studies of morbidity rather than mortality, external comparative data are unlikely to exist, as virtually no systematic measurements of sickness have been made in general populations. Moreover, the ascertainment of respiratory symptoms and signs is notoriously dependent on the methods used to detect them. In studies of occupational bronchitis, for example, it would be necessary to have information from a large and truly representative sample of the general population using standard questionnaires and measurements of respiratory function. As few surveys of this kind have been done, internal comparisons cannot be avoided.

In practice, therefore, an external standard can only be considered in surveys of mortality. The usual procedure is to calculate the numbers of "expected" deaths by applying age-, sex-, cause-specific death rates for the national or regional population, year by year, to the cohort. However, specific occupational groups are likely to differ from the general population in several important ways:

1. Socioeconomically and geographically
2. In level of medical care and frequency of autopsy diagnosis
3. As a result of the physical requirements of the particular industry.

There is no rule-of-thumb solution to these difficulties; they must be recognized and dealt with on their merits.

B. Cross-Sectional Studies

Longitudinal designs, though well suited to studies of the incidence of accidents, acute illness, and death, are less easily applied to disease which is chronic, progressive, or insidous in onset. Moreover, longitudinal studies are generally time consuming and expensive. Whether the cohort is defined in the past or in the present, observation has still to be maintained over large numbers for long periods of time. Many epidemiological questions in occupational medicine are concerned with the natural history and causes of chronic respiratory disorders in which neither clinical manifestations nor etiological hypotheses are sufficiently well defined to justify a cohort study. In these circumstances, it may be better to take the cross-sectional approach and study disease associations over a very limited time period. Such investigations are termed *prevalence surveys* and, strictly speaking, focus on the situation as it exists at a defined point of time. Any longitudinal component then rests on verbal histories and available records. The most serious constraint lies in the fact that the data usually relate only to persons and places presently in view, and various steps may have to be taken to improve the time dimension. Two examples, one short and one extensive, may help to illustrate the uses and limitations of this approach.

Example 1

An apparent increase in histoplasmosis in Montreal, in 1963 to 1964, threw suspicion on large-scale demolition and construction work then in progress for the 1967 International Exposition, EXPO 67. In 1966, almost 3000 first-year university students in the city were asked to participate in a histoplasmin survey; 2666 (95%) agreed and were given an intradermal test; 94% of those tested returned for reading, and 12% were found positive. The test results are shown in Table 3, by students' home address before arrival at the university and, in Figure 4, by district in urban Montreal [16]. This simple and inexpensive survey provided much interesting information on the epidemiology of Histoplasma infection but raised as many questions as it answered. How representative were students of the areas from which they came? What about the 5% untested and the 6% unread? Can present rates be interpreted without knowledge of *when* the infections were acquired? What was the subsequent incidence of infection in the negatives? What are the clinical implications of histoplasmin sensitivity? Some but not all these questions were tackled subsequently. Tests were repeated on the same "cohort" a year later to determine conversion rates, estimated overall at 2%. An attempt was made to test a random sample of those who failed to attend with results which suggested that there had been no serious bias. Converters were followed clinically and radiologically; only three showed any abnormality, none serious.

Table 3 Histoplasmin Test Results in Students at McGill University According to Previous Home Address

Previous address	Tested	Positive	Percentages
Montreal			
Urban	1157	201	17
Suburban	443	27	6
Rest of Quebec	164	12	7
Rest of Canada	314	13	4
USA	135	11	8
Asia	157	10	6
Rest of world	136	24	18
Trinidad and Tobago	23	15	*65*
Other countries	113	9	*8*
Total	2496	298	12

Source: After MacEachern and McDonald (1971)[16].

Example 2

In 1966, it become urgently necessary to measure the long-term health effects of occupational exposure to chrysotile asbestos. Mortality could be and was studied in a defined cohort (as already mentioned), but effects on respiratory function, radiographic change, and symptomatology could not, except by the initiation of a survey which would have taken a working lifetime to complete. We chose, instead, a series of feasible though scientifically less certain inquiries, designed to exploit the accumulated experience of past employment in the industry.

In 1967, a typical prevalence survey of orthodox design was conducted among current workers in the industry, using an age-stratified random sample of over 1000 men selected from a total workforce of some 6000 employed on October 31, 1966. The sampling system was rather too complex and there were problems in its application [17]. Representativeness was sought, at the same time trying to ensure that a high proportion of older men with long exposure would be examined, and that comparison could be made among eight mining comparies which differed in size. The men selected were invited to attend for respiratory function tests and completion of a standard respiratory symptom questionnaire, in French or English, and the most recent routine chest x-ray for each man was selected for reading. Work histories were again used to estimate dust exposure in duration and concentration. We succeeded

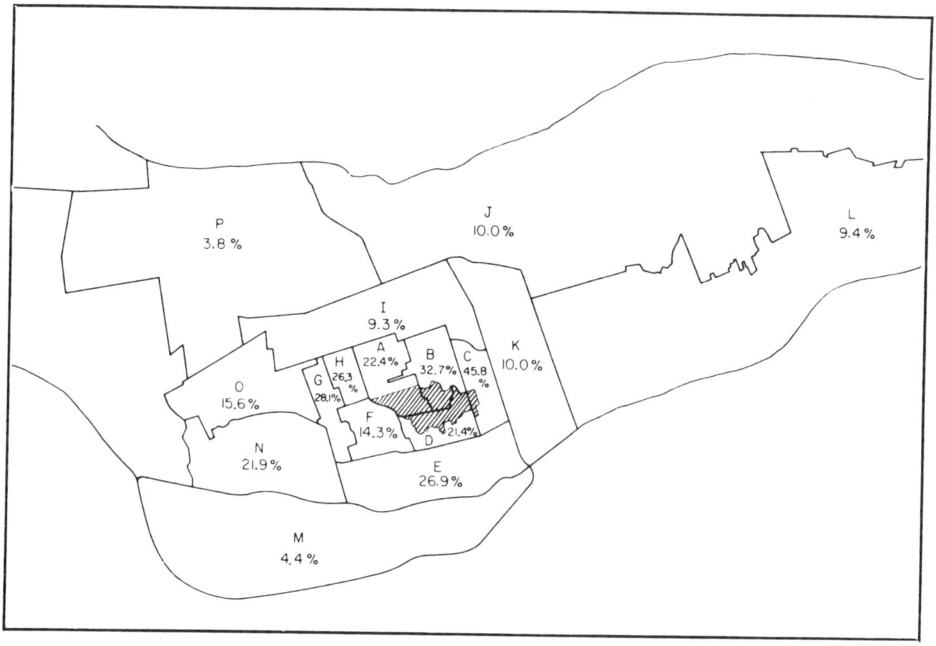

Figure 4 Urban Montreal: Percentage of positive reactors by district. Mount Royal Park occupies the shaded area. (Reproduced from MacEachern and McDonald, 1971 [16].)

in examining 84% of the sample but, because of deficiencies in work histories or test results, the analysis was reduced to 80%.

Simultaneously, a second main survey, also loosely cross-sectional, was initiated [18]. Routine annual chest x-rays had been taken on all chrysotile miners and millers for many years. Sets of x-rays, numbering about a quarter of a million in all, were on file in the clinics for nearly 16,000 workers, most of whom were no longer employed. The most recent radiograph for each man was selected for reading. To avoid bias, the films were first thoroughly mixed into random order and then the identifying information on each was covered with an opaque label bearing only a serial number. The assessment was carried out by an international panel of six readers working independently. This was the first occasion on which the UICC/Cincinnati (later ILO/UC) classification system [19] was used. The analysis was limited to data on some 13,000 men with complete work histories, who had been at least 1 month in the industry. The prevalence of radiological changes was studied in six age groups against a variety of exposure indices, calculated from duration of employment, dust concentration, and effort at work. This analysis suffered from all the problems of corss-sectional studies, with these additional complications: (1) the period of observation covered 20 to 30 years, and (2) men immediately before leaving a job may be atypical of all employees who achieve the same length of employment. The effect of these two selective factors is quite unknown and, in retrospect, it might have been wiser to pick films for study from men still at work, at three or four points in time.

Data from these two main prevalence surveys made possible a considerable number of analyses which related various measures of health to each other and to indices of exposure, taking account of age, physique, and smoking habit. The nature and degree of bias introduced by selection of current workers for the main study of respiratory symptoms and function and by the peculiar sampling procedure in the x-ray survey could only be guessed at the time. In fact, the biases were in opposite directions, as a recent follow-up indicated; the sick and disabled are probably underrepresented in cross-sectional samples of current workers, but overrepresented among men selected shortly before termination of employment. Despite these weaknesses, the results remained useful. They demonstrated that the main effects of chrysoltile exposure—breathlessness on exercise [17], reduced lung volume and flow rates [20], and small irregular parenchymal lung opacities and pleural thickening [18]—are all directly related to accumulated dust exposure. On the other hand, bronchitic symptoms were related primarily to smoking habit and only in light smokers and nonsmokers to dust. The necessity to postulate some other etiological factor than chrysotile for pleural calcification was also shown. Finally, the correlation between radiological and functional changes [21] provided the first validation of the ILO/UC classification.

A further problem inherent in the cross-sectional approach is that it lacks any longitudinal time component, particularly related to outcome. To make good this deficiency, four more studies were later added, as follows.

From those whose radiograph was read in 1967 to 1968, a sample of men was selected, each with five chest films spanning an average of 20 years. These pentads were assessed in known temporal order by four readers and the results related to age, smoking habit, duration of employment, and average dust concentration before and between films [22]. The correlations between various measures of exposure and both occurrence and progression of radiological change were low, suggesting that other factors including susceptibility were also important determinants.

A sample of men who had left the industry (1950–1967) and been x-rayed before leaving, were brought back in 1972 for a medical examination and further x-ray. The film pairs from each man were read for evidence of increased radiographic abnormality and this was found in 29%. A proportion of the parenchymal changes (but not pleural) were considered attributable to the earlier occupational exposure to chrysotile [23].

Two cohorts were selected in order to study how radiological changes predicted mortality. One cohort comprised 988 men from the 1967 to 1968 prevalence survey, for whom there were also data on pulmonary function and respiratory symptoms; 130 of these had died before 1976. The other cohort comprised all 4559 men in the main mortality cohort (excluding the 988 just mentioned) for whom there was an x-ray reading; 1453 of these had died before 1976. Relative risks for each main cause of death were then calculated for each radiographic feature [24]. Excess mortality from cardiorespiratory causes was well predicted, malignant disease less so. The findings thus provided further validation of the ILO/UC classification.

In 1975, an effort was made to find and retest all men examined in 1967 to 1968. Some 800 of the 1045 were seen; most of the remainder had died or left Quebec. The resulting paired data for each man were analyzed to measure the incidence and progression of asbestotic changes over the 7 year period, in relation to dust exposure, allowing for age and smoking habit. Once again it was found that the correlation between clinically detectable manifestations of change and indices of exposure were poor, emphasizing the importance of environmental control rather than biological monitoring in the protection of the worker [25].

The main weakness of the cross-sectional design is survivor bias, and this is almost insuperable. It was said of the original survey in 1938 by Dreesen et al. [26], on which the first threshold limit value for asbestos dust was based, that the dead were buried and the sick in hospital. Despite this, the results had considerable value for even an imperfect survey is better than none. The only way of dealing with the problem is to find and examine those who should by rights have been included or at least a representative sample of them. Even for the living, this is difficult, and for the dead impossible. This source of bias gives rise to real difficulty in the interpretation of cross-sectional results, as the following example shows. It was found in the prevalence survye of chrysotile workers that, in men with radiological evidence of asbestosis, obstructive and restrictive patterns of pulmonary function were equally common [27]. This ran counter to the conventional view of asbestosis, that restrictive disease predominates. In discussing their finding, the authors correctly recognized, "This may be a consequence of our subjects being drawn exclusively from a working and therefore survivor population, without taking into account retired individuals who may be more disabled, a more than likely explanation if this profile [i.e., restrictive pattern] was associated with greater disability."

C. Case-Control Studies

The strength of the two survey designs which have been discussed lies in the fact that cases of disease are ascertained after definition of the population at risk. Because of the scale on which they have generally to be conducted, such surveys tend to require considerable resources of many kinds. The more rare the disease under investigation, the larger must be the survey. In the cohort study of chrysotile miners and millers, it was only after 10 years operation and a total of 4500 deaths, that the number of cases of mesothelioma rose to ten. In the cross-sectional survey of the same mining population, despite almost excessive age-weighting, the number of cases in the higher categories of radiographic change was too few for separate study. When resources are limited or the disease uncommon a more economical strategy is required; a case-control design may then be the answer. This approach is a simple one derived from the traditions of clinical medicine and everyday life; events are examined and interpreted against other comparable experience. This was how Macbeth [28] reasoned on becoming aware of 20 cases of cancer of the paranasal sinuses in an English town (High Wycombe), 15 associated with the making of wooden chairs; and Wagner and colleagues [29], on noting the remarkable concentration of pleural mesotheliomas in one area of the Cape Province of South Africa. Both discoveries called for, and later received, carefully designed studies of further case series, with parallel observations on comparable controls. After the event, some may question whether confirmatory investigations were really necessary, but few causal associations are as strong as those cited, and false alarms cannot otherwise be dispelled. The need for controls stems from the fact that, in any universe of cases, only a proportion come to light, and these will reflect a host of selective and local factors. Thus, it would be expected that a relatively high proportion of cases of any disease, in High Wycombe, would be in furniture workers, since making chairs is the major industry; and proximity to asbestos mines might well be a feature of mesotheliomas in the Cape Province, for analogous reasons. If etiological hypotheses are to be tested on highly selected cases, the degree of association with the suspected cause must also be measured in similarily selected persons, but without the disease. Principles for conducting such case-control surveys have been developed to produce a reliable estimate of the "normal" expectation in these circumstances.

Selection of Cases

Diagnostic criteria, and the procedure for finding and registering cases, must be precisely defined. Generalizable results are wanted, so unduly narrow geographical and time limits are to be avoided. Cases of farmer's lung, for example, should probably be drawn from more than one season and climatic zone. Cases registered in ignorance of the causal hypothesis are clearly preferable to those collected later, when the diagnoses could well be biased as a result.

Selection of Controls

Patients chosen for study will differ from the general population in two ways: in respect of factors which relate directly or indirectly to the cause of the disease, and in selective factors which lead to their registration. In selecting controls, the aim must be to match for the second group of factors and not for the first—a difficult task. Human behavior is complex and its determinants numerous and interrelated; it is all too easy, therefore, to overmatch controls with cases in selective characteristics and so obscure real differences in the frequency of the suspected cause. It is fortunate that close matching by more than three simple factors, of which two must almost always be age and sex, is seldom feasible. This leaves room only for the important issue of how each case came to light. Thus, cases diagnosed in the hospital, at autopsy, in the doctor's office, by routine screening, etc., should be matched by controls (i.e., noncases) drawn in like manner. A difficulty arises where exposure to the agent may take place at work and/or in the neighborhood. This is not uncommon, as industries tend to be located close to their source of raw materials and, at the same time, pollute the local environment. In assessing the occupational component, we must match for locality, because specific industries are only in certain places. However, the controls thus selected clearly cannot be used to investigate the effect of local pollution.

An analogous problem, common in lung disease, is the need to take smoking into account, both as an independent cause of the disease in question and also as a factor which may interact in some way with the agent under review. If we do not match for smoking, we cannot measure the effect of the agent alone; if we do match for smoking, we cannot assess interactions. For these reasons, it is often desirable to select more than one series of controls, matched to the cases in different ways. It has been suggested that the various control series selected should be unrelated, to ensure that spurious results are not obtained from overmatching or undermatching. Unfortunately, this approach may lead to conflicting findings which cannot be resolved. It may be more sensible, therefore, for the two or more control series to differ only in respect of single matching factors, deliberately chosen to discriminate between alternative hypotheses.

Data Collection

In case-control studies, accurate and unbiased information is particularly difficult to obtain. Subjects are often hard to trace, records may well be scanty or nonexistant, and memories faulty. Appropriate records are invaluable, provided that they are available equally for cases and controls. In questioning subjects or relatives, the interviewer should, if possible, be kept ignorant of the identity of cases and controls. Within reasonable standards of honesty, the respondents' attention should be directed at several questions, and not only at the critical one, to reduce suspicion and the coloring of fact with opinion. Interviewing procedures require care and judgment, since details of occupational history may be impossible to obtain without considerable probing. The essential points are first, to ensure that cases and controls are treated identically, and second, to leave very few of either untraced, as only matched pairs should be used in the analysis.

Coding and Analysis

The end is not reached with the recording of information: it has still to be classified and analyzed. These procedures are also susceptable to bias. In assessing the data, there are decisions to be made at every stage. Is the subject the right person? Which, if any, of conflicting statements, should be accepted? What level of exposure did this job entail? If we settle for "not known" when there is any shadow of doubt, the study is doomed and, anyway, how is "doubt" to be defined? Most questions can be dealt with by exercise of reasonable judgment, but only if they are made "blind" as to the identity of cases and controls. Similar problems are encountered during analysis; it is all too easy to modify the hypothesis under test, to meet better the recorded data. To do so is scientifically dishonest—a challenge to the investigator's conscience, nevertheless, since only he or she need ever know. It is perfectly legitimate, of course, to report and discuss the effect of modifying the hypothesis, but no statistical tests can then be applied to the findings.

An Example

Some of the principles and problems may be better appreciated in the light of experience with an actual survey. In 1967, we thought it important to examine the association between mesothelioma and asbestos in broader context by studying a nationally representative series of cases and controls in Canada and, later, in the United States [30]. Cases were registered by writing to all practicing pathologists, and controls were selected from the pathology files in the same hospitals. The controls were chosen from fatal cases of nonpulmonary malignant disease with lung metastases, matched for sex, age, and year. Interviewers, mainly nurses, visited relatives without knowledge of which were cases and controls. A four-page standard questionnaire was completed for each subject on occupation, residence, and smoking habits, and the data were classified "blind." Points to note were:

1. *Registration of cases.* Emphasis was put on wide geographical cover, within specified time limits, and on a clearly defined case-finding procedure. However, possible bias due to pathologists' increasing awareness of the association with asbestos could not be removed.
2. *Controls.* These were selected from deaths with a similar terminal illness, and comparable emotional impact on relatives to cases. Although this was so for pleural mesothelioma, the same could not be claimed for the peritoneal cases. A second control series was used during part of the study, comprising deaths from primary lung cancer, similarly matched. These were chosen to evaluate the importance of cigarette smoking, and this was successfully achieved.
3. *Data collection.* This was satisfactory in terms of objectivity, but has been criticized on the ground that nurses were not sufficiently familiar with industrial jobs and processes, and so did not probe adequately. As work and environmental histories were obtained only from relatives, supplementary inquiries would have been valuable, but this was beyond our resources.
4. *Data classification.* Although this was satisfactorily blind, it was at first unduly subjective and dependent on personal opinion. This was somewhat improved by arranging for the classification of all jobs possibly associated with asbestos exposure, by four independent experts.

IV. Descriptive Studies

The conduct of purely descriptive studies of disease incidence and prevalence is a less exciting role for epidemiology than those so far described, but one which is certainly useful. Such studies may also throw light on questions of cause and control of disease, but their aim is primarily to give a balanced picture of a situation at a point in time, or at intervals along the way. These studies are generally cross-sectional in type. Even when intended for continuous surveillance, they are seldom truly longitudinal, in that the same subjects are not deliberately followed forward. Cross-sectional inquiries are needed for planning of services, definition of research priorities, and resource allocation. The "monitoring" variety are made to detect changes in frequency, as a guide for control measures. Some studies of the natural history and out-

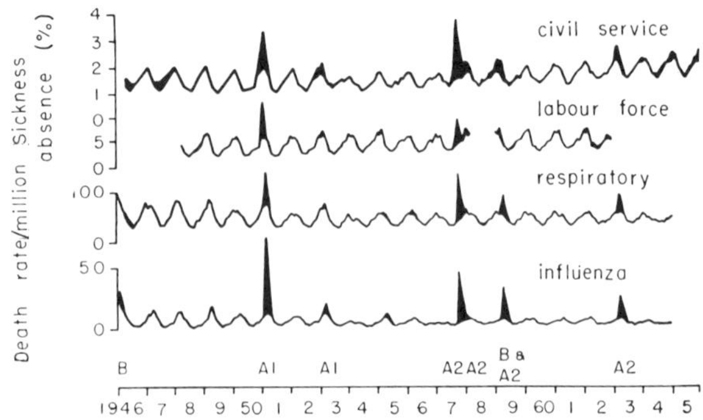

Figure 5 Excess sickness and mortality in Canada attributable to influenza, 1946–1965. (Originally published in *Canadian Medical Association Journal,* 97:522–527, September 2, 1967 [31].)

come of disease, treated and untreated, are also essentially descriptive. They yield information basic to the clinical needs of diagnosis, prognosis, and (subjective) assessment of treatment.

There are no special principles of design and data collection for descriptive studies which have not been mentioned already in this chapter. They must interfere with the natural order of things as little as possible and, financially, have often to be conducted for next to nothing. This calls for opportunism, and a willingness to modify classic designs and methods to achieve practical objectives. This free-style type of epidemiological inquiry makes greater demands on skill and judgement than set piece investigations, to ensure that various compromises are kept within the bounds of scientific validity.

It is not easy to set down rules of guidance for varied and *ad hoc* field studies. Definitions and denominators must be given the highest priority. The working population under study or "at risk" must be clearly specified in terms of age, sex, space, time, and other relevant aspects. The same applies to methods for case detection and to diagnostic criteria. Avoidance of bias, particularly due to incomplete information, is important as elsewhere. It is worth remembering that it is always better to have all the required data for a 10% sample of subjects than some of the data for all of them. The great virtue of deliberate sampling is that it allows effort and resources to be concentrated on quality rather than quantity. Since the object is usually to *estimate,* rather than to determine precisely, the considerable gain in reliability, which sampling offers, is well worth a slight loss in precision.

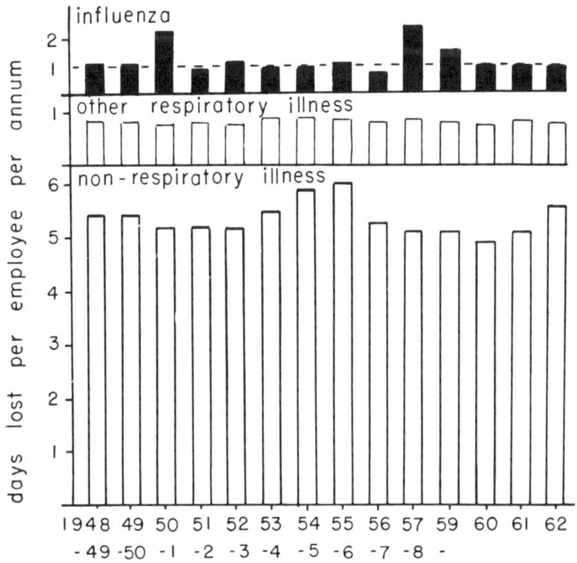

Figure 6 Sickness absence in Canadian male civil servants, 1948–1962. (Originally published in *Canadian Medical Association Journal,* 97:522–527, September 2, 1967 [31].)

Another concept to be exploited, whenever possible, is the remarkable regularity of many natural events. This often permits stable baseline rates and proportions, to be set for a variety of health indices. An example, illustrated in Figures 5 and 6, shows the impact of epidemic influenza on sickness absence and mortality from respiratory causes in Canada [31]. Estimates derived from Figure 6 of days lost from this disease per male employee in the Federal Civil Service, are presented in Table 4.

This general approach has many possible applications in occupational epidemiology. Systematic recording of specific events in defined populations can provide norms against which the unusual may show itself quite clearly. Were this kind of data on disease frequency and outcome widely available, evidence could be obtained more readily on the effectiveness of new methods of control and treatment.

An extremely simple monitoring technique which deserves to be better known requires the use of graph paper. The baseline is divided into sections, of length proportional to the size of each population subgroup under review. As events or diseases of interest occur, they are plotted on the appropriate section of the baseline. Columns are gradually built up which quickly reveal anything unusual. This visual method can, of course, be made quite complex, by allowing for additional variables, such as age, type of job, and duration of

Table 4 Sickness Absence Attributable to Influenza in Male Civil Servants (Canada 1951–1960)

Epidemic months	Excess absence (%)	Days lost per employee
1951 Jan.–Feb.	8.8	0.65
1953 Feb.–April	2.0	0.15
1955 Feb.–May	2.4	0.18
1957 Sep.–Dec.	7.6	0.56
1958 Jan.–Feb.	1.9	0.14
1959 Mar.–May	3.7	0.27
Total (10 years)	26.4	1.95

Source: After McDonald (1967)[31].

employment, on separate sheets of graph paper. A limiting factor in all surveillance methods is population size; large groups and/or common events are needed to produce stable rates.

V. Principles of Measurement

The skeleton of survey design must now be given body, in the form of observations and measurements. Other chapters of this book deal at length with particular aspects of physical measurement, but some points of special epidemiological relevance deserve brief mention here. There are a number of time-honored criteria against which it is useful to judge any observations made for scientific purposes. These separate themselves into three main groups.

A. Sensitivity-Specificity Issues

A sensitive indicator will pick up a high proportion of what it is desired to detect; false negatives are not acceptable, though there may well be many false positives. High specificity is usually achieved at the cost of many false negatives, or low sensitivity. The desired balance depends on the objective, but the problem is complicated by the issue of representativeness. Tests of high specificity are unfortunately liable to yield unrepresentative findings. For example, the tuberculin test is a very sensitive but relatively nonspecific indicator of *active* tuberculosis. On the other hand, isolation of *M. tuberculosis* from sputum, although less sensitive and highly specific, will detect only certain types of active disease. Parallel situations are encountered when measuring the environment. The mass assay of airborne particles versus electron-microscope analysis of filter samples illustrate two opposite extremes.

B. Reliability—Error Problems

Every test is liable to some error and resulting variation and, thus, is more or less reliable (reproducible or repeatable). The errors characteristic of any test are derived from two sources: the subjects observed and the observer; hence the terms subject variation and observer error. Observers vary in their ability to repeat identical measurements (intraobserver variation) and also between themselves (interobserver variation). Unlike the sensitivity-specificity issue, errors present no dilemma; whatever their cause they must be reduced to an absolute minimum. Failure to do so endangers the sensitivity of the investigation as a whole or, worse still, leads to bias and incorrect conclusions.

No measurements in epidemiology have received more attention from the standpoint of reliability than the chest radiograph (see Chapter 3). In order to minimize error, something akin to a code of practice has evolved [32], most features of which establish principles which apply equally to other measurements made for survey purposes:

1. Standardization of radiological technique
2. Classification, whereby the shadows observed can be recorded qualitatively and quantitatively, without diagnostic interpretation
3. Scoring of each film by more than one reader, each working alone, with results averaged (or considered separately), unmodified by consensus
4. Readers ignorant of the identity and provenance of the films, except in general terms
5. Admixture of a proportion of "normal" films into the series
6. Standard films available to each reader for ready reference
7. Rereading of a subsample of films in each survey, to assess intra- and interobserver error.

C. Questions of Validity

The inventions of physical and biological scientists enable measurements to be made with increasing precision, elegance, and reliability. However, this is no guarantee that health and disease can be better described. The chest x-ray is a case in point; opacities *per se* are not disease and may or may not well reflect it. This is evident in the chest films of coal, asbestos, and barium miners. Tests of respiratory physiology can describe structure and function in some detail, but how well do they measure disability compared, say, to a simple exercise tolerance test? These questions relate to the characteristic of "validity," by which is judged the capacity of a test to describe the quality we want described. While validity is clearly to be sought, it must sometimes taken second place to reliability; witness, the general preference for function tests and x-rays, rather than symptom questionnaires. However, it may well be that in assessing disability, too much emphasis is now being put on indirect tests of low and uncertain validity.

D. Measurements of Exposure

Failure to specify exposure, save in terms of duration, is the most common and serious weakness in occupational epidemiology. The causes are clear enough. Either measurements of concentration were not made in the workplace over the relevant period, or not recorded, or were of poor quality, or not relatable to specific jobs, etc. These deficiencies are a fact, and cannot be corrected, but investigators must also take some blame for a degree of defeatism. Some have failed to appreciate how limited in value are studies which make no attempt, even to guess, the severity of exposure. Others, more perfectionist in temperament, have allowed the best to be enemy of the "better than nothing"—always a mistake in epidemiology. It follows that some grading of exposure should be attempted unless it is totally impossible, but such grading, when subjective, must be carried out in complete ignorance of outcome.

In the future, we shall do better by seeing to it that environmental measurements of potential use in epidemiology are made and recorded in the major sectors of industry. As before, there is the danger of being handicapped by perfectionism. For instance, it may be argued that unless we measure each particular agent separately, something of importance will be missed, or that exposure of the individual worker cannot be estimated adequately without constant use of personal monitors. There is some truth in these statements, but their total acceptance would be a serious setback for epidemiological research in occupational lung disease. Epidemiology requires a different strategy, with emphasis on the following:

1. Aerodynamic studies in workplaces of varied size and shape, so that distribution patterns of gases, aerosols, and vapors can be estimated from measurements of concentration at a limited number of index sites
2. Periodic and detailed qualitative and quantitative analyses, based on air sampling, at the more important index sites
3. Maintenance of good work history records, not for the purpose of pay, but with attention to *place* of work, so that approximate levels of past exposure for individual workers can be rationally assessed at a future date

At the present time, this strategy must compete with priorities, usually given both by industrial hygienists and government inspectors, to monitoring the sources of pollution for the purpose of control. Important though these measurements are, they give little idea of most workers' day-to-day experience.

VI. Summary

Epidemiology seeks to put disease in proper perspective so that its importance can be assessed and its causes identified among coincidental associations. Everything depends on the application of simple principles of logic to study design and on the collection of reliable data, for errors in these cannot be corrected by sophisticated measurement techniques, computer programes or statistical analyses. There is no basic difference between evaluation of suspected causes and testing methods of treatment or prevention. Either way, the aim is to obtain a sound estimate of what would have happened without the factor (or treatment) and to make comparisons which are generalizable. Strictly controlled trial designs are occasionally possible and always a model against which the validity of less rigid experimental and observational surveys can be judged. The controlled experiment is longitudinal, with the outcome recorded in defined populations and comparability in respect of confounding variables assumed by virtue of randomization. Cohort and time-series designs are also longitudinal, but as the study groups are selected or self-selected in a nonrandom manner they may or may not be comparable. Cross-sectional surveys have two further shortcomings: observed time sequences are replaced by histories and records, and findings are based on survivors and not on the original population at risk. Finally, in case-control designs, even the cases are selected and, in ignorance of the population from which they come, "controls" must be chosen from "noncases" by mimicking the selection process. Epidemiology is a practical science which inevitably entails compromise with perfection, acceptable only if there is insight into the nature of resulting errors; but clinical and social decisions must be made and it is the medical investigator's job to provide the best possible guidance.

References

1. Campbell, D. T., and J. C. Stanley, *Experimental and Quasi-experimental Designs for Research.* Chicago, Rand McNally, 1966, pp. 5–6.
2. Greenberg, B. G., and B. F. Mattison, The whys and wherefores of program evaluation, *Can. J. Publ. Health,* **46**:293–299 (1955).
3. Report of MRC Committee on Influenza and Other Respiratory Virus Vaccines, 1960–3, *Br. Med. J.,* **2**:267–271 (1964).
4. Weiss, C. H., *Evaluation Research.* Englewood Cliffs, New Jersey, Prentice-Hall, 1972.
5. Cochrane, A. L., *Effectiveness and Efficiency. Random Reflections on Health Services.* Abingdon, Nuffield Provincial Hospitals Trust, 1972.
6. Hill, A. B., *A Short Textbook of Medical Statistics.* London, Hodder and Stoughton, 1977, p. 294.
7. Loosli, C. G. (Ed.). *Conference On Newer Respiratory Disease Viruses.* Bethesda, USPHS, 1972, pp. 120–148.
8. McDonald, J. C., A. J. Zuckerman, A. S. Beare, and D. A. J. Tyrrell, Trials of live influenza vaccine in the Royal Air Force. *Br. Med. J.,* **1**: 1036–1042 (1962).
9. Pepys, J., and B. J. Hutchcroft, Bronchial provocation tests in etiologic diagnosis and analysis of asthma, *Am. Rev. Respir. Dis.,* **112**:829–859 (1975).
10. Liddell, F. D. K., J. C. McDonald, and D. C. Thomas, Methods of cohort analysis: Appraisal by application to asbestos mining. *J. Roy. Stat. Soc., A,* **140**:469–491 (1977).
11. McDonald, J. C., A. D. McDonald, G. W. Gibbs, J. Siemiatycki, and C. E. Rossiter, Mortality in the chrysotile mines and mills of Quebec, *Arch. Environ. Health,* **22**:677–685 (1971).
12. McDonald, J. C., and F. D. K. Liddell, Mortality in Canadian miners and millers exposed to chrysotile, *Ann. N.Y. Acad. Sci.,* **330**:1–10 (1979).
13. Jones, J. S. P., F. D. Pooley, and P. G. Smith, Factory populations exposed to crocidolite asbestos—a continuing survey. *IARC Scientific publications, INSERM,* **52**:117–120 (1976).
14. McDonald, A. D., and J. C. McDonald, Mesothelioma in persons exposed to crocidolite in gas-mask manufacture, *Environ. Res.,* **17**:340–346 (1978).
15. McDonald, J. C., and A. J. Zuckerman, ABO blood groups and acute respiratory virus disease, *Br. Med. J.,* **2**:89–90 (1962).
16. MacEachern, E. J., and J. C. McDonald, Histoplasmin sensitivity in McGill University students, *Can. J. Publ. Health,* **62**:415–422 (1971).

17. McDonald, J. C., M. R. Becklake, G. Fournier-Massey, and C. E. Rossiter, Respiratory symptoms in chrysotile asbestos mine and mill workers of Quebec, *Arch. Environ. Health,* **24**:358–363 (1972).
18. Rossiter, C. E., L. J. Bristol, P. H. Cartier, J. G. Gilson, T. R. Grainger, G. K. Sluis-Cremer, and J. C. McDonald, Radiographic changes in chrysotile asbestos mine and mill workers of Quebec, *Arch. Environ. Health,* **24**:388–400 (1972).
19. International Labour Office, *ILO/UC international classification of radiographs of the pneumoconioses, 1971.* Occupational Safety and Health Series No. 22 (revised), Geneva, ILO, 1972.
20. Becklake, M. R., G. Fournier-Massey, C. E. Rossiter, and J. C. McDonald, Lung function in chrysotile asbestos mine and mill workers of Quebec, *Arch. Environ. Health,* **24**:401–409 (1972).
21. Becklake, M. R., G. Fournier-Massey, J. C. McDonald, J. Siemiatycki, and C. E. Rossiter, Lung function in relation to chest radiographic changes in Quebec asbestos workers, *Bull. Physiopathol. Respir.,* **6**:637–659 (1970).
22. Liddell, F. D. K., G. E. Eyssen, D. Thomas, and J. C. McDonald, Radiological changes over 20 years in relation to chrysotile exposure in Quebec. In *Inhaled Particles,* Vol. IV. Edited by W. H. Walton. Oxford, Pergamon, 1977, pp. 799–812.
23. Becklake, M. R., F. D. K. Liddell, J. Manfreda, and J. C. McDonald, Radiological changes after withdrawal from asbestos exposure, *Br. J. Ind. Med.,* **36**:23–28 (1979).
24. Lidell, F. D. K., and J. C. McDonald, Radiological findings as predictors of mortality in Quebec asbestos workers, *Br. J. Med.,* **37**:257–267 (1980).
25. Becklake, M. R., Clinical measurements in Quebec chrysotile miners: Use for future protection of workers, *Ann. N.Y. Acad. Sci.,* **330**:23–29 (1979).
26. Dreesen, W. C., J. M. Dallavalle, T. I. Edwards, J. W. Miller, R. R. Sayers, H. F. Easom, and M. F. Trice, A study of asbestosis in the asbestos textile industry, Publ. Health Bull No. 241, Washington, D.C., 1938.
27. Fournier-Massey, G., and M. R. Becklake, Pulmonary function profiles in Quebec asbestos workers, *Bull. Physiopathol. Respir.,* **11**:429–445 (1975).
28. Macbeth, R., Malignant disease of the paranasal sinuses, *J. Laryngol.,* **79**:592–612 (1965).
29. Wagner, J. C., C. A. Sleggs, and P. Marchand, Diffuse pleural mesothelioma and asbestos exposure in the north-western Cape Province, *Br. J. Ind. Med.,* **17**:260–271 (1960).
30. McDonald, A. D., Mesothelioma registries in identifying asbestos hazards, *Ann. N.Y. Acad. Sci.,* **330**:441–454 (1979).
31. McDonald, J. C., Influenza in Canada, *Can. Med. Assoc. J.,* **97**:522–527 (1967).
32. Weill, H., and R. Jones, The chest roentgenogram as an epidemiologic tool, *Arch. Environ. Health,* **30**:435–439 (1975).

14

Worker Surveys

GEOFFREY B. FIELD

The Prince Henry Hospital
Sydney, New South Wales, Australia

This chapter outlines the principles governing the conduct of surveys in industry and draws attention to some of the pitfalls encountered in converting an idea for a study into a reality. Its purpose is not to bind investigators to a set of rules but to provide a framework upon which they can fashion their studies. Unlike laboratory experiments, epidemiological surveys, particularly in industry, often present problems beyond the control of the investigator. A good design anticipates these as far as possible and avoids them when they can be circumvented and compromises when they can not. The study must be tailored to the conditions as they exist; if the conditions fall short of the ideal, as they inevitably will, the design will be less than ideal but this does not justify abandoning the study if it is basically sound and its limitations are acceptable. There is room for imagination and flair in the design of surveys; if circumstances rule out the conventional approach, the unconventional should be tried if it will meet the aims of the survey.

Surveys in industry, like other scientific studies, should start with an hypothesis. The translation of that hypothesis into an investigation which will yield scientifically valid results is the function of the survey design. The design embraces all aspects of the survey from a precise statement of its purpose to the minutiae of measurement techniques. The aim of the study is the focus upon which all other aspects of the design are centered; the structure of the survey must be developed with this central theme constantly in mind. Practical considerations may force a departure from the optimum design but they should never dominate it. If the aims of the survey cannot be achieved with the facilities available, they must be modified. The data-gathering exercise with, at best, a nebulously defined purpose and no hypothesis to test is to be deplored. The argument that "we shall see what comes out of the data" runs contrary to the basic principles of scientific method and is no justification for an uncritical approach to survey design.

The classic pneumoconioses, such as coal workers' pneumoconiosis and silicosis, present fewer problems in survey design than the hazards associated with asbestos, cotton dust, and the complex chemical processes of modern industrial technology. The main thrust of respiratory surveys in industry is now directed at these latter hazards whose effects on the health of the workforce are often insidious or simulate conditions which are common in the community such as asthma and the bronchial disease of cigarette smoking. This chapter is concerned primarily with the investigation of these hazards, although the principles of survey design apply equally to the classic pneumoconioses.

I. The Survey Protocol

The protocol is a statement of the survey design. It should be factual and contain all the details necessary for the conduct of the survey. Preparation of a protocol forces the investigator to be specific about both the theoretical and the practical aspects of the design. The discipline of writing a protocol does much to ensure that an ill-conceived design is not put into practice and that preoccupation with the overall concept of the survey does not lead to neglect of the pedestrian details. A clearly presented protocol also allows management to define its role in the survey and to anticipate any problems with production schedules.

The protocol should begin with a brief outline of the background to the survey and the reason for doing it. The theoretical aspects of the design are then described in detail under the following broad headings: aims of survey, definition of population, sampling techniques, type of survey, and measurement techniques. A copy of all questionnaires should be included. The practical aspects of running the survey and enlisting the cooperation of the workforce are equally important to the success of the study. The initial approach to the workforce, the administrative organization, the testing schedule, and the location of survey personnel and instruments must be considered. Finally, a statement must appear in the protocol regarding the distribution of the report on the survey findings, the confidentiality of individual data, and the right to publish the results in scientific journals. These latter points are often taken for granted by academically based survey teams, but management and unions often hold strong views on these matters and considerable ill will may be generated if a mutually satisfactory arrangement is not negotiated in advance of the actual survey.

II. Defining the Population

The work environment is only one of the features distinguishing an industrial workforce from the general population and from workforces in other industries. Selection factors influencing the composition of the workforce will ensure that it differs from the community from which the employees are drawn. Communities in turn have their own characteristics which distinguish one from another. An expanding, progressive community will attract a different type of person to one geographically isolated from the mainstream of industry and associated with limited job opportunities. Industry can also influence the community with which it is associated by pollution of the atmosphere or by returning to the community employees who have been retrenched or retired because of occupational disability. Selection factors also operate within a workforce, creating differences between employee groups engaged in different jobs or working in different sections of the plant. A workforce must therefore always be treated as a biased sample of the general population and inhomogeneous within itself. This bias and inhomogeneity has to be accepted in industrial surveys but it must not be ignored. Every effort should be made to estimate its influence on the population prior to the survey by appropriate enquiries and, if necessary, a pilot study of the workforce. This information is essential for a precise description of the population and for defining the limits of the total population and relevant subgroups.

Surveys should be designed around a single wworkforce unless the syndrome under investigation has such a low incidence that it is essential that more than one be studied. The inclusion of several workforces in a survey population has two undesirable effects. It obliges the investigator to neglect bias and community differences in the composition of individual workforces when interpreting the data, and it obscures real differences in the response of the workforces to their environment unless these differences are specifically sought by a separate analysis of each workforce. Combining a number of workforces in a single study does not necessarily make the findings more applicable to the industry in general. If one is interested only in establishing the prevalence of disease in a particular occupation, then the more workforces that can be included in the study the more likely are the findings to be representative of the industry as a whole, but this is rarely a worthwhile exercise.

The survey population must be defined in the protocol with sufficient precision for there to be no doubt which members of the workforce are included and which are not. No deviation from the criteria should be permitted and no alteration made subsequently unless indicated for reasons independent of the survey findings. The temptation to delete individuals or to alter population criteria after examining the survey data must be strictly avoided.

A. Sources of Bias

The extent to which the composition of a workforce differs from the community from which it is drawn depends mainly on the method of selecting new employees and on labor turnover. Most industries insist that new employees pass a preemployment or preplacement medical examination. The magnitude of the bias generated by this requirement will depend on the standard of health demanded by the industry relative to that existing in the community. The usual effect is to produce a workforce whose health is superior to that of the community, especially in areas or periods of unemployment, but where there is competition for available labor the opposite may occur. The age structure, ethnic background, socioeconomic status, and urban or rural location of the community will influence its general standard of health and therefore the difference in standard between the community and the industry.

The many reasons an employee chooses to leave an industry almost all result in a biased loss from the workforce. If the work is heavy, the less healthy tend to leave; if the work is poorly paid, the more healthy tend to leave as they have a better chance of finding alternative employment. The turnover rate will be influenced by the prevailing economic climate and employment opportunities and may therefore vary with age and length of service in the industry. If the work environment itself is affecting the health of the workforce, a significant bias occurs in the labor turnover, and the employees who remain represent a survivor population. The paradoxical situation then arises that the longer the length of service the less likely is there to be evidence of occupationally induced disease. This is particularly true of an industry with an asthma hazard, where the greatest loss from the workforce tends to occur in the younger age groups with a relatively short length of service.

Heterogeneity within a workforce can result from preplacement medical requirements or from labor turnover if the medical standards for entry into different sectors of the workforce vary or the turnover rates are different. Transfer and promotion of personnel inevitably create bias within a workforce. Many industries, particularly those with a recognized occupational hazard, follow a policy of relocating employees with health problems in lighter or less hazardous jobs within the industry. In one industry with an asthma hazard, nine men, transferred to other sections of the plant because of respiratory symptoms, were found to have an FEV_1 0.7 liters less and a histamine reactivity 3 times greater than the remainder of the workforce. This indicates the magnitude of the bias which may be created by such transfers. Promotion is always selective, and health is likely to be a major consideration. However, the advancement of an employee may be influenced by more subtle judgments. This was well illustrated in one survey in industry in which the foremen were found to be 8 cm taller on average than the remainder of the workforce. The same type of bias was encountered in another industry where the average height of new employees increased abruptly following the introduction of stricter preemployment health criteria which made no reference to height.

B. Identifying Sources of Bias

Evidence of bias in the composition of the workforce should be sought during the planning stages of a survey as it may have a considerable bearing on the design ultimately adopted. Medical and personnel officers can provide valuable information on potential sources of bias. The policy regarding medical examinations is particularly relevant. How strict are the preemployment criteria? Are they the same for all sectors of the workforce? Are there any specific exclusions, e.g., a history of asthma? Has there been any change in the criteria, perhaps following the recognition of a respiratory hazard in the industry? Is there regular medical surveillance of the workforce, and if so, what action is taken on the findings? Does the firm relocate or retrench medically unfit employees? The personnel officer can give an opinion on the desirability of the industry as a place to work in the eyes of the community and the degree to which employees strive to remain in the industry. He or she should be asked to supply details of the labor turnover, preferably in the form of a cohort analysis extending back sufficiently far to include the longest serving employee. The reasons for fluctuation in the labor turnover, and if retrenchments have occurred during periods of reduced production, the basis for selecting those dismissed should be sought. Some industries keep a record of the reasons given by employees for resigning. They are unlikely to be accurate but may point to a selective loss from the workforce for health reasons.

These enquiries indicate whether the survey population is likely to differ materially from the community or from other workforces included in the study. They also allow the homogeneity of the population to be assessed with respect to factors unrelated to the work environment. However, important sources of bias may not be detected unless specifically sought in the analysis of the survey data. Figure 1 shows a highly significant trend in diffusing capacity with increasing length of service in the potroom workers of an aluminium smelter in which less than 5% of the original workforce was still employed after 10 years. The trend was not explained by differences in age, height, smoking habit, or work environment. The most likely explanation of this trend was that employees with more than 4 years service represented a survivor population.

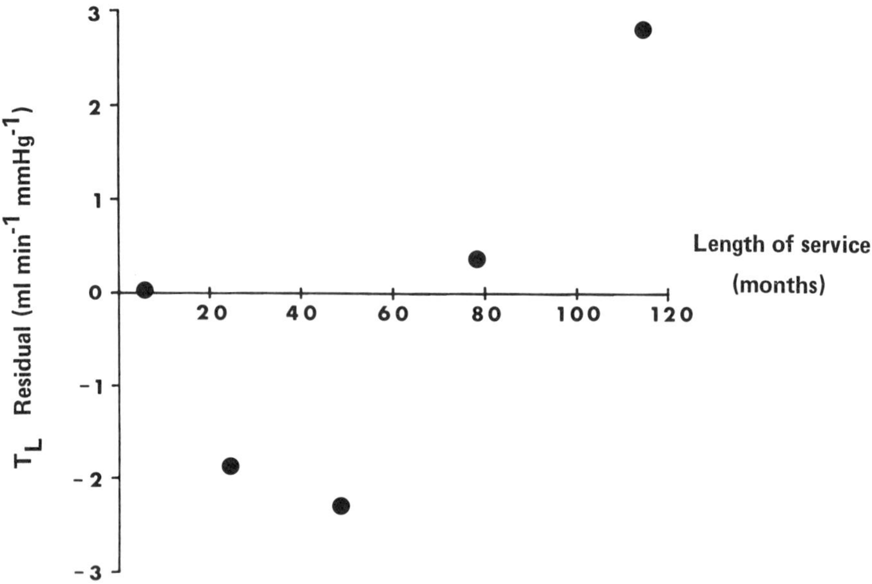

Figure 1 The relationship of transfer factor, after adjustment for age, height, and smoking habit, to length of service in the potroom of an aluminum smelter. The data are derived from 100 potroom employees divided into five length-of-service categories, each containing 20 men. The points indicate the mean T_L of each category expressed as the difference from the overall mean for the smelter workforce.

C. "Control" Populations

There is a widely held belief that the effect of a respiratory hazard in industry cannot be assessed without reference to a control population. This attitude has arisen through the almost universal use of control populations in animal studies. By definition, the control population must be identical in all respects to the study population except for exposure to the respiratory hazard under investigation. This is readily achieved in animal experiments by randomly allocating specially bred animals either to the study or to the control group. Such precise matching is impossible in surveys in industry in which the populations are predetermined and cannot be manipulated in this fashion. No matter how carefully the control population is chosen, the fact that its composition is predetermined must prejudice its comparibility and therefore its value as a control. An inappropriate control population can seriously affect the survey findings either by obscuring a real effect of the work environment or by generating a spurious one. Great care must therefore be exercised in the choice of a control population. Often, the need for a control population can be avoided by subdividing the population on the basis of exposure to the respiratory hazard and then looking for trends between high- and low-exposure groups. When a workforce has been uniformly exposed to a respiratory hazard there may be no alternative to the use of a control population, but this is an unusual situation. Considerable thought must be given to the selection of control subjects and their suitability should be tested by specifically examining the survey data for population differences not attributable to the work environment, e.g., economic status, age and sex distribution, and smoking habit.

Published prediction tables for lung function are a special instance of a control population. Their use as a standard against which to compare survey data must be condemned. They are almost always based on volunteer populations which have been culled to eliminate all but the most healthy and they are often limited to nonsmokers from a narrow range of occupations and socioeconomic backgrounds. The bias in their composition makes them unsuitable for standardizing group data although their use in assessing individual results is acceptable as the bias is then small in relation to the "normal" range of lung function. The more sophisticated the lung function test the less likely are normal standards to be representative, and the more likely they are to be based on bizarre samples of hospital employees, medical and technical staff, and patients with no evidence of respiratory disease.

III. Population Sampling

Sampling is a useful procedure for reducing the number of subjects included in a study when the survey population is large, or for modifying the structure of the original population to increase the representation of specific subgroups. The sample must be either representative of the population or precisely defined in a way which allows the survey findings to be applied to the population as a whole. Four sampling techniques are commonly used in occupational respiratory surveys.

A. Random Sampling

Random sampling allows survey numbers to be reduced to a level which permits the study to be completed in a reasonable time with the available staff and facilities. The decision to study a random sample rather than the total population should not be taken lightly. It avoids the cost and logistic difficulties of a large-scale survey but introduces other problems which may frustrate the aims of the survey. The precision of the findings will depend on the size of the sample; if the sample is too small, real trends may be obscured or may not reach conventionally accepted significance levels. The choice of sample size, therefore, assumes prior knowledge of the magnitude of the expected trends. Alternatively, a decision must be made on what constitutes a trend of "practical significance" and the sample size chosen accordingly.

It is difficult to convey the concept of random sampling to a workforce. The selection of some members and the exclusion of others generates suspicion and destroys a major incentive to participate—the fact that all other members are participating. The default rate is usually higher in surveys based on random sampling and may be sufficient to jeopardize the success of the survey. A compromise is to involve all subjects in some part of the survey, and a sample in the critical or complex phases.

B. Stratified Sampling

One of the functions of surveys in industry is to examine the relationship between population variables such as lung function and the degree of exposure to a respiratory hazard. Bias is likely to occur if other variables are not evenly distributed in relation to exposure or if the population is not evenly distributed over the range of exposure values. This requirement is seldom present in industrial populations. The problem is overcome by stratified sampling. The population is divided into subgroups defined by one or more variables. For example, the population might be divided into male and female, and each sex further subdivided into groups with different degrees of exposure. A random sample is then taken from each group to obtain a composite sample with the desired characteristics. The population may be stratified for one or more variables, but there is a multiplicative relationship between the number of variables and the number of subgroups generated. It is therefore rarely possible to stratify for more than three variables in an industrial population without the numbers in each subgroup becoming unacceptably small.

Stratified sampling is also useful for eliminating a correlation present in the original population. For instance, cumulative exposure to a respiratory hazard is usually correlated with age. Regression of lung function on cumulative exposure will therefore contain an aging effect. This can be eliminated by stratifying the population with respect to age and length of service and then taking random samples of the same size from each subgroup to form a composite sample.

Stratified sampling can be performed before the survey and data collected only on those subjects contained in the sample. However, this will lead to the same problems of worker participation as random sampling. If the workforce is not prohibitively large, it is preferable to collect data on the whole population and draw the sample subsequently according to criteria set out in the protocol.

Table 1 Cough Frequency in Nonsmokers

Score	Oil refinery, n = 58 (%)	Other industries, n = 151 (%)
1	57	57
2	21	14
3	14	8
4	2	4
5	3	5
6	3	12
	100	100

C. Matched Pairs

Matching is a technique applicable particularly to workforces comprising a small exposed population and a large nonexposed one. The latter serves as a source of controls which can be matched individually with members of the exposed group. The number of variables for which each pair can be effectively matched will depend on the relative size of the two groups. Age, sex, smoking habit, and length of service are the variables most commonly selected, but others may be indicated by the requirements of individual surveys.

Where the numbers are insufficient for individual matching, it may be possible to select a control sample in which each of the relevant variables has the same mean and distribution as in the exposed population. The major limitation of this approach is that matching is achieved only for the total population and not for subgroups within it.

Matched samples may be used in all types of surveys but are particularly appropriate to retrospective surveys where they provide the best solution to the problem of obtaining a suitable control group. In prospective surveys, matched pairs suffer from the disadvantage that attrition of the sample due to labor turnover or nonresponse is approximately twice as great as in unmatched samples, because for each dropout two subjects are lost to the analysis.

Matching for specified variables usually ensures reasonable matching for other correlated variables. However, anomalies will arise if the correlations within the exposed and the control populations are different. In a survey of oil refinery workers, it was found that the prevalence of nonsmokers was greater than in other Australian industries which we have studied. The prohibition on smoking at work was clearly an important factor in determining smoking habits in the refinery. Table 1 shows the distribution of cough frequency scored on a ranked scale [1] for nonsmokers in the refinery and in a variety of other industries. The greater prevalence of high cough scores in the latter industries suggests that in these industries a significant proportion of nonsmokers did not take up the habit because of respiratory symptoms. Had the refinery population been matched for smoking habit with a control population from these other industries, there would have been a strong probability of mismatching with respect to a past history of respiratory illness.

D. Volunteer Samples

Few surveys are compulsory, and the term *volunteer* is here applied to surveys where willingness to participate is the major or only criterion for selection. In general, such samples are heavily biased and have nothing to recommend them. The value of the information obtained from them depends on the response rate. For example, if the prevalence of a respiratory symptom in a 70% sample of the workforce is found to be 5%, the true prevalence must lie between 3.5% and 33.5%, assuming on the one hand that none of the defaulters have symptoms and on the other that they all have symptoms. The sample prevalence is a poor estimate of the true prevalence and furthermore the conventional methods for calculating the sample error of this estimate are not applicable.

IV. Types of Survey

Surveys in industry can be broadly classified into two types: cross-sectional and longitudinal (prospective). They are not mutually exclusive, and a particular survey design may incorporate features of more than one type. The aim of the survey, the incidence and the natural history of the syndrome under investigation, and the specificity of the diagnostic criteria must be taken into consideration when choosing an appropriate design. The optimum design from a theoretical viewpoint may present logistic problems which force a compromise. Inadequate medical records, high labor turnover, interference with production schedules, and poor motivation of the workforce are common problems for which allowance must be made when designing the survey.

A. Cross-sectional Surveys

Cross-sectional surveys are the most popular probably because they give the highest yield of data relative to the effort of planning and execution. The simplest objective of a cross-sectional survey is to establish the prevalence of a syndrome in a workforce. Unless the syndrome is unique to the industry, this information is not particularly useful. Alternatively, the prevalence of the syndrome can be compared with that in a control population. Provided the control population is truly appropriate, a higher prevalence in the industry indicates a cause-and-effect relationship. If there is no suitable control population, the workforce can be grouped according to severity or duration of exposure to the respiratory hazard, and an association sought between the prevalence of the syndrome in each group and the degree of exposure. This technique avoids the difficulty of finding a control population but it does require assessment of the environment.

Measurements of lung function are extensively used to complement questionnaire data in surveys in industry. Prevalence estimates can only be obtained from lung function results if they are specified as normal or abnormal. Since no clear distinction can be made between normal and abnormal lung function, such estimates depend solely on the chosen criteria for abnormality. However, prevalence estimates may be made from questionnaires and radiographs, and the lung function data used to evaluate the questionnaire responses or the radiographic classification.

Because of the unreliability of symptom questionnaires in an industrial setting, lung function studies are assuming a greater role in detecting the effects of a respiratory hazard in the work environment. Instead of merely validating questionnaire responses, they are used in cross-sectional surveys to demonstrate trends in respiratory function in relation to environmental measurements or differences between exposed and control populations. The tests must be appropriate to the syndrome under investigation and allowance must be made either in the design or in the analysis for variation in age, height, and cigarette consumption. Unfortunately, adjustment for these factors rarely accounts for more than 60% of the irrelevant variation between subjects. In cross-sectional surveys, this detracts considerably from the value of lung function tests in the detection of early disease.

B. Short-Term Longitudinal Surveys

The sensitivity of lung function tests is greatly enhanced if each subject can be used as his or her own control. This is possible only in a longitudinal design, but if serial measurements are made over a period of days, most of the problems of long-term prospective surveys are avoided. This type of longitudinal survey has proved very effective in the study of occupational respiratory syndromes characterized by transient changes in lung function such as occupational asthma, byssinosis, and extrinsic allergic alveolitis. Measurements are usually made at the beginning and end of the working day or working week. Alternatively, the they can be repeated on several occasions throughout a work shift to determine the time course of any change in respiratory function or to relate such a change to specific work procedures. The latter technique is particularly useful in the study of occupational asthmatic syndromes. In a recent survey in an aluminum smelter, serial measurements of spirometry were made on a sample of the workforce throughout several work shifts. Asthmatic reactions on exposure to smelting fumes were demonstrated in several employees, and a greater average variation in lung function over a work shift was found in employees with heavy exposure to fumes than in those with light exposure. Although this type of design is far superior to questionnaire techniques for documenting acute respiratory reactions to the work environment, it is subject to a number of sources of error which, if neglected, may obscure real trends or generate spurious ones. The normal diurnal variation in respiratory function may produce changes of the same order as the reaction to the work environment. One solution is to make the measurements over a period of the day when diurnal variation is minimal; alternatively, the magnitude of the variation may be estimated from an appropriate control sample. Training effects present a more serious source of bias and have been almost completely neglected in the literature. This problem is greater with effort-dependent measurements such as vital capacity and peak expiratory flow rate. The error can be minimized by obtaining sufficient replicate measurements at each testing session to ensure that the subject is giving his or her best performance. Even so, a small but statistically significant improvement may occur between testing sessions due wholly to training effects.

Ambient temperature and calibration drift in measuring equipment must be controlled as strictly as possible in a longitudinal survey. Systematic variation in these factors will not bias a properly randomized cross-sectional study but will inevitably produce a spurious trend in a longitudinal study. This problem is discussed in more detail later.

The need for repeated measurements at relatively short intervals throws a considerable strain on the cooperation of the subjects. This may lead to an unacceptable default rate even when testing is confined to simple spirometry. The problem is considerably magnified with more complex tests which take longer to perform. If repeated measurements are required throughout a shift, the subject may spend a large proportion of his or her time in the laboratory. The response to the work environment will then be distorted by the intermittent pattern of exposure. There is no simple way of avoiding these problems, and in general, the short-term longitudinal study does not lend itself to detailed measurements of lung function. If simple spirometry will not suffice, an alternative design must be sought.

We were faced with this difficulty when designing a survey to determine the time course of the acute reaction to cotton dust using spirometry and maximum expiratory flow-volume curves breathing air and helium as indices of airway function. The employees of a large cotton-spinning mill were stratified by sex and length of service and then randomly allocated to half hourly time slots throughout the working week. Each employee was studied only once but, with 12 subjects in each time slot, it was possible to show statistically significant trends in lung function over a work shift and over the working week. Although adjustments were made for differences in age, height, and smoking habit, this design is inevitably less sensitive than one in which serial measurements are made on each subject. However, it is the only practical method for the detailed study of short-term trends and is comparable in sensitivity to a cross-sectional design in which an exposed population is compared with a control population.

C. Prospective Surveys

A prospective morbidity survey can be regarded as a series of cross-sectional studies on the same population at widely separated intervals, usually a year or more. Theoretically, the prospective survey is a powerful epidemiological tool as it provides all the information of a cross-sectional study and, more importantly, it indicates the incidence of disease in a workforce. Because serial measurements are obtained on each employee, it is a more sensitive technique for determining the effect of the work environment on respiratory function than a cross-sectional study. In practice, these advantages often prove illusory [2].

There are two essential requirements for a successful prospective survey: a stable population and reproducible measuring techniques. It is rare in these days of increased population mobility to find a stable industrial workforce. A labor turnover of 15% per year is reasonably typical of Australian workforces and a figure in excess of 25% per year not rare. The loss of employees from the workforce depletes the number available for follow-up and is never random. Health is an important reason for self-selection out of the workforce; hence the remaining members of the population are biased in a way that will lead to an underestimate, or occasionally an overestimate, of the incidence of disease. This problem can be avoided either by establishing ongoing medical surveillance in which each employee is examined immediately prior to leaving the job, or by locating all employees who have left during the period of the survey and examining them as part of the follow-up. The former solution is logistically difficult and the latter usually feasible only in a closed community [3].

It is extremely difficult to maintain standard measuring techniques over a period of years. Even though the wording of a questionnaire is not altered, the original interviewer may not be available or the same question may be interpreted differently by employees on a second occasion when they have had a chance to consider its implications or when their attitudes have been influenced by management, unions, or media coverage. Although lung function tests have the advantage of objectivity, it is difficult to maintain their repeatability over an extended period. This is true even of simple spirometry. The calibration of portable spirometers is rarely exact, and systematic differences are commonly observed in the results obtained by different technicians on the same subject. Although the absolute magnitude of the errors may be small, they may well be sufficient to invalidate the findings of a 3 year follow-up when the annual decrements attributable to age in the one second forced expiratory volume and vital capacity are of the order of only 20 ml. Complex tests present greater difficulties as it is often not possible to defer improvements in instrumentation and procedures for the duration of a prospective survey and older equipment must be replaced. In a 4 year follow-up of employees in the asbestos industry, we found that batch differences in the characteristics of the esophageal balloons introduced a 10% error into the measured transpulmonary pressure. Smaller errors occurred in a number of other "standardized" tests due to minor changes in instrumentation. It is essential that such errors be quantitated. Ideally, this should be done by comparing the results of the old and the new procedures in trained subjects, but this can prove time consuming as a hundred or more such comparisons may be needed to obtain sufficiently precise estimates. Provision must be made in the survey design for detecting these errors. The most practical method is to compare the results of a sample of unexposed employees at the time of the follow-up survey with a similar sample from the initial survey. Any residual difference in lung function after adjustment for age, height, and smoking habit may then be attributed to differences in technique. This method, which we used in the asbestos survey referred to above, is not ideal, as the standard error of the estimates of technical difference will inevitably be inflated by between-subject differences not removed by adjustment for age, height, and smoking habit. When these estimates are used to adjust the follow-up data, the standard error of the latter will be considerably increased, so destroying one of the major advantages of the prospective design. However, it will lessen the risk of drawing invalid conclusions.

None of the difficulties associated with prospective surveys is insuperable and this design remains the most sensitive for detecting the long-term effect of the work environment on the lungs. The problems are stressed because prospective surveys often appear deceptively simple and definitive. They require careful planning and the potential value of the study must be weighed against the difficulties that are likely to be encountered.

D. Retrospective Approach

The case-control study is generally unsuited to worker surveys due to its "retrospective" nature. It identifies cases by the "effect" and then with a suitable comparison or control group, works backward toward establishing cause. This type of study is most useful when the incidence of the disease under study is low and/or the latency period is long, such as with cancer. The case-control study is fully discussed in Chapter 13.

E. Historical Prospective Surveys

These surveys draw their data from records of past events but otherwise resemble prospective surveys. They are uniquely suited to studies of occupational lung disease in industries which have kept comprehensive personnel records and have maintained regular medical surveillance of the workforce over an extended period. This information permits the investigator to follow the medical history of each employee and to determine the incidence of disease in the workforce. The major advantages of this type of survey are that the data are immediately available and can be acquired at a fraction of the cost of a prospective survey. However, it is subject to the limitation of all retrospective surveys, namely that the investigator has no control over the data which are recorded and must work within the constraints of the information available.

F. Pilot Studies

A pilot study is a small-scale survey with limited objectives and is usually a preliminary to a full-scale survey. The two common reasons for doing a pilot study are to obtain environmental data with which to subdivide the population according to exposure to the respiratory hazard, and to obtain basic information on the population so that random, stratified, or matched samples can be chosen for more detailed study. In general, the same rules apply to pilot studies as to other types of survey but as their purpose is to provide data rather than to answer an hypothesis, their design presents less difficulty.

It is important to limit the information sought in this initial approach to the employees to the minimum necessary for planning the main survey. The reason for this is that the default rate tends to increase with each successive approach to a workforce, particularly if measurements have been made on the previous occasions. The purpose of a pilot study should be explained in advance to the workforce and the information obtained by simple, and preferably self-administered, questionnaires. Often much of the information required is available from other sources such as company records; these sources should be checked before making a direct approach to the workforce.

V. Choice of Measurements

The measurements made in a survey must be appropriate to the aims of the survey. This simple principle can easily be overlooked in the desire to conform with standard practice or "make the most of the survey" by collecting as much data as possible. Two questions should be asked when choosing the measurements. "What measurements will provide the information required of this survey? What additional measurements are necessary to avoid ambiguity and uncertainty in the interpretation of the data? It is sometimes reasonable to include measurements which permit comparison with other studies, but in general, if a measurement contributes little or nothing to the aims of the study it should be rejected. Worthless measurements waste the company's time and strain the cooperation of the employees.

A. Diagnostic Criteria

The more specific the objectives of a survey, the more discriminating the information must be. A broad enquiry into the respiratory health of a workforce calls for measurements which cast a wide net and is best served by a standard respiratory symptom questionnaire supplemented by "screening" tests of respiratory function such as spirometry. The selection of appropriate measurements is more difficult when the survey is concerned with a particular disease. It is here that confusion between epidemiological and clinical diagnosis commonly occurs. An epidemiological diagnosis should be independent of the observer performing the measurements and interpreting the data. Clinical diagnosis, on the other hand, is very much a function of the observer and is based on undefined judgments whose reliability depends on the experience and acumen of the observer. In surveys, diagnosis must be based on epidemiological principles, and appropriate diagnostic criteria defined in terms of data obtained from measurements which are themselves defined in the protocol. The diagnostic criteria adopted may have a profound influence on the findings; it follows that comparison with the results of other surveys may not be valid unless identical criteria have been used.

The simplest diagnostic classification consists of two categories, positive and negative. More ambitious classifications subdivide the positive diagnoses into further categories defined by the stage and severity of disease as in the ILO classification of pneumoconiosis by chest radiograph. The criteria defining the categories must meet two requirements. First, they must ensure that the categories accurately represent the presence, absence, and, if appropriate, the severity of the disease in question. Second, they must leave no doubt to which category each subject belongs. It is extremely difficult to define a disease by criteria which are infallible. The possibility of incorrect classification may have to be accepted and the criteria formulated to minimize either false positive or false negative diagnoses, whichever is most appropriate to the aims of the study.

The measurements made in the survey are dictated by the diagnostic criteria and must be chosen so that the data can be expressed unequivocally in terms of these criteria and each individual allocated to his or her correct category. Conceptually, the choice of measurements is therefore the final, not the first, step in the design of the survey.

Surveys in industry are increasingly directed at the detection of respiratory impairment before the emergence of overt disease in the workforce. The use of diagnostic criteria is unsatisfactory in these studies as it is usually impossible to formulate adequate criteria. Instead, exposure-related trends in respiratory impairment are sought in the workforce as a whole or in defined subgroups. In this type of study, the individual loses his or her identity and the question of individual diagnosis does not arise. It has the advantage that the results of the survey are not expressed in terms of individual measurements so inferences regarding diagnosis cannot influence the findings of the study. The disadvantage is that prevalence and incidence have no meaning in this context and the results will not initially give an accurate indication of the probability of an individual developing disease.

B. Type of Measurement

A wide variety of measurements has been used in respiratory surveys in industry but the four most common types are questionnaires, physical signs, chest radiographs, and lung function tests. It is not the purpose of this chapter to discuss their individual merits, but each has features which are relevant to survey design.

Questionnaires are widely used in surveys because they provide an easy method of collecting data on large populations at minimal cost. Their lack of objectivity is not usually a problem except where emotional issues are involved. However, emotional issues commonly lie behind an invitation to conduct a survey in industry. Employees who are convinced that their work environment is hazardous cannot be expected to give reliable or objective responses to a symptom questionnaire. Also, some will not admit to respiratory symptoms out of fear of jeopardizing their jobs even though they are assured that the questionnaire results are confidential. Nevertheless, symptom questionnaires are useful in the investigation of certain occupational respiratory diseases, particularly occupational asthma, but they should be supported by objective data. It has been our practice to use the questionnaire data to subdivide the population into symptom groups and then to use respiratory function data to compare the groups. The workforce is told in advance that this will be done and they are warned that incorrect answers to the questions will blur comparisons based on the lung function tests and may obscure the effects of a respiratory hazard.

Although physical signs are more objective than questionnaire data, their value depends on the experience of the observer and the extent to which bias can be avoided. The same criticisms apply to chest radiographs, but the latter have the advantage of providing a permanent record whereas physical signs cannot be reviewed at a later date. Physical signs and radiological criteria should be precisely defined in the survey protocol and the data recorded independently by at least two observers. The use of more than one observer not only allows the observer error to be quantitated but also enhances the discriminatory power of the measurements [4].

Lung function tests are objective and applicable to a wide range of occupational respiratory syndromes but they must not be credited with a specificity which they do not possess. Abnormal lung function may be used as a diagnostic criterion but never the only one. Even in asthma, where airway obstruction is probably the most important criterion, it is not diagnostic unless it can be shown to be present on one occasion and absent on another. The choice of lung function tests is crucial to the success of a survey and requires careful thought in the planning stages. No tests is specific for a particular morphological lesion but a suitable combination of tests can reflect the site and severity of physiological impairment with reasonable accuracy. Single tests cannot localize the site of the lesion and may underestimate the degree of physiological impairment. The forced expiratory volume in one second is often useful as a screening test but it does not indicate where the lesion lies in the airways and is relatively insensitive to impaired function in the peripheral airways. A reduction in transfer factor (diffusing capacity) may be an early indication of pulmonary asbestosis but is unpredictable, and many subjects with a marked increase in lung elastic recoil suggestive of pulmonary fibrosis have a transfer factor within the normal range. Where the effects of a respiratory hazard are unknown or poorly documented, the tests selected for the survey must provide adequate coverage of the different types of physiological impairment likely to be encountered; hence the initial investigation requires a battery of tests but follow-up studies can be confined to those which prove the most informative. The tests which are most useful in clinical practice are often neither the best nor the most sensitive for epidemiological surveys. Extrapolation from clinical experience may result in the omission of a valuable test in favor of one which contributes little or nothing to the detection of early disease.

The survey design must take into account the extraneous sources of variation which affect lung function tests. Random changes make the tests less discriminatory while systematic changes may introduce spurious trends into the results. It is important to minimize this variation and to quantitate it. All tests should be performed at least in duplicate. Not only does the mean of the replicates provide a better estimate of the true value but also the variation between replicates is a measure of the repeatibility of the test. Where a judgment is required of a person measuring the test record, as in the closing volume test, two observers should measure the record independently. Short-term variation is usually, but not always, random; variation over a period of hours is more likely to be systematic and due to identifiable sources such as temperature and calibration changes. The effect of temperature fluctuation on tests requiring complex instrumentation is unpredictable and standard correction factors may not be applicable. It is better to conduct the tests in a room with a constant ambient temperature, but if this is impractical the ambient temperature should be recorded regularly and introduced as a covariate into the subsequent analysis of the data. Calibration drift in electronic instruments can be minimized by using high-quality equipment left switched on for the duration of the survey. The conventional method of dealing with calibration drift is to recalibrate the equipment at specified times and to make a linear correction for the effect of drift over the intervening periods. This approach ignores the fact that calibration procedures are themselves subject to variation. It has been our practice in recent years to obtain calibration data at regular intervals but to make no alteration to the instrument settings. We have found the variation to be random and within the error of the calibration procedures except on rare occasions when a fault has developed in an instrument. Should a systematic drift occur, it can be quantitated by fitting a curve to the calibration data or, if linear, it can be included as a covarate in the analysis of the survey data.

VI. Practical Aspects of Survey Design

A. Enlisting Worker Participation

All surveys in industry should aim for 100% participation by the workforce; in general, we regard a response rate of less than 95% as unacceptable. Considerable effort is needed on the part of the survey team to achieve this level of participation and many otherwise well conceived surveys have foundered because the cooperation of the workforce was taken for granted. The employees must be convinced that the survey is being done primarily for their benefit—to safeguard their health or to identify and estimate the effect of a respiratory hazard in their work environment. They are not interested in academic objectives nor do they look favorably on projects that might be construed as management oriented. The first step in enlisting their cooperation is therefore to make certain that the survey will be of direct and practical benefit to the worker on the shop floor. The proposed survey must then be conveyed to the workforce by someone whom they consider has their interests at heart and whose opinion they respect. In Australia, and probably in most other countries, this person will usually be a senior trade union official. A recommendation from a trade union carries an authority which neither management nor the survey personnel can hope to match. We have found that the active support of the trade union virtually guarantees a satisfactory response rate.

Once the survey has been approved in principle by management, we ask that a trade union representative be invited to all subsequent discussions and be given the opportunity to express an opinion regarding the aims of the survey and to take an active part in planning the practical aspects. This approach helps to allay suspicions and promote an atmosphere of mutual cooperation.

Once the protocol has been prepared and approved by management and trade union, management officially informs the workforce that the survey will go ahead and union officials discuss the proposals with the delegates from the shop floor, who in turn explain the survey to the other employees. Shortly after, and as close to the start of the survey as possible, the head of the survey team addresses the assembled workforce and briefly describes the aims of the survey and the measurements to be made. It is essential that a senior trade union official be present to speak in support of the survey and a senior member of management to demonstrate the firm's interest in the project. If complex lung function tests involving body plethysmography and esophageal balloon measurements are to be made, the trade union's appeal for cooperation will carry far more weight if the official has already been through the complete testing procedure and can speak from personal experience.

All measurements must be made in company time. Any survey design which requires employees to present for tests in their own time will have a high default rate and the responders will be a very biased sample of the population. If measurements are required before the start or on completion of the work shift, management must officially notify the workforce that this will be regarded as extra working time and will be paid for at the appropriate rates. This not only ensures a satisfactory response but also indicates to the workforce that management is actively concerned to ensure a thorough and successful survey.

Survey personnel must be instructed to inform a senior member of the team if an employee is upset in any way by a survey procedure, particularly lung function tests or invasive procedures such as blood sampling. The situation must be handled promptly with tact and understanding as one disgruntled employee can rapidly destroy the team's rapport with the workforce. Some men have an exaggerated fear of procedures such as blood sampling, swallowing esophageal balloons, or sitting in a body plethysmograph but may still present for their tests as they do not wish to lose face with their fellow workers. Their chances of tolerating the procedures successfully are remote. This problem can be avoided if the workforce are told that senior members of the team are always available to discuss in private any queries regarding the procedures used in the survey. We have found that it pays to overlap appointments for complex lung function tests as employees are reassured by the sight of a colleague successfully negotiating them.

B. Confidentiality of Results

We issue a report of the survey findings to management on the understanding that it will be passed on to the union without undue delay. No employee is identifiable from the data presented in the report and no reference is made to individuals. The workforce is assured in advance of the survey that individual results will be regarded as confidential. It is essential to the success of the survey that this assurance be given unequivocally and honored without exception. However, employees are given the opportunity to authorize in writing the release of their personal results to the industry's medical officer or to their own family doctors. If employees are found to be in need of medical advice or treatment but have not signed a release form, they are advised confidentially to consult their doctors or to discuss the matter with a medically qualified member of the survey team. Often a return visit is paid after analysis of the results and presentation of the report to allow informal discussion of the findings, and to discuss individual problems.

C. Logistics

The cost of running a survey will almost always be small by comparison with the cost to the firm of lost workhours and production. Particular attention should therefore be paid in the design to minimizing disruption of production schedules. Whenever possible the survey should be conducted on-site in the industry so avoiding the unwieldy and time-consuming exercise of transporting employees to another location. A mobile laboratory, requiring only an electricity and water supply [5], can be installed in a convenient location on the industrial site and allows the survey team to work under optimal conditions.

Employees should be interviewed and tested by appointment. The appointments should be spaced sufficiently to allow for minor delays and to avoid employees queueing for their tests. Where the industry operates 24 hr a day, the testing schedule must cover all shifts and the survey team must be large enough to mount a 24 hr roster.

Acknowledgments

The research activities of the Division of Thoracic Medicine, The Prince Henry Hospital, have been supported consistently by the Workers' Compensation (Dust Diseases) Board of New South Wales and for special purposes by the National Health and Medical Research Council, the Asthma Foundation of New South Wales, and the Australian Tobacco Research Foundation, as well as by industry and trade unions.

References

1. Field, G. B., The application of a quantitative estimate of cough frequency to epidemiological surveys, *Int. J. Epidemiol.*, **3**:135–143 (1974).
2. Cochrane, A. L., Rhondda Fach, South Wales. In *Comparibility in International Epidemiology*. Selected papers from the International Conference

on Comparibility in Epidemiological Studies, fourth scientific conference of the International Epidemiological Association, Princeton New Jersey, 1964. Edited by R. M. Acheson. Milbank Memorial Fund, 1965, pp. 326–332.
3. Bouhuys, A., A. Barbero, R. S. F. Schilling, and K. P. Van De Woestijne, Chronic respiratory disease in hemp workers, *Am. J. Med.,* **46**:526–537 (1969).
4. Oldham, P. D., Numerical scoring of radiological simple pneumoconiosis. In *Inhaled Particles III,* Vol. 2. Proceedings of an international symposium organized by the British Occupational Hygiene Society in London, September 14–23, 1970. Edited by W. H. Walton. London, Unwin Brothers, 1971, pp. 621–630.
5. Field, G., P. Owen, and B. Gandevia, Mobile laboratory for respiratory surveys in industry, *Med. J. Aust.,* **1**:867–869 (1976).

15

Statistical Analyses

GEOFFREY BERRY

MRC Pneumoconiosis Unit
Penarth, South Glamorgan
Wales, United Kingdom

I. Introduction

It would not be possible to describe adequately all the statistical methods likely to be useful in research into occupational lung diseases in a single chapter and no attempt will be made to do so. Instead, some of the techniques available for particular types of problems will be described and illustrated by example. These techniques will be mainly those which, in the author's experience, are not as widely known or used as they could be.

Similarly, it would be neither possible nor desirable to make this chapter self-contained in the sense that it would be comprehensible to anyone without previous statistical knowledge. It will be assumed that readers understand statistical terms such as mean, standard deviation, estimate, and standard error of estimate, that they are familiar with the concept of significance tests, the normal (Gaussian) distribution, with the Student's t test for the comparison of two means and the assessment of the significance of a regression coefficient, and with the chi-squared (χ^2) test for the analysis of 2 $\times$ 2 or larger contingency tables. There are many statistical textbooks which cover this basic knowledge but in this chapter, where reference is made to a statistical text for fuller details, it will usually be to the book by Armitage [1].

An important distinction which arises in most research into occupational lung diseases is that between experimental and observational studies. Suppose it is required to evaluate the efficacy of a drug in the treatment of a disease. Then a way of proceeding would be to compare a group of, say, 26 patients treated with the drug with a group of 26 patients not so treated but otherwise observed in the same way. This is an experiment, usually referred to as a clinical trial, and its basic ingredient should be that the 26 patients who received the drug were chosen out of the total of 52 patients by some random process. We could imagine this process as consisting of shuffling a standard pack of playing cards and dealing them out, one to each patient, and those patients with a red card would receive the drug and those with the black card would not, i.e., they would be controls. Now, suppose that 20 of the patients receiving the drug improved but that only 6 of the controls improved. Then, provided the trial has been conducted properly, there are two possible conclusions:

1. That the drug had some effect
2. That the drug had no effect and the observed difference was due to chance

It can be calculated that if the drug had no effect then the probability of a difference at least as large as was observed occurring by chance is only 0.0002. This is the test of significance, and since the probability is so low it could confidently be concluded that the drug had some effect.

Now suppose that instead of testing a drug we were investigating exposure to an industrial pollutant. Suppose we observed that out of 26 persons exposed, there were 20 with a particular sign of effect compared with only 6 out of 26 nonexposed controls. A significance test could be carried out exactly as in the case of the clinical trial and it would be concluded that it was unlikely that the observed difference could be due to chance. However in this case, in contrast to a clinical trial, there is more than one possible interpretation of the observed effect. One possibility is that the exposure has had some effect, but an alternative is that the exposed and control groups differ in some other way. The latter possibility can be raised only because the individuals in the exposed and control groups have not been allocated to these groups by a random process. In some cases it is clear that the exposed and treated groups do differ; for example, the age distributions may differ, the smoking habits may differ, or the control group may consist of office workers and therefore not be comparable with a group of manual workers. In such cases then it is clearly valid to argue that the observed difference in the numbers with the sign of interest could be due, either partly or wholly, to other observed differences between the groups. But even if the two groups have been shown to be similar in all other measured respects the possibility remains that the observed difference could be due to differences between the groups in some features of which we are not aware. Fisher [2] criticized the attribution of causation to the discovery of an association between smoking and lung cancer over 20 years ago. One of his arguments was that the association could be due to differences in genotype between smokers and nonsmokers. Even now this subject is not free from controversy [3].

Since it is impossible to allocate individuals to different occupations by a random process then all studies of occupational lung disease must be observational rather than experimental. It might therefore be considered that it is impossible to establish that occupational exposure to a particular substance *caused* a particular effect, however well designed had been a study showing a statistically significant effect. It is certainly impossible to establish causation simply on the basis of a significance test in an observational study. Hill [4] listed aspects of an association which should be considered "before deciding that the most likely interpretation of it is causation." He summarized the position as follows:

> What I do not believe–and this has been suggested–is that we can usefully lay down some hard-and-fast rules of evidence that *must* be obeyed before we accept cause and effect. None of my nine viewpoints can bring indisputable evidence for or against the cause-and-effect hypothesis and none can be required as a *sine qua non.* What they can do, with greater or less strength, is to help us to make up our minds on the fundamental question–is there any other way of explaining the set of facts before us, is there any other answer equally, or more, likely than cause and effect?

The basic observations constituting a set of data are of two types. In one the observation consists of a measurement made on a continuous scale such as height or forced expiratory volume (FEV). In the other the observation is a statement of which, of two or more categories, an individual belongs to. Examples of this are sex, cause of death, and the grade of bronchitis on a four point scale, 0, 1, 2, or 3. There are differences in the statistical methods appropriate for the analysis of these types of data. A group of measurements might be summarized by the mean and standard deviation and the significance of the difference between two groups assessed using Student's t test. In contrast, categorized data would be summarized by the proportion in each category and the comparison between two groups could involve the analysis of a contingency table using a χ^2 statistic.

Although there is a fundamental difference between the analyses appropriate to the two types of data it is important to realize that this difference is restricted to the way that variation comes to be present in the data, i.e., to the error structure. For a continuous variate, such as FEV, it might be valid to assume that after allowing for other variables which may affect the value, the observations are distributed normally within a group. If all variables which may affect the value have been allowed for, there will be nothing left to affect it but a multitude of unspecifiable sources of disturbance, and this is just the situation where the normal distribution is produced. Such an assumption could never be justified for a variable taking one of two classes, such as the presence of a disease. Instead, the corresponding situation is that, if all relevant variables have been allowed for, each person in the group shares the same chance of having the disease, and the frequencies in the two classes are given by a binomial distribution.

If we are interested in the relationship between a variable and other variables then the situation is similar for the two types of data. For example, suppose we had available estimates of the exposure of individuals to some environment. Then the relationship of FEV and exposure could be examined by fitting the linear regression of FEV on exposure. Similarly, the probability of disease could be related to exposure, and with a suitable transformation of the probability scale, it could be appropriate to consider a linear relationship. This has been recognized for a long time; the classic probit analysis of biological assay is essentially a linear regression of the probit transformation of the proportion of animals affected on the logarithm of the dose [5]. However it is only recently, as powerful and general computer programs have become available [6,7], that is has been possible to take full advantage of this common feature of the analysis of different types of data.

Nevertheless, although it should be recognized that there is much to be gained by regarding the analysis of continuous and categorical data as parts of a unified method, rather than as distinct methods, it is convenient to discuss the two types of data separately.

Statistical analyses are often carried out on a computer and, by removing much tedious calculation from the researcher, this is a good thing, provided that it is remembered that the analyses should be carried out with the *help of* and not *by* the computer. The most important parts of an analysis are making sure that the data are correct and deciding which statistical methods are appropriate. In order to use a computer it must have the necessary statistical software. There are several statistical packages, systems, or languages available but this is not the place for a discussion of their relative merits. Most researchers will, of necessity, use what is readily available to them. Some of the examples given later have been analyzed using GLIM [6] or GENSTAT [7], which are the statistical systems I regularly use, but identical results could be produced using other software.

II. The Analysis of Continuous Data

In this section methods of analyzing continuous data are considered. Some commonly used methods are based on the normal distribution; these include Student's t test, analysis of variance, analysis of covariance, fitting constants, and regression analysis. Although these methods are sometimes thought of as distinct methods they are all special cases of the more general method of fitting a linear model to the data. In this method a variable y is analyzed in terms of its relationship with a number of other variables, $x_1, x_2, x_3, \ldots, x_k$. The latter variables may be continuous or categorized; some will be those of direct interest while others may be nuisance variables, i.e., variables of no direct interest but which have to be taken into account because it is known or suspected that they are associated with y, e.g., height for FEV.

A. Sources of Variation

The general linear model takes the form

$$y = b_0 + b_1 x_1 + b_2 x_2 + \cdots + b_k x_k + e \tag{1}$$

where e is the residual, or the deviation of the observed from the fitted value of y. The methods of analysis under discussion are valid if, and only if, the distribution of residuals is normal with constant variance and if the residuals are mutually independent. It will often be obvious that this last condition is fulfilled, but in other cases care is necessary to ensure that it is. Consideration of the different sources of variation contributing to the residuals will usually enable an appropriate analysis to be constructed; this is best illustrated by an example.

Suppose the forced expiratory volume (FEV) is measured on a group of men on two occasions a year apart. Then it would be incorrect to analyze the pairs of measurements with a single error term. Such an analysis would ignore that the two residuals for each man are not independent, since a man with an above-average FEV on the first occasion would probably be above average on the second occasion also, and vice versa. There are several sources of variation in the data, including variation due to technical causes, but two sources have to be carefully distinguished. First, there is variation between different men; part of this variation may be removed by making allowance for age and height but this is incidental to the point under discussion. Second, there is variation in the change in FEV between the two occasions. These two sources of variation lead to two separate analyses. The first analysis is of absolute level of FEV and uses the mean of the two measurements for each man. The second analysis is of the change in FEV and uses the differences between the first and second measurements. As is well known, it is necessary to allow for age and height in the first analysis but this is probably not necessary in the analysis of change, since the effect of age and height on absolute level of FEV are eliminated when the differences are calculated.

The distinction is the same as that between a paired and an unpaired t test. The two analyses are referred to as the between and within men analyses, respectively, and as long as the two are separated no difficulty arises.

Difficulties in interpretation arise if the change is related to the absolute level. Oldham [8] warned that relating the change to the measurement on the first occasion introduces spurious correlations and recommended using the mean of the two values for the absolute level. Although this removes the spurious correlation, difficulties in interpretation still remain because of what Fletcher et al. [9] call the "horse-racing effect;" i.e., there is an inevitable correlation between absolute level and rate of change because those with the higher rates of change will, on average, have declined to lower absolute levels. Thus it cannot be inferred from the correlation that a low FEV causes a high rate of decline.

B. Reference Values

The relationship of lung function to age and stature is well documented and it is sometimes convenient to eliminate the unwanted variation due to age and height before starting the main analysis. This may be achieved using published reference relationships (Ref. 10, p. 381), and standardizing to a constant age and height. For example, using the reference relationship for Caucasian males, the FEV of a man aged a years and of height h meters would be standardized to age 50 years and height 1.7 m by adding

$$0.031(a - 50) - 3.62(h - 1.7)$$

to the measured value. As far as comparisons between groups are concerned it makes no difference what standard age and height are used. However, so that the final results are not too far removed from the data, standardization should be to an age and height near to the mean age and height of the study.

An alternative method of standardizing for height arises from the work of Cole [11], who showed that for both FEV and the forced vital capacity (FVC) the mean values are approximately proportional to the height squared.

Thus standardization to a height of 1.7 m is accomplished by multiplying the measured FEV or FVC by $(1.7/h)^2$.

Sometimes standardization is effected by dividing the measured values by the predicted values, calculated from a reference relationship, and expressing the results as percentages of predicted.

The reference relationships are dependent on ethnic group (Ref. 10, p. 356) and for a given ethnic group vary from country to country and between different regions of the same country. Often, therefore, there will be good reason to suppose that a published reference relationship is not completely appropriate for the group being studied. The purpose of standardizing for age and height is to eliminate the bias resulting from small differences in mean age and height between groups, and to increase the precision of comparisons by removing the variation due to age and height from the residual variation, which is used to estimate standard errors. The use of a published reference relationship, provided it is an approximation to the true relationship, will contribute toward these objectives. Cox [12] showed that standardizing for a single variable using an appoximate regression coefficient leads to a gain in precision provided that the approximate coefficient does not exceed twice the true value.

Except in small studies the use of a published reference relationship can be avoided completely by working within the data themselves. For example, in a study of cotton workers [13], the relationship of FEV with age and sitting height was calculated from the subjects in the study who had neither byssinosis nor bronchitis. Alternatively, the variables age and height could be included as variables in a regression analysis, and this meets Oldham's [14] criticism that using reference values to eliminate age and height from further consideration could give an incomplete analysis.

C. Analysis of Variance

The analysis of variance is a general method in which the total variation of a variable is divided into that part which can be explained in terms of other variables and that part which remains unexplained, the residual variation. Thus the fundamental equality of the method is

$$\text{Total variation} = \text{variation due to other variables} + \text{residual variation}$$

The variation is measured as a sum of squares of differences between the observed and mean or expected values.

The method will be illustrated using the data of Constantinidis et al. [15]). Lung function measurements were available on 60 coal workers; 36 of these had progressive massive fibrosis (PMF) and the other 24 had Caplan's syndrome. For each type of disease the category of disease (A, B, or C), defined in terms of the total size of the opacities on the chest radiograph, had been determined. The individual values of the FVC are shown in Figure 1 for each of the six groups, and the mean values are given in Table 1. These values have all been standardized to a height of 1.7 m and to age 55 years, near to the mean age of the men in the study, 55.85 years.

The purpose of the study was to compare the values of lung function between the six groups of subjects. Since the mean FVC is not relevant to comparisons between groups the total variation is measured about the mean and has a sum of squares of 35.9538 with 59 degrees of freedom (df). The analysis determines how much of this variation may be attributed to differences between the six disease groups and the residual variation, which is the variation

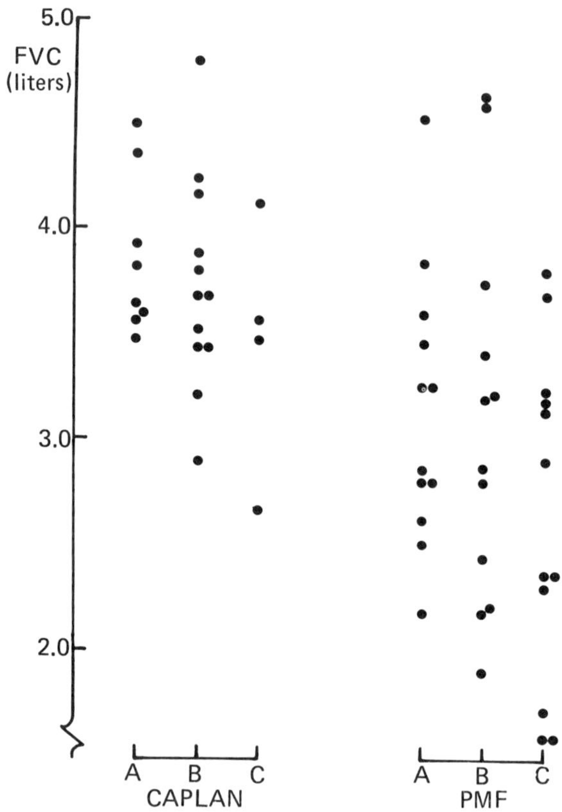

Figure 1 Values of forced vital capacity, standardized to age 55 years and height 1.7 m, by type and category of disease. (Data from Constantinidis et al. [15].)

Table 1 Summary of FVC for Six Groups

Type of disease	Category	Number of subjects	Sum of FVC (liters)	Mean FVC (liters)	Standard error of mean FVC
Caplan	A	8	30.78	3.85	0.24
	B	12	44.52	3.71	0.20
	C	4	13.80	3.45	0.34
PMF	A	12	37.59	3.13	0.20
	B	12	36.95	3.08	0.20
	C	12	31.58	2.63	0.20
Total		60	195.22	3.25	

Source: Data from Constantinidis et al. [15].

within groups. The analysis of variance is given in Table 2. If the FVC was not related to the disease group then the mean square between groups would have a similar value to that within groups; otherwise the mean square between groups would be larger. This is the case, and the ratio of the two mean squares is 4.55. The significance of this variance ratio is assessed by reference to tables of critical values of the variance ratio, sometimes referred to as the F ratio. These are published in sets of statistical tables (e.g., Ref. 16) and in statistical texts (e.g., Ref 1, Table A4). The value is significant at the 1% level, indicating that there are real differences between the groups. Discussion of the nature of these differences will be deferred to the next section.

The square root of the residual mean square is 0.68 and this is an estimate of the within-group standard deviation. The standard errors of the group means are obtained by dividing this standard deviation by the square root of the number of men in each group (Table 1).

Table 2 Analysis of Variance

Source of variation	Sum of squares	df	Mean square	Variance ratio
Between groups[a]	10.6584	5	2.1317	4.55
Within groups	25.2954	54	0.4684	
Total	35.9538	59		

[a]The sum of squares between groups = $30.78^2/8 + 44.52^2/12 + \ldots + 31.58^2/12 - 195.22^2/60$. (See Ref. 1, p. 189.)
Source: Data from Constantinidis et al. [15].

D. Fitting Constants

The analysis in the last section was restricted to comparisons between six groups and did not utilize the fact that the groups represent the combinations of two factors, one with two categories and the other with three categories. Where the groups have structure then the sum of squares between groups should be divided into components representing the different aspects of the structure. There are three distinct aspects: the main effect of disease type, the main effect of disease category, and the interaction of disease type and category. A main effect is an average effect of a factor where the averaging is over the levels of the second factor. The interaction of two factors represents the difference in one factor's effect according to the level of the other factor. (It should be noted that the word *effect* is used in accordance with accepted statistical terminology and does not necessarily imply causation.)

In a designed experiment it is often arranged that the main effects of two factors can be estimated independently of one another, i.e., they are orthogonal. In the example being considered this would have been the case if there had been 12 subjects in the Caplan A and the Caplan C groups. Then it would make no difference whether the Caplan effect was estimated as the average of the separate effects for categories A, B, and C or simply as the difference of the means of the Caplan subjects and the PMF subjects, i.e., ignoring disease category. But in the actual case it would be incorrect to estimate the Caplan effect ignoring disease category. It would be incorrect because, whereas one-third of the PMF subjects belong to each of the categories A, B, and C, the fractions of the Caplan subjects in the three categories are 1/3, 1/2, and 1/6. When the different effects cannot be estimated independently, then the analysis is nonorthogonal, and this will be the case in most studies in occupational medicine since these rarely take the form of designed experiments.

From Table 1 the difference between the Caplan and PMF groups, the Caplan effect, is 0.72 liters for category A, 0.63 liters for category B, and 0.82 liters for category C. The main Caplan effect is an average of these three values where the averaging process takes account of the fact that the three effects are estimated with different precisions because they are based on different numbers of subjects; the details are given by Armitage (Ref. 1, p. 264) but the calculations may be carried out more conveniently by fitting a regression equation (Ref. 1, p. 331) and this is the approach adopted here. The interaction of disease type and category is a measure of the difference between the three effects given above.

With two factors the analysis of variance is constructed by evaluating four separate sums of squares, these due to:

1. The first factor ignoring the second
2. The second factor ignoring the first
3. The two main effects fitted together
4. The two main effects and the interaction fitted together

Sums of squares (1), (2), and (4) are easily calculated; (4) is given in Table 2. The third sum of squares (3) is calculated by the method of fitting constants, originally described by Yates [17]. The main effect of disease category can be described in terms of two constants, one representing the difference between categories B and A, and the other the difference between categories C and A. The Caplan effect is described by one constant. Thus if both main effects are being fitted simultaneously, but with no interaction term, then these three constants are to be estimated. The calculations will usually be carried out on a computer and are equivalent to the fitting of a multiple regression with three independent variates. These three variates are dummy variates defined as follows:

x_1 = 1 for a subject in category B and zero otherwise

x_2 = 1 for a subject in category C and zero otherwise

x_3 = 1 for a subject with Caplan's syndrome and zero otherwise

The regression coefficients then correspond to the three constants defined above. An additional two dummy variates may be defined to represent the interaction terms

$x_4 = x_1 x_3$ = 1 for a subject with Caplan category B and zero otherwise

$x_5 = x_2 x_3$ = 1 for a subject with Caplan category C and zero otherwise

Table 3 Sums of Squares for Analysis of Variance

Effects fitted	Variables in regression	Sum of squares due to regression (df)
1. Disease category	x_1, x_2	3.8078 (2)
2. Disease type	x_3	8.4211 (1)
3. Category and type (main effects)	x_1, x_2, x_3	10.5867 (3)
4. Category, type and interaction	x_1, x_2, x_3, x_4, x_5	10.6584 (5)

Source: Data from Constantinidis et al. [15].

Table 4 Analysis of Variance

Source	Sum of squares	df	Mean square		Variance ratio
Category, ignoring type	3.8078	2			
Type, eliminating category	6.7789	1	6.7789		14.96[b]
Type, ignoring category	8.4211	1			
Category, eliminating type	2.1656	2	1.0828		2.39[b]
Category and type	10.5867	3			
Interaction, type and category	0.0717	2	0.0359	0.4530[a]	0.08
Residual	25.2954	54	0.4684		
Total	35.9538	59			

[a]Combined since there is no evidence of interaction.
[b]Calculated using the combined residual mean square.
Source: Data of Constantinidis et al. [15].

and then the whole analysis may be carried out using regression methods. While this may seem wasteful of computing power it may be the most convenient approach.

The necessary sums of squares are given in Table 3 and the analysis of variance in Table 4. The sum of squares used to test the effect of disease type must be that calculated after eliminating the effect of category. Fitting disease category alone accounts for a sum of squares of 3.8078 (Table 3) and if in addition disease type is fitted then the sum of squares accounted for is 10.5867. The sum of squares due to disease type, after allowing for disease category, is obtained by subtraction. Similarly, the interaction sum of squares is the difference between (4) and (3). There is clearly no evidence of any interaction between disease type and category; in fact, the interaction variance ratio may appear surprisingly low but is not significantly so. Therefore the interaction terms may be excluded, and this is achieved by adding the interaction sum of squares to the residual sum of squares to form a residual sum of squares with 56 df; the main effects of category and type are then assessed in relation to the combined residual. The differences between the three categories are not significant ($P = 0.1$), while disease type has a highly significant effect ($P < 0.001$).

Since there is no interaction the results may be summarized more concisely than by the six mean values given in Table 1 (although the six separate means would also be essential in a report of the analysis). The estimates of the effects are given in Table 5. The men with Caplan's syndrome had, on average, an FVC 0.70 liter greater than men with PMF. Men with categories B and C had lower FVC than those with category A by 0.09 and 0.48 liter, respectively. The latter effect is significant at the 5% level but

Table 5 Summary of Effects

Effects	Estimate of effect (l) and standard error
Caplan	0.70 ± 0.18 ($P < 0.001$)
Category B	-0.09 ± 0.20
Category C	-0.48 ± 0.23 ($P < 0.05$)

Source: Data from Constantinidis et al. [15].

this cannot be taken at face value since it is not sensible to consider the difference between categories A and C without taking account of the intermediate category B. The categories A, B, and C form an ordered set and, so far, no account has been taken of this in the analysis. A formal approach is to fit a linear trend of FVC through the categories A, B, and C. This may be done by replacing x_1 and x_2 by

$$x_6 = \begin{cases} 0 \text{ for category A} \\ 1 \text{ for category B} \\ 2 \text{ for category C} \end{cases}$$

The sum of squares due to fitting the linear trend, allowing for disease type, is 1.8753. This gives a variance ratio of 4.14 and 1 with 56 df which is significant at the 5% level. By subtraction (from 2.1656; see Table 4) the sum of squares due to deviations about a linear trend is 0.2903 which is clearly not significant. Therefore the association of FVC with disease category is consistent with a decline of 0.23 liter in FVC for each increase in category.

E. Regression

Regression methods are used to analyze the association between one variable, measured on a continuous scale, and a number of other variables. The variable being analyzed is usually referred to as the dependent variable and the others as the independent variables. This latter terminology is misleading in that the validity of the method does not require that they be independent of one another. Except in experimental studies, it will rarely, if ever, be the case that the independent variables are uncorrelated.

The general linear regression equation is

$$y = b_0 + b_1 x_1 + b_2 x_2 + \cdots + b_k x_k + e \quad (2)$$

where e is the residual or error term. This equation is identical to Equation (1), since regression and the methods previously discussed are all examples of a general method of analysis.

There are two reasons for including an independent variable in the equation. One is that the relationship of y to x_i may be of direct interest. For example the relationship of FEV to length of exposure in a factory, or between FEV and concentration of dust, provides evidence on the effect of the factory environment on respiratory health. The second reason is that there is a relationship between y and x_i and it would be inefficient, and possibly misleading, to exclude this relationship from the analysis. The variable x_i is then referred to as a nuisance variable. It would be grossly misleading to analyze the relationship between FEV and length of exposure without taking account of age; it may or may not be misleading to analyze the relationship between FEV and dust concentration ignoring age and height. It would not be misleading if the correlations between dust concentration and both age and height were low. But such an analysis would certainly be inefficient because the residual variation would be higher than it would be after taking account of age and height.

Since the independent variables are intercorrelated the analysis is nonorthogonal so that the effect of each variable has to be assessed after allowing for all the other variables. This is done by fitting the regression containing all the independent variables and assessing each variable by its estimated regression coefficient and the standard error of the estimate, and the significance is determined by a t test. This test is identical to, but much more convenient than, the variance ratio test that would be obtained by fitting the regression containing all the other independent variables and then including the variable being assessed.

Step-Down Procedures

If some variables have no significant effect then caution is needed in simplifying the analysis by excluding them. It is not valid to exclude all nonsignificant variables in one step because excluding one variable alters the significance of all the remaining variables, and possibly to a marked effect. To take a trivial example: if both standing height and sitting height were included in an analysis of FEV then it would be possible that neither would be significant. The interpretation of this is that if standing height is included then there is no significant effect due to also including sitting height, and vice versa. But if either variable is excluded then the other will assume significance.

An approach to the problem is to work systematically starting with the regression containing all the independent variables. The least significant variable is then excluded and the regression recomputed. Again, the least significant variable is excluded and the process continues until all the included variables are significant at some level. This approach would be tedious and inefficient without a suitable computer program; GENSTAT [7] makes provision for selecting and excluding the least significant variable. An alternative procedure is to work the other way round (step-up) adding the most significant variable at each stage, but neither method necessarily leads to the optimum set of independent variables.

Regression in Groups

If the subjects form a number of groups then it is relevant to examine whether the regressions differ between the groups. If they do not the analysis may be simplified. There are three possibilities. First, completely separate regressions are necessary for each group and no simplification is possible. Second, the regression coefficients, $b_1, b_2, \ldots, b_k$, do not differ significantly between the groups but the constant term b_0 is dependent on group. In this case the regressions are parallel and the differences in position estimate the differences between groups after allowing for the regressor variables. The analysis is then equivalent to the analysis of covariance. Third, neither the coefficients nor the constant terms differ between groups and a single regression ignoring groups is adequate.

These three possibilities can only be explored in sequence, since it obviously would not make sense to assess the differences between the constant terms unless it had already been established that the regression coefficients did not differ between groups, and parallel regressions had been fitted. The calculations can be conveniently carried out by defining dummy variables to represent groups. For simplicity, suppose there are two groups and define

$$g = 1$$

for group 2, zero otherwise.
Also define variables $z_1, z_2, \ldots, z_k$

$$z_i = g\, x_i$$

Then the full regression is

$$\begin{aligned} Y = {} & b_0 + b_1 x_1 + b_2 x_2 + \cdots + b_k x_k \\ & + c_0 g + c_1 z_1 + c_2 z_2 + \cdots + c_k z_k \end{aligned} \tag{3}$$

Fitting this is equivalent to fitting separate regressions for each group; $b_0, b_1, \ldots, b_k$ are the coefficients for the first group and $b_0 + c_0, b_1 + c_1, \ldots, b_k + c_k$ for the second group. Omitting $z_1, \ldots, z_k$ from the regression gives parallel regressions with c_0 estimating the difference between groups. Finally, omitting g results in a single regression independent of group. An analysis of variance may be constructed to correspond to this procedure. In the general case of m groups this has degrees of freedom as follows:

Due to common regression	k
Gain due to separate constants	$m - 1$
Gain due to separate slopes	$k(m - 1)$
Residual	$n - m(k + 1)$

where there are n subjects.

There are intermediate possibilities between parallel and separate regression; some regression coefficients may depend on groups while others may not. The step-down procedure can be used to simplify the regression but it is necessary to take account of the structure of the variables in Equation (3). If variable x_i were eliminated while z_i remained then this would be equivalent to including x_i for subjects in group 2 but not for those in group 1, and, although there may be circumstances in which this is a sensible thing to do, this is not part of the procedure under discussion. Therefore the step-down procedure starts with the full regression of Equation (3) but only the variables $z_1, z_2, \ldots, z_k$ are eligible for elimination. If z_i is eliminated then x_i may be added to the set of variables eligible for elimination. Finally, g may only be eliminated if all of $z_1, z_2, \ldots, z_k$ have been eliminated. This procedure was followed by Miller et al. [18] except that for computing convenience they eliminated as many of the z variables as possible before considering the x variables.

Transformations

The methods under discussion depend on three properties. First, the dependent variable is, for fixed values of the independent variables, normally distributed. Second, the variance of the normal distribution is constant. Third, the regression model may be specified in a linear form. If the relationship is nonlinear it may be possible to overcome this by including additional or modified independent variables. For example y may be linearly related to log (x) rather than x. However if there is nonnormality or a nonconstant variance (heteroscedasticity) then a transformation of the dependent variable may result in normality and homoscedasticity.

The most common transformation is the logarithmic. This is used when the standard deviation increases in proportion to the mean of the observations. A warning sign that a logarithmic transformation might be appropriate is if the standard deviation of the dependent variable is more than half the mean value, or if the mean is not approximately midway between the minimum and maximum. These effects could be produced by one or two gross errors in the data so that it is important to check for outlying measurements; a plot, such as Figure 1, is useful for this purpose. It has been argued that the "lognormal distribution will almost always improve the description of the observations" (Oldham, Ref. 19, p. 189).

Another useful transformation is the reciprocal. This is sometimes used, for example, for the duffusing capacity of the pulmonary capillary membrane (DM) and the volume of blood in the alveolar capillaries (Vc). The use of the reciprocals in these cases corresponds to the method of deriving the measurements.

Often in practice a transformation which stabilizes variance also produced linearity but this need not occur. Methods of analysis are available for the case where one transformation is necessary to produce normality or a constant variance and another to produce linearity [20]. These methods involve more complex calculations than those that have been considered so far but are practical with suitable computer software. The calculations are in fact no more complex than those required for categorical data (to be considered in the next section).

III. The Analysis of Categorical Data

The most familiar form of categorical data is the fourfold, or 2 X 2, contingency table of frequencies. The χ^2 test, which should be calculated with Yates's correction for continuity, and the exact test, necessary when an expected frequency is small, are well known (Ref. 1, p. 134–136).

The exact test gives an unambiguous calculation of the one-tailed probability of observing the given table or any more extreme one. Usually a two-sided test is required, and here there is some ambiguity of practice. The logic of the test requires that it is calculated by including the more unlikely tables in the other tail (Oldham, Ref. 19, p. 97), but Armitage (Ref. 1, p. 137) considers that doubling the one-sided probability is "probably to be preferred on the grounds that a significant result is interpreted as strong evidence for a difference *in the observed direction,* and there is some merit in controlling the chance probability of such a result to no more than half the two-sided significance level." In this case there seems to be no objection to stating the one-sided significance level as such.

These tests are applicable to the problem of testing the difference of a proportion between two independent populations. When the populations are not independent but consist of matched pairs then a different test is required. Matched data are considered in section F, but first more complicated situa-

Table 6 Incidence of Bronchitis

	Bronchitis		
Type of mill	Yes	No	Total
Synthetic fiber	13	83	96
Cotton	102	335	437
Total	115	418	533

Source: Data from Berry et al. [21].

tions will be discussed for unmatched data; in particular, the combination of several 2 X 2 tables, the examination of trends in contingency tables classified by a factor with more than two ordered levels, and the analysis of contingency tables classified by more than two factors. Before turning to these topics, methods of measuring the size, rather than the significance, of an association in a 2 X 2 table are considered.

A. Association in 2 X 2 Tables

Table 6 gives some data from a survey of workers in the cotton industry. There were 437 men and women working in cotton mills who did not have bronchitis, as established by questionnaire, at the beginning of the survey. The questionnaire was repeated 2 years later, and 102 of those workers were then recorded as having bronchitis. As controls a group who worked in mills processing synthetic fiber were taken; 13 of 96 developed bronchitis in the 2 year period. The χ^2 test for the 2 X 2 table gives a value of 3.91, so that there is a significant association ($P < 0.05$).

Although it is important to test the significance of the association it is more important to estimate its size. The natural way of doing this is to express the incidences as percentages in each type of mill. Thus, 23.3% of workers in cotton mills developed bronchitis compared with 13.5% of workers in synthetic fiber mills. The difference of 9.8% has a standard error of 4.6% (Ref. 1, p. 129).

Now consider the data of Table 7. A group of 201 men with bronchial carcinoma was studied and it was established that 58 had been exposed to asbestos. A control group of patients with no evidence of bronchial carcinoma was chosen.

The association in Table 7 is highly significant ($\chi^2 = 11.5$). One way of expressing the association is to say that 29% of the men with cancer gave a history of exposure to asbestos compared with only 14% of the controls. However, it is of more interest to compare the percentage of asbestos-exposed

Table 7 Asbestos Exposure and Bronchial Carcinoma

	Exposed	Not exposed	Total
Patients with cancer	58	143	201
Controls	29	172	201
Total	87	315	402

Source: Data from Martischnig et al. [22].

men with cancer with the percentage of nonexposed with cancer, but it is impossible to do this with the data of Table 7. Of men with asbestos exposure in the study 67% have cancer, but this percentage has no meaning since it depends on the arbitrary choice of the size of the control group.

Relative Risk

In general terms the situation is as follows. Suppose that in a population there are individuals with and without some factor, and that a proportion P have the factor. Suppose that a proportion p_1 of those with the factor have a particular disease and for those without the factor the proportion with disease is p_2. Then the proportions of the total population may be classified in a 2 X 2 table as follows:

		Disease +	Disease −	
Factor	+	Pp_1	$P(1 - p_1)$	P
	−	$(1 - P)p_2$	$(1 - P)(1 - p_2)$	$1 - P$
				1

Now suppose a study is carried out and the number of individuals are classified in 2 X 2 table:

		Disease +	Disease −	
Factor	+	a	b	a + b
	−	c	d	c + d
		a + c	b + d	n

The interpretation of the frequencies depends on the way the study was carried out. If groups with and without the factor were defined first and then observations were made on the disease status (the prospective approach, as for Table 6) then

$$\frac{a}{b} \text{ estimates } \frac{Pp_1}{P(1 - p_1)} = \frac{p_1}{1 - p_1}$$

and

$$\frac{c}{d} \text{ estimates } \frac{p_2}{1 - p_2}$$

In this case the unknown proportion P cancels out for each factor level and both p_1 and p_2 can be estimated.

If the study was carried out by first selecting a group with disease and choosing a comparison group without disease, and then establishing the factor status of each subject (the retrospective or case-control approach, as for Table 7) then

$$\frac{a}{c} \quad \text{estimates} \quad \frac{Pp_1}{(1 - P)p_2}$$

and

$$\frac{b}{d} \quad \text{estimates} \quad \frac{P(1 - p_1)}{(1 - P)(1 - p_2)}$$

Neither ratio has a useful interpretation and both contain the unknown proportion P. However, if the two ratios are divided we obtain

$$R = \frac{a/c}{b/d} = \frac{ad}{bc} \quad \text{estimates} \quad \frac{p_1(1 - p_2)}{p_2(1 - p_1)} \tag{4}$$

This expression is known as the *odds ratio* because it is the ratio of the odds in favor of disease at each factor level. It is also referred to as the approximate *relative risk* because if the disease is rare, i.e., if $1 - p_1$ and $1 - p_2$ are near unity, then the ratio is approximately equal to p_1/p_2. In the retrospective type of study the odds ratio is the only function of the proportions of interest p_1 and p_2 which can be estimated. In a prospective study p_1 and p_2 can be estimated separately but it should be noted that the cross-product ad/bc estimates the odds ratio in this case also.

The sampling variation of R is given approximately by

$$\text{Variance}(\ln R) = \frac{1}{a} + \frac{1}{b} + \frac{1}{c} + \frac{1}{d} \tag{5}$$

where ln represents the natural logarithm (which is usually included as a function on a scientific calculator).

Returning to the data of Table 7

$$R = (58 \times 172)/(29 \times 143) = 2.41$$

$$\ln R = 0.878$$

$$\text{Variance } (\ln R) = 0.0645 = (0.254)^2$$

Thus approximate 95% confidence limits of ln R are 0.88 ± 1.96 × 0.254, or 0.380 and 1.376, which are equivalent to limits for R of 1.46 and 3.96. The above method of calculating the confidence limits for R would breakdown if any of the frequencies were zero and the approximation would be worst for low frequencies. Alternative methods are reviewed by Fleiss [23].

The Logit Transformation

A proportion lies within the finite range 0 to 1 and as a result many types of analysis are unsatisfactory particularly when there are observations near to either extreme. For example, if it was required to relate the proportion p with disease to a continuous measure of exposure x then it would be natural to think in terms of a regression of p on x. However a linear relationship would be unsatisfactory since the fitted line would extend above p = 1, and possibly also below p = 0, for positive values of x. This disadvantage can be overcome by transforming p so that the range becomes unbounded.

A suitable transformation in common use is the logit, or logistic, transformation defined by

$$y = \ln \frac{p}{1 - p}$$

(Sometimes the definition includes a factor of ½ so that the logits are half those given in the above equation.)

As p varies from 0 to 1, y varies from $-\infty$ to ∞ and the transformation is symmetrical about p = 0.5, i.e., logit (p) = −logit (1 − p). Equal changes on the logit scale correspond to smaller changes in p at the extremes than at values in the middle of the range. Thus a change in p from 5% to 10% is equivalent on the logit scale to a change from 41% to 59%.

The fact that when p = 0 or 1 the logit is infinite is inconvenient in graph plotting but the method of analysis is such that no difficulty arises.

Other transformations are used for proportions and discussions of the various options are given by Armitage (Ref. 1, pp. 355–359) and Oldham (Ref. 19, pp. 5–13).

Table 8 Asbestos Exposure, Bronchial Carcinoma, and Smoking

Smoking (cigarettes/ day)		Exposed	Not exposed	Relative risk (R)	ln R	Weight (w)[a]
0–14	Cancer	7	28	1.08	0.080	3.56
	Controls	12	52			
15–24	Cancer	25	66	2.92	1.070	5.95
	Controls	10	77			
⩾25	Cancer	26	49	3.26	1.182	4.45
	Controls	7	43			

[a]w is the reciprocal of the variance of ln R: $\Sigma w = 13.96$, $\Sigma w \ln R = 11.91$, $\Sigma w (\ln R)^2 = 13.05$. Test of combined effect: $(11.91)^2/13.96 = 10.16$ (χ^2 1 df). Test of heterogeneity: $13.05 - 10.16 = 2.89$ (χ^2 2 df). Combined estimate of $\ln R = 11.91/13.96 = 0.853$ ($R = 2.35$). Standard error of combined estimate $= 1/\sqrt{13.96} = 0.268$. 95% limits of ln R, 0.328, and 1.378 ($R = 1.39$ and 3.97).
Source: Data from Martischnig et al. [22].

The logit is the logarithm of the odds, and so the logarithm of the odds ratio [Eq. (4)] is simply the difference of two logits, one calculated for each row (or column) of a 2 × 2 table.

B. Combining 2 × 2 Tables

Often there are several 2 × 2 tables which all provide evidence on a particular association. For example, similar studies might have been carried out by different investigators, or within one study it might be prudent to divide the groups into subgroups according to the level of a third factor. Each 2 × 2 table provides an estimate of the association of interest and it may be possible to combine the separate estimates into a single estimate. Where this is possible it has the advantages, first, that the conclusions are simplified, and second, that the combined estimate will be more precise than its separate constituents. It could be that none of the separate 2 × 2 tables provides convincing evidence of an association but that the combined estimate is clearly significant.

It will only be possible to combine the separate estimates in a meaningful way if it is reasonable to suppose that they are all estimates of the same quantity, and a test of the strength of the evidence contrary to this supposition should be included in the analysis. If there is evidence that the associations are heterogeneous a single figure should not be used to summarize them.

In Table 8 the data of Martischnig et al. [22] are shown again with the subjects divided into three groups according to smoking habits. The data have been combined using the method of Woolf [24]. The method involves the calculation of a weighted mean of the three estimates of the logarithm of the relative risk. A weighted analysis is necessary because the estimates have different precisions and the weights are the reciprocals of the variances of ln R as calculated from Equation (5). Details of the calculations are given in the lower half of Table 8. The test of heterogeneity of relative risk between smoking groups is nonsignificant. Of course it cannot be concluded from this that there are no important differences between the groups since the relative risk varies markedly from 1.1 to 3.3. The study is not large enough to demonstrate whether this variation is real.

The combined estimate of relative risk is 2.35 with 95% confidence limits of 1.39 and 3.97, which are similar to the calculations based on Table 7 (relative risk 2.41, limits 1.46 and 3.96). This may appear surprising in view of the known association between bronchial cancer and smoking, which was also demonstrated within this study, but the similarity occurred because the men exposed to asbestos had similar smoking habits to the nonexposed. If this had not been the case conclusions based solely on Table 7 could have been very misleading. In spite of the similarity of the estimates, the conclusions from Table 8 are much stronger than those from Table 7. The latter conclusion is that there is a significant association, with a relative risk of 2.4, between bronchial carcinoma and asbestos exposure. This could be criticized on the grounds that part of the apparent effect was a hidden effect of smoking. This criticism cannot be leveled against the conclusion from Table 8.

Another frequently used method is that of Mantel and Haenszel [25]. Suppose the frequencies in the ith table are

		Factor		
		+	–	Total
Disease	+	a_i	b_i	$a_i + b_i$
	–	c_i	d_i	$c_i + d_i$
	Total	$a_i + c_i$	$b_i + d_i$	n_i

Then in the absence of any association between the factor and disease the expected value of a_i, $E(a_i)$, and the variance of a_i, $V(a_i)$, are given by

$$E(a_i) = \frac{(a_i + b_i)\,(a_i + c_i)}{n_i}$$

$$V(a_i) = \frac{(a_i + b_i)\,(c_i + d_i)\,(a_i + c_i)\,(b_i + d_i)}{n_i^2\,(n_i - 1)}$$

The difference between a_i and $E(a_i)$, when judged against its variance, measures the evidence for an association between the factor and disease within the ith table. The basis of the test is to combine the differences, giving equal weights to each difference. The test statistic, which includes a continuity correction and is approximately distributed as a χ^2 with 1 degree of freedom, is

$$\frac{(|\Sigma a_i - \Sigma E(a_i)| - \tfrac{1}{2})^2}{\Sigma V(a_i)}$$

The Mantel-Haenszel combined estimate of relative risk is

$$\frac{\Sigma(a_i d_i/n_i)}{\Sigma(b_i c_i/n_i)}$$

The methods of Woolf [24] and Mantel and Haenszel [25] usually give similar answers (e.g., for the data of Table 8 the Mantel-Haenszel estimate of relative risk is 2.38 and the χ^2 test statistic is 10.39), and the choice between them is to some extent a matter of personal taste. Woolf's test has the advantage of comparing, as well as combining, the relative risks, but this advantage is illusory in some cases since, as the data of Table 8 demonstrate, it may be impossible to discriminate between quite large differences. If any of the frequencies are zero then Woolf's test breaks down but the Mantel-Haenszel test remains viable.

Another method of combining 2 X 2 tables, due to Cochran [26], is appropriate to the case where the data are of the prospective type, so that it is possible to estimate for each table the proportions of subjects with disease at each level of the classifying factor. The difference between these two proportions is a measure of the association within a table and a weighted analysis of these differences is carried out to combine the separate measures. The weights are such that the procedure works best if the differences are constant on the logit or probit scales. The method is set out and illustrated by Armitage (Ref. 1, p. 370).

The method of Woolf [24] is a weighted analysis of the logarithms of relative risk, and, as discussed earlier, the logarithm of a relative risk is the difference between two proportions on a logit scale. Also Cochran's method [26] is designed for the case when the differences between proportions are constant on the logit scale. A natural extension is to carry out the whole analysis after a logit transformation and use a method similar to that of fitting constants. The optimum method of estimation using this approach is that of maximum likelihood which includes the proper weighting of the proportions being analyzed according to the sampling variation. Such an analysis

Table 9 Incidence of New Cases of Byssinosis in Women by Dust Concentration

Dust concentration range	Mean (mg/m^3)	Number at risk	Number of new cases	Incidence (%)
0.25–0.49	0.34	61	2	3.3
0.50–0.74	0.58	83	8	9.6
0.75–0.99	0.84	71	13	18.3
1.00–1.24	1.17	47	13	27.7
1.25–2.38	1.48	60	13	21.7

Source: Compiled from Berry et al. [21].

would not break down for a zero frequency, as Woolf's method does, since the weights used are fitted weights not empirical weights. An example of this approach, but using the probit transformation, is given by Oldham (Ref. 19, p. 110). A fuller discussion of this topic will be deferred to a later section where contingency tables classified by more than 2 factors are considered. A set of k 2 X 2 tables may quite properly be thought of as a single k X 2 X 2 table.

C. Trends in Contingency Tables

The data in Table 9 are the incidences of byssinosis in a 2 year period. The subjects at risk are divided into groups on the basis of the concentration of dust to which they were exposed in the cotton mill where they worked. There is an apparent increase in incidence with increasing dust concentration, and the question considered in this section is how to test the significance of the trend.

Now in this example the subjects have been subdivided according to an objective measure of dust concentration. Often in data of this sort the subdivision is not so well determined. For example, the dustiness could have been expressed as very low, low, average, high, and very high. Then the five categories occur in a definite order but no other information on the relative dustiness is necessarily available.

Most of the methods of fitting trends involve the assignment of scores to the ordered categories. In the absence of any information to the contrary it is reasonable to choose these scores to be equally spaced so that in the example of Table 9, if measured dust levels had not been available, then scores of −2, −1, 0, 1, and 2 could have been assigned. Cochran [26] described a test which is essentially an approximate calculation of the regression of the proportion with disease on the score. Details of the necessary calculations are given by Armitage (Ref. 1, p. 363). Applying the test to the data of Table 9 gives a χ^2 of 13.67 with 1 df for the trend which is therefore significant ($P < 0.001$). Analyses of this sort are often criticized or mistrusted on the grounds that they depend on an arbitrary system of scoring which it is impossible to justify. However, provided only that the scores are allocated without reference to the data, the analysis provides a valid test, in the sense that if there is no real trend the probability of obtaining a significant result is controlled by the significance level. The scores will not be optimum and this leads to a decrease in sensitivity of the test, i.e., a real trend will not be found significant as readily as if the true scores were known. In practice this reduction in sensitivity is often small.

Sometimes the data are such that it is the response factor which consists of ordered categories. For example, the amount of disease might be compared in two populations and the disease may be classified as absent, mild, moderate, or severe. In this case it would be more natural to calculate and compare the mean disease score in each population. It happens that this approach leads to exactly the same test as considered in the last paragraph when the problem was the other way round [27]. An alternative method of analysis when the response variable consists of ordered categories is given by Clayton [28]. This method treats the problem as determining the difference in location between the two populations where each is regarded as a multinomial distribution. It is assumed that the logit transformation of the cumulative distribution function differs between the two populations by a constant, and this assumption makes it unnecessary to allocate scores to the ordered categories.

In the particular case of Table 9 it is not necessary to allocate scores arbitrarily; the actual dust levels may be used. Then the test described by Cochran [26] involves the approximate fitting of a linear regression of the proportion developing byssinosis on dust level. If a regression is to be fitted the method of fitting could be exact, rather than approximate, and the regression chosen could be such as to avoid the possibility of absurd consequences such as a proportion becoming negative. If the proportions are transformed to logits and the dust concentrations to logarithms then a linear regression will ensure that the fitted proportion always lies within the range 0 to 1 and in addition that it will be zero for zero dust level. This seems a reasonable condition to apply to a dust-related disease. The exact method of fitting is by maximum likelihood. The details will not be described and involve an iterative calculation. The calculations will usually be carried out on a computer and suitable programs are available (e.g., GLIM [6]).

The fitted relationship is shown in Figure 2 and the test statistic of the regression is 15.66. This is approximately distributed as a χ^2 with 1 df (note that, although the method of fitting is exact, it is only approximate to consider the test statistic as a χ^2). The fitted relationship is not much different

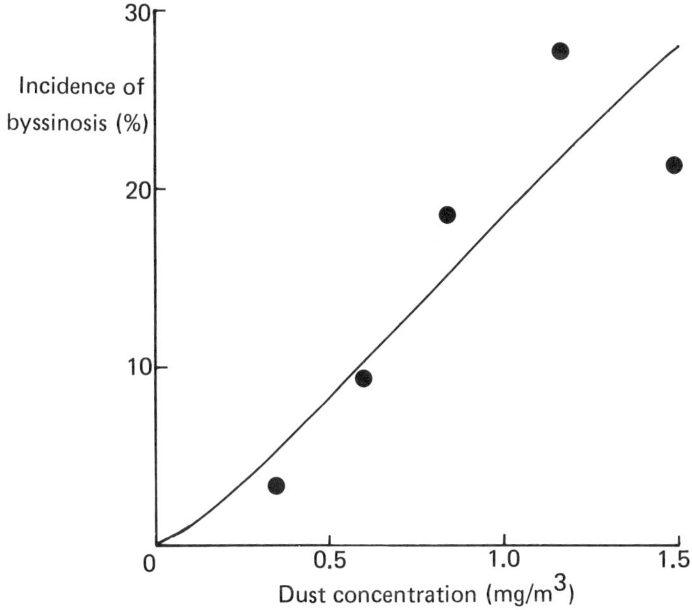

Figure 2 Incidence of byssinosis in 2 year period and dust concentration. The fitted curve is the linear relationship between the logit of incidence and the logarithm of dust concentration.

from a linear regression of incidence on dust concentration constrained to go through the origin.

D. Higher Order Contingency Tables

In Table 10 the prevalence of byssinosis is shown in relation to sex, smoking, dust concentration, and length of exposure in the cotton industry. Thus subjects are classified by four factors in addition to their disease status. An analysis is needed to establish the association of each factor with disease and also to see if there are any interactions between the factors. As an exploratory device it is useful to calculate the crude prevalences, and these are shown in Table 11. They give the impression that all the factors are associated with disease but this could be misleading because of correlations between the factors. For example a higher proportion of men than women were smokers, a higher proportion of women than men had completed 20 years' service, and a higher proportion of women with short service smoked than those with long service.

Table 10 Byssinosis: Relationship with Sex, Smoking, Dust Concentration, and Length of Exposure

Dust concentration (mg/m^3)	Nonsmokers and exsmokers[a]			Smokers[a]		
	Length of exposure (years)					
	0–9	10–19	20+	0–9	10–19	20+
Women						
0.25–0.74	0/23	1/28	24/111	1/36	9/33	23/89
0.75–1.24	2/20	4/23	16/63	7/54	11/43	22/65
1.25–2.38	0/12	4/14	23/42	12/44	10/27	27/45
Men						
0.25–0.74	0/3	1/6	3/3	1/16	4/6	5/9
0.75–1.24	0/7	4/11	2/6	7/25	21/40	12/24
1.25–2.38	1/14	3/4	3/4	6/24	12/22	8/10

[a]No. with byssinosis/no. of subjects.
Source: Data from Berry et al. [21].

There are several ways of proceeding to disentangle the effects of the separate factors. One would be to take each factor in turn and to calculate prevalences after standardizing for the other three factors. The indirect method of standardization could be used with the total survey population treated as the standard. Statistical tests of each factor could be constructed

Table 11 Crude Prevalences (%) of Byssinosis

Smoking	Women	Men	Both sexes
Non and exsmokers	22.0	29.3	23.1
Smokers	28.0	43.2	32.4
Dust concentration (mg/m^3)			
0.25–0.74	18.1	32.6	19.8
0.75–1.24	23.1	40.7	28.3
1.25–2.38	41.3	42.3	41.6
Length of exposure (years)			
0–9	11.6	16.9	13.3
10–19	23.2	50.6	32.7
20+	32.5	58.9	35.7
Total	25.4	39.7	28.7

Source: Data from Berry et al. [21].

using the Mantel-Haenszel procedure, i.e., a test of the sex effect could be regarded as the combination of eighteen 2 X 2 tables [29]. This approach will not be pursued here.

If the data had consisted of measurements on a continuous scale, say the FEV of each subject had been measured, then the method of analysis would have been to fit constants for main effects and interactions with the significance of the effects assessed by a nonorthogonal analysis of variance. The method to be adopted with the data consisting of proportions with disease is a generalization of this method [20]. The methodology has been known for over 25 years [30] but in spite of this has not been widely used. One reason for this has been the lack of a general computer program but this problem is solved by GLIM [6]. The method consists of fitting a linear model of the main effects and interactions of the four factors to the logit of the proportion with disease.

The analog of the analysis of variance is the analysis of deviance. The deviance is a measure of the lack of fit of the model and is therefore the analog of the residual sum of squares. The deviance has a number of degrees of freedom associated with it, equal to the number of independent observations less the number of independent terms fitted, just as in the familiar analysis of variance.

The analysis of deviance is shown in Table 12. The main effect of each factor is assessed, after allowing for the main effects of the other three fac-

Table 12 Analysis of Deviance

Effects included[a]	Deviance	df	
Sex, Sm, D, L	37.98	29	
Sm, D, L	58.00	30	
Reduction due to sex	20.02	1	$P < 0.001$
Sex, D, L	49.28	30	
Reduction due to Sm	11.30	1	$P < 0.001$
Sex, Sm, L	78.94	31	
Reduction due to D	40.96	2	$P < 0.001$
Sex, Sm, D	123.30	31	
Reduction due to L	85.32	2	$P < 0.001$
Sex, Sm, D, L, L X Sm	30.79	27	
Reduction due to L X Sm interaction	7.19	2	$P < 0.05$

[a]Sm = smoking, D = dust concentration, L = length of exposure.
Source: Data from Berry et al. [21].

tors, by calculating the reduction in deviance due to including the factor under consideration to a model which already includes the other factors. So, for example, the deviance after fitting smoking, dust concentration, and length of exposure is 58.00 with 30 df. If in addition sex is fitted then the deviance is reduced to 37.98 with 29 df. Therefore the effect of sex is to reduce the deviance by 20.02 with 1 df. The significance of this is established by reference to the χ^2 distribution. The same procedure is carried out for the other three factors and all four factors are highly significant. The deviance after fitting all four main effects is 37.98 with 29 df, and this measures the lack of fit of the model. Since the value is not significant ($P > 0.1$) it could be concluded that the model provides a satisfactory fit to the data. However, the deviance includes contributions from all the interactions and it is possible for some real interactions to be masked by the other null interactions. To check this possibility six more models were fitted including all four main effects and each two-factor interaction in turn. The smoking × length of exposure interaction is significant ($P < 0.05$, Table 12) but all of the other two-factor interactions are nonsignificant. Therefore it may be concluded that the prevalence of byssinosis is significantly associated with sex, smoking, dust concentration, and length of exposure and also that the association with length of exposure differs for nonsmokers and smokers.

So far the significant factors affecting the prevalence of byssinosis have been identified but the most important part of the analysis remains. That is the presentation of the results to reveal the established effects. Since the analysis was carried out on the logit scale the most obvious presentation is in terms of the fitted constants of that analysis. Since these constants are not readily comprehensible their antilogarithms have been taken to convert them to odds ratios or relative risks. These constants are shown in the first column of Table 13. Thus the effect of sex is such that men have an odds ratio 2.3 times that of women. The form of the interaction of smoking and length of exposure is also clear from this presentation; the length of exposure effect is less in smokers than in nonsmokers so that smoking has little effect in those with long exposure.

An alternative presentation [31] is in terms of standardized prevalences calculated by the direct method on the fitted prevalences in each cell of the original classification. These standardized prevalences are shown in the second column of Table 13. The standardized prevalences, although valid for the internal interpretation of the results of the survey, have the disadvantage of being dependent on the particular distribution of factors which happened to occur within the survey. Thus the standardized prevalence for women of 25.1% is the prevalence which would have been expected to occur if the

Table 13 Summary of Effects

Sex		Odds ratio	Standardized prevalence (%)
Women		1.0	25.1
Men		2.3	41.3
Dust concentration (mg/m^3)			
0.25–0.74		1.0	20.2
0.75–1.24		1.5	27.2
1.25–2.38		3.4	43.4
Smoking and length of exposure			
Non/exsmokers	0–9	1.0	3.2
	10–19	8.8	20.7
	20+	21.0	36.7
Current smokers	0–9	5.7	14.7
	10–19	18.8	34.4
	20+	27.1	42.2

Source: Data from Berry et al. [21].

women had had the same distribution of dust concentration, smoking, length of exposure, and all combinations of these factors, as occurred in the population of men and women combined. These prevalences are unlikely to be comparable with estimates from other studies but those of the odds ratio would be.

E. Log-Linear Models

The method discussed in the last section is a special case of a more general methodology which involves the fitting of log-linear models. These models are such that the logarithms of the expected frequencies in the cells of a multidimensional table are sums of constants representing the main effects and interactions of the factors forming the table. In the last section, the data of Table 10 were regarded as a 2 X 2 X 3 X 3 table of proportions. The more general method would be to regard the data as a 2 X 2 X 2 X 3 X 3 table of frequencies. However if this had been done, and a log-linear model fitted, then the analysis would have yielded identical results. Great care would have been necessary to ensure that the analysis of byssinosis was carried out conditionally on all the total numbers of subjects given in Table 10; this would have involved including terms in the model for all the main effects and interactions of the four classifying factors, i.e., 35 extra terms of no direct interest. Clearly there would have been no advantage in complicating the analysis by regarding the data as a five-factor table of frequencies.

Two features of the data of Table 10 make the logit approach possible. First, only one factor (disease) is of direct interest; this is referred to as the response factor and the other factors as classifying factors. Second, the response factor has just two levels. If either or both of these conditions do not hold then the more general approach may be called for. Two cases may be distinguished. In the first there is a single response factor which has more than two levels. In the second there is more than one response factor. An example of the first case is given by Nelder and Wedderburn [20], and Everitt [32] gives an example of the second case in which all three factors of a 2 X 4 X 4 contingency table are of direct interest.

F. Matched Samples

In case-control studies it is common practice to match each case with one or more controls, where the matching is for one or more factors which are not of direct interest but which are thought to be associated with the disease under investigation. Such matching has two purposes. First, it eliminates the possibility of bias which would occur if there was an association between the matching factors and the factor under investigation. Second, the variation due to the matching variables is removed and so the study is more precise.

Matched samples of categorical data have often been analyzed ignoring the matching. This is clearly inefficient, unless the matching is irrelevant, but has been done for two reasons. First, the correct methodology has not been widely known, and, except for the simplest case, has only been developed recently. Second, an unmatched analysis would usually yield a conservative test of significance so that it was known that the analysis would not result in false claims of significant results.

Single Control-Dichotomous Factor

The simplest case is that of one control per case and the factor under investigation having just two levels. There are four possibilities for each pair and the data should be considered in the form

		Control		
	Factor	+	−	
Case	+	a	b	a + b
	−	c	d	c + d
		a + c	b + d	m

Although this has the appearance of a 2 X 2 table its construction is quite different; the entries are not individuals but pairs, so that there are a pairs where both the case and the control are positive for the factor. These a pairs, as well as the d pairs whose members are both negative for the factor, provide no evidence on the association between disease and factor so that the test must be restricted to the b and c dissimilar pairs. If there is no association then it would be expected that b = c and an exact test of this is based on the binomial distribution with probability parameter ½. The normal approximation to the test is sometimes referred to as McNemar's test (Ref. 1, p. 126).

If it is assumed that the relative risk is independent of the matching variables then it is estimated by b/c. Confidence limits for the relative risk can be calculated based on the confidence limits of the binomial parameter giving b positive cases out of b + c dissimilar pairs [33].

Multiple Controls—Dichotomous Factor

It is sometimes good practice to choose more than one control per case. By these means the precision of a study in which it is not possible to obtain more cases may be increased; however, it will rarely be worthwhile having more than four controls per case. Where the factor has just two levels then the test is an extension of the test mentioned in the last section. The method is described by Pike and Morrow [34] and by Miettinen [35], who also [33] gives details of methods of estimating the relative risk and its confidence intervals.

Single Control—Factor with Multiple Levels

Pike et al. [36] consider the analysis of matched pairs where the factor under investigation has more than two levels which are not ordered. If the factor has k levels then there are [k(k − 1)]/2 relative risks but these would only be consistent if they could all be expressed in terms of k − 1 independent relative risks. A method of testing evidence of association, of estimating the relative risks and their confidence intervals and of testing their consistency is given by Pike et al. [36].

It the multiple levels are ordered then McCullagh [37] has extended the method of Clayton [28] to matched pairs; he illustrates the method by application to the change in the radiological category of pneumoconiosis in the period between surveys.

Multiple Controls—Factor(s) with Multiple Levels

The analysis of multiple matched controls where the factor under study has just two levels was discussed. However, frequently the situation is more complicated. For example, Liddell et al. [38] investigated the association between lung cancer and asbestos exposure. For each of a number of lung cancer cases five age-matched controls were chosen and estimates were made of the asbestos exposure. The measure of asbestos exposure was on a continuous scale but was grouped into ordered categories. In addition, smoking habits were recorded and, since smoking is associated with lung cancer, it was required to take account of smoking in the assessment of the asbestos effect. Thus there were two factors to take account of simultaneously. Both factors had multiple levels and one of them could be regarded as a continuous variable instead of a multileveled factor. A method for analyzing data of this type has been developed only recently and stems from an important paper by Cox [39], who considered the analysis of a prospective study in which it is required to assess the relationship between the risk of some event, such as death due to a specific cause, and a number of covariates known for each individual in the study. Suppose the covariates are $x_1, x_2, \ldots, x_k$ and each of these may be either continuous variables or dummy variables taking the values 0 or 1 to indicate the absence or presence of a factor. Then Cox [39] proposed a model in which the death rate at time t is $\lambda(t) \exp(\Sigma b_i x_i)$, where $\lambda(t)$ is an unspecified function of t. Therefore the relative death rates of different individuals are proportional to their values of $\exp(\Sigma b_i x_i)$, at all values of t, provided that the x_i are not time dependent.

It is at first sight surprising that this method extends to a retrospective study, but regarding a retrospective study as a sample of a prospective study makes the extension a natural step. The application to case-control studies has been described by Thomas (Addendum to Ref. 38) and by Breslow and his colleagues [40–42]. Suppose that a particular case has c controls and that x_{oi} is the value of x_i for the case and x_{ji} for the jth control. Then it is known that just one of the c + 1 individuals is a case, and the probability that this one is the observed case is

$$\exp\left(\sum_{i=1}^{k} b_i x_{oi}\right) \Big/ \sum_{j=0}^{c} \exp\left(\sum_{i=1}^{k} b_i x_{ji}\right)$$

The likelihood is the product of the probabilities over all the cases and the method of maximum likelihood provides estimates of the b_i and significance tests. In this representation the b_i are the logarithms of relative risks; if x_i is a dummy variable representing a factor then $\exp(b_i)$ is the relative risk due to the factor, while if x_i is a continuous variable then $\exp(b_i x_i)$ is its relative risk.

In some situations a different type of parametrization may be required but the basic method may be extended to cope with alternative expressions for the relative risks (e.g., see Ref. 43). The method is general and includes some of the methods discussed earlier as special cases, e.g., the method for a factor with multiple levels and a single control [36].

The general method is "conceptually straightforward although computationally somewhat involved" [42], but as it becomes more widely known, and computer programs become available, then it will no longer be necessary to analyze matched data ignoring the matching.

Acknowledgments

I am grateful to Dr. P. D. Oldham and Mr. C. E. Rossiter for their comments on an earlier draft, to Miss C. Heywood for preparing the figures, and to Mrs. J. A. Bolan for typing the script.

I am also grateful to the editors of *Thorax, British Journal of Industrial Medicine,* and the *British Medical Journal* for permission to use some of the data given in papers [15,21,22], and to the authors of those papers.

References

1. Armitage, P., *Statistical Methods in Medical Research.* Oxford and Edinburgh, Blackwell, 1971.
2. Fisher, R. A., *Smoking–The Cancer Controversy.* Edinburgh, Oliver and Boyd, 1959, pp. 11–25.
3. Burch, P. J., Smoking and lung cancer: The problem of inferring cause, *J. R. Stat. Soc. A,* **141**:437–477 (1978).
4. Hill, A. B., The environment and disease: Association or causation, *Proc. R. Soc. Med.,* **58**:295–300 (1965).
5. Finney, D. J., *Probit Analysis.* Cambridge, University Press, 1947, p. 28.
6. Baker, R. J., and J. A. Nelder, *The GLIM System, Release 3.* Oxford, Numerical Algorithms Group, 1978.
7. Alvey, N. G., C. F. Banfield, R. I. Baxter, J. C. Gower, W. J. Krzanowski, P. W. Lane, P. K. Leech, J. A. Nelder, R. W. Payne, K. M. Phelps, C. E. Rogers, G. J. S. Ross, H. R. Simpson, A. D. Todd, R. W. M. Wedderburn, and G. N. Wilkinson, *GENSTAT–A General Statistical Program.* Harpenden, Statistics Department, Rothamsted Experimental Station, 1977.
8. Oldham, P. D., A note on the analysis of repeated measurements of the same subject, *J. Chron. Dis.,* **15**:969–977 (1962).
9. Fletcher, C., R. Peto, C. Tinker, and F. E. Speizer, *The Natural History of Chronic Bronchitis and Emphysema.* Oxford, University Press, 1976, pp. 71–73.
10. Cotes, J. E., *Lung Function,* 3rd ed. Oxford, Blackwell, 1975.
11. Cole, T. J., Linear and proportional regression models in the prediction of ventilatory function, *J. R. Statist. Soc. A,* **138**:297–337 (1975).
12. Cox, D. R., The use of a concomitant variable in selecting an experimental design, *Biometrika,* **44**:150–158 (1957).

13. Berry, G., C. B. McKerrow, M. K. B. Molyneux, C. E. Rossiter, and J. B. L. Tombleson, A study of the acute and chronic changes in ventilatory capacity of workers in Lancashire cotton mills, *Br. J. Ind. Med.*, **30**:25–36 (1973).
14. Oldham, P. D., The uselessness of normal values. In *Introduction to the Definition of Normal Values for Respiratory Function in Man.* Proceedings of an International Symposium of the Societas Europae Physiologiae Clinicae Respiratoriae held in Alghero, 15–19 May, 1969. Edited by P. Arcangeli. Torino, Panminerva, 1970, pp. 49–56.
15. Constantinidis, K., A. W. Musk, J. P. R. Jenkins, and G. Berry, Pulmonary function in coal workers with Caplan's syndrome and non-rheumatoid complicated pneumoconiosis, *Thorax*, **33**:764–768 (1978).
16. Fisher, R. A., and F. Yates, *Statistical Tables for Biological, Agricultural and Medical Research*, 6th ed. Edinburgh, Oliver and Boyd, 1963.
17. Yates, F., The Analysis of multiple classifications with unequal numbers in the different classes, *J. Am. Statist. Assoc.*, **29**:51–66 (1934).
18. Miller, G. J., M. J. Saunders, R. J. C. Gilson, and M. T. Ashcroft, Lung function of healthy boys and girls in Jamaica in relation to ethnic composition, test exercise performance, and habitual physical activity, *Thorax*, **32**:486–496 (1977).
19. Oldham, P. D., *Measurement in Medicine–The Interpretation of Numerical Data.* London, English Universities Press, 1968.
20. Nelder, J. A., and R. W. M. Wedderburn, Generalized linear models, *J. R. Statist. Soc. A*, **135**:370–384 (1972).
21. Berry, G., M. K. B. Molyneux, and J. B. L. Tombleson, Relationships between dust levels and byssinosis and bronchitis in Lancashire cotton mills, *Br. J. Ind. Med.*, **31**:18–27 (1974).
22. Martischnig, K. M., D. J. Newell, W. C. Barnsley, W. K. Cowan, E. L. Feinmann, and E. Oliver, Unsuspected exposure to asbestos and bronchogenic carcinoma, *Br. Med. J.*, **1**:746–749 (1977).
23. Fleiss, J. L., Confidence intervals for the odds ratio in case-control studies: The state of the art, *J. Chron. Dis.*, **32**:69–82 (1979).
24. Woolf, B., On estimating the relation between blood group and disease, *Ann. Hum. Genet.*, **19**:251–253 (1955).
25. Mantel, N., and W. Haenszel, Statistical aspects of the analysis of data from retrospective studies of disease, *J. Natl. Cancer Inst.*, **22**:719–748 (1959).
26. Cochran, W. G., Some methods of strengthening the common χ^2 tests, *Biometrics*, **10**:417–451 (1954).
27. Yates, F., The analysis of contingency tables with groupings based on quantitative characters, *Biometrika*, **35**:176–181 (1948).
28. Clayton, D. G., Some odds ratio statistics for the analysis of ordered categorical data, *Biometrika*, **61**:525–531 (1974).
29. Mantel, N., Chi-square tests with one degree of freedom; extensions of the Mantel-Haenszel procedure, *J. Am. Statist. Assoc.*, **58**:690–700 (1963).
30. Dyke, G. V., and H. D. Patterson, Analysis of factorial arrangements when the data are proportions, *Biometrics*, **8**:1–12 (1952).

31. Berry, G., Parametric analysis of disease incidences in multiway tables, *Biometrics,* **26**:572–579 (1970).
32. Everitt, B. S., *The Analysis of Contingency Tables,* London, Chapman and Hall, 1977, pp. 94–99.
33. Pike, M. C., and R. H. Morrow, Statistical analysis of patient-control studies in epidemiology—factor under investigation an all-or-none variable. *Br. J. Prev. Soc. Med.,* **24**:42–44 (1970).
34. Miettinen, O. S., Individual matching with multiple controls in the case of all-or-none responses, *Biometrics,* **25**:339–355 (1969).
35. Miettinen, O. S., Estimation of relative risk from individually matched series, *Biometrics,* **26**:75–86 (1970).
36. Pike, M. C., J. Casagrande, and P. G. Smith, Statistical analysis of individually matched case-control studies in epidemiology: Factor under study a discrete variable taking multiple values, *Br. J. Prev. Soc. Med.,* **29**:196–201 (1975).
37. McCullagh, P., A logistic model for paired comparisons with ordered categorical data, *Biometrika,* **64**:449–453 (1977).
38. Liddell, F. D. K., J. C. McDonald, and D. C. Thomas, Methods of cohort analysis: Appraisal by application to asbestos mining, *J. R. Statist. Soc. A,* **140**:469–491 (1977).
39. Cox, D. R., Regression models and life-tables, *J. R. Statist. Soc. B,* **34**: 187–202 (1972).
40. Breslow, N. E., The proportional hazards model: Applications in epidemiology. *Commun. Statist. Theor. Meth.,* **A7(4)**:315–332 (1978).
41. Prentice, R. L., and N. E. Breslow, Retrospective studies and failure time models, *Biometrika,* **65**:153–158 (1978).
42. Breslow, N. E., N. E. Day, K. T. Halvorsen, R. L. Prentice, and C. Sabai, Estimation of multiple relative risk functions in matched case-control studies, *Am. J. Epidemiol.,* **108**:299–307 (1978).
43. Berry, G., Dose-response in case-control studies, *J. Epidemiol. Community Health,* **34**:000–000 (1980).

16

Scientific Basis for Public Policy Decisions

HANS WEILL

Tulane University School of Medicine
New Orleans, Louisiana

In elegant fashion, the contributors to this monograph have set out the manner in which new knowledge can be obtained which relates inhalant exposures in the workplace to the spectrum of disordered respiratory health and how (or when) this relationship is modified by personal characteristics (host factors) and disease mechanisms. Their presentations amply illustrate the increasing complexity of methods which are being applied to the investigations of the working populations which are at potential or actual risk for development of respiratory disease. The ultimate goal of this research is the prevention of occupational lung disease; it should be clear how this scientific activity leads to the stated objective.

First, the research efforts *establish* that a hazard exists, relying on methods that optimally balance sensitivity with specificity. This of course depends upon the demonstration of *causation* which is not the same as showing an *association* between an environmental factor and disease, as splendidly discussed by Hill [1]. He indicates that the factors to be considered before deciding that the association is one of causation include strength (of the association), consistency of the observed association, specificity, temporality, biological gradient (dose-response relationship), plausibility, coherence (in accordance with generally known facts regarding the disease), experimental evidence, and analogy (circumstances similar to another previously proven causal association).

Science also helps in *quantifying* the risk associated with a specific workplace exposure. It has been amply demonstrated that all risks are not equal nor should they be treated as such [2]. As difficult as it may be at times, risk judgments must be made in relation to benefit, while improving science and technoloty leads to enhanced sensitivity in the measurement of both risk and benefit. Risk assessment leads to the rational setting of priorities, and in turn the optimal allocation of resources, not simply economic but, perhaps of even greater importance, research and technological.

Third, science will provide clues (or evidence) leading to high yield prevention or intervention strategies. For example, pulmonary physiological and radiographic evidence of dose-related effect secondary to exposure to mineral dusts can (and has) led to reduced levels of airborne particulates to a point where risk of adverse lung effects is either minimal or absent. Demonstrating another approach, research may make possible the identification of workers who are susceptible to inhalants which produce occupational asthma, information which obviously can lead to their exclusion from such exposure. It has also become apparent that recognition of critical interactions and their modifications on the biological response leads not only to a better understanding of the occupationally induced disease but to its more effective management from the standpoint of individual workers as well as large industrial populations. Brief examples of such interactions include multiple carcinogens, both occupational and nonoccupational, and smoking-exposure-atopy interactions in acute and chronic airways obstruction. Many of the methods discussed in this monograph will also be useful in monitoring the consequences of implementing public health policy directed toward the prevention of these diseases, confirming the desired favorable outcome.

How may the methods discussed have potential impact on the decision-making process which establishes public health policy? If, for example, tissue mineral analysis revealed that a great proportion of the asbestos fibers seen with the electron microscope represents a "survivor population" and such fibers were predominantly of the amphibole type, one might conclude that there is less peripheral lung deposition and/or retention of the more widely used chrysotile asbestos fibers, a conclusion which could lead to their differing treatment in the regulatory process.

Radiographic findings possess little specificity, their value being derived from correlations with other biological and exposure data. External validation will ultimately provide the basis for assessing the level of radiographic abnormality which indicates a specific disease process. Recognizing the important inter- and intraobserver variability found with independent reading of x-rays using the ILO International Classification, particularly when the profusion of small opacities is at the lower levels, will hopefully result in rational judgments concerning the use (or nonuse) of this or other classifications (designed for epidemiological purposes) in deciding individual workers' compensation awards.

Most of the respiratory disorders which are causally related to an adverse workplace exposure do not exhibit specific markers indicating their etiology; these conditions also appear in the nonexposed general population. We must rely on epidemiological investigations to sort out the contributions of multiple influencing variables, as, for example, smoking and certain industrial chemical exposures in chronic bronchitis or atopy and organic dust exposure in occupational asthma. When an occupational exposure has long been recognized as causing lung disease, exposure dose may gradually have been reduced by control of airborne inhalants. If the exposure-related health effect has a long latent period, the indicators of current disease will reflect higher exposures in the past. How then can permissible exposure limits be set in such circumstances and how will we know if the lower levels existing today carry an acceptably low risk? The answer is: with great difficulty. Epidemiology can help, and inevitably assumptions must be made concerning the shape of the dose-response curve [3,4], and since observations on long-term, low-level exposure are usually not available, extrapolations will be made using biological data associated with higher exposures.

The least controversial, or conversely, the most widely accepted policy decisions on environmental issues are based on epidemiological studies. This in no way minimizes the important role of animal models in the early recognition of certain environmental hazards, particularly in carcinogenesis. Several chapters in this monograph deal with study design, data collection, analysis, and interpretation of results from studies of working populations which may be at risk for development of occupational lung disease. It will be apparent to the reader that varying epidemiological approaches and techniques result in evidence or "proof" which also varies in strength or power. Ultimately, those responsible for public policy decisions must weigh the strength of the evidence. How epidemiological evidence can influence such decisions may be inferred from these chapters.

Work in our own unit on the health risks associated with dust exposure in asbestos cement manufacturing illustrates how varying epidemiological study designs have added to our knowledge concerning this important occupational health problem. Utilizing retrospective dust dose estimation for each of almost 1000 currently employed workers in a cross-sectional investigation, radiographic and physiological evidence of asbestosis was found to be dose related and, in addition, demonstrated which functional measurements were most sensitive and how their sensitivity compared to radiographic evidence of pneumoconiosis [5]. A mortality study of past employees in this industry demonstrated a dose-response relationship between excess risk of respiratory malignancy and asbestos exposure, using both the cohort and case-control approaches [6]. In both the morbidity and mortality investigations, low levels of exposure were identified where an adverse biological effect was not detectable. Comparison of these "no demonstrable effect" levels has led to the preliminary conclusion that in this type of asbestos exposure, a fibrogenic dose and carcinogenic dose are similar (in a population, not necessarily an individual), a finding which may have implications in decisions regarding whether bronchogenic carcinoma is "asbestos attributable" for compensation and other legal purposes as well as to the setting of permissible exposure standards for prevention of cancer in addition to pulmonary fibrosis.

A longitudinal cohort study of asbestos cement workers focusing on the determinants of progression in asbestosis has revealed that progression of small irregular opacities (likely to be due to asbestosis) is related to cumulative asbestos dust exposure, while progression of pleural abnormalities is related to time since first exposure but not to total dose [7]. We have therefore concluded that workers exposed to asbestos who have early but definite evidence of parenchymal fibrosis should be removed from further exposure since adding to their total dust burden may in the future increase their risk of progressive lung fibrosis. Our findings, however, suggested that this course is probably not necessary in workers exhibiting only benign pleural abnormalities.

While these studies are cited for illustrative purposes, it can be appreciated that occupational health standards may be partially based on these kind of data, particularly when results are replicated, estimation of individual dose is improved, and enhanced sensitivity and specificity are available for the methods used to detect an adverse health response.

It is the responsibility of the scentific community to provide the public with dispassionate presentation of data and reasonable interpretation of research results. Estimation of risk will be derived from new knowledge obtained by biomedical scientists and their statistical colleagues. Characterization of exposure must come from data generated by industrial hygienists and environmental chemists, whose techniques are fully described in this monograph. The public interest in environmental characterization used in research also lies in the probability that methods ultimately utilized for regulation (compliance with standards) will have been proven valid and efficient by the investigators in this field.

Measurement of benefit, however, comes not only from scientists but will depend upon the input of economists, social scientists, and public health experts. In the weighing of risks and benefits, whether by scientists or nonscientists, it is the responsibility of each to fully recognize and communicate the limitations of the methcds used to generate the information on which public policy is based. Uncertainties, however, must not be used to delay unduly decisions of great importance for the protection of the health of workers. Both uncommunicated results or misinterpretation of data can result in substantial public disservice primarily for the reasons indicated previously, i.e., risk of misallocating limited resources with failure to maximize health benefits.

We have not in the past, nor can we hope to in the future, live in the vacuum of a completely "safe" or "risk-free" society. Risk assessment is not only the responsibility of statisticians and their models; biologists must not abdicate their duty to introduce biological (health) relevance into ultimate judgments concerning the magnitude and acceptability of risks. Such risks when quantifiable should be compared to other risks which are well known and accepted by the public [8].

In this sensitive and frequently polarized area of scientific inquiry, there must be safeguards to assure that new knowledge can be developed, free of extraneous pressures from special interests, while peer analysis, with its implicit acceptance or rejection, proceeds in an orderly fashion. It is counterproductive at that stage to attribute political, economic, or similar motives to evolving scientific judgments. Upon the completion of research and the timely communication of its results, public interest will then be served by extensive nonscientific contributions to the discourse leading to decision making. It is, of course, extremely difficult to reach agreement concerning when this point is reached. It is only if the scientist fully discharges the responsibilities suggested above that this early "prepublic" scientific debate will not be misconstrued as a "cover-up." As in other fields, the credibility of investigators must be established by their integrity, which will properly be continually scrutinized by an interested public. The methods reviewed in this monograph will add to the data base upon which the public can make needed informed decisions which will lead to the protection and conservation of society's most important resource—its productive members.

References

1. Hill, A. B., The environment and disease: Association or causation? *Proc. R. Soc. Med.*, **58**:295 (1965).
2. Gilson, J. C., Asbestos cancers as an example of the problem of comparative risks. In *Environmental Pollution and Carcinogenic Risks.* INSERM Symposia Series 52, 1976, IARC Sci. Pub. No. 13, p. 107.
3. Crump, K. S., D. G. Hoel, C. H. Langley, and R. Petro, Fundamental carcinogenic processes and their implications for low dose risk assessment, *Cancer Res.*, **36**:2973–2979 (1976).
4. Cornfield, J., Carcinogenic risk assessment, *Science,* **198**:693–699 (1976).
5. Weill, H., M. M. Ziskind, C. Waggenspack, and C. E. Rossiter, Lung function consequences of dust exposure in asbestos cement manufacturing plants, *Arch. Environ. Health,* **30**:88–97 (1975).
6. Weill, H., J. Hughes, and C. Waggenspack, Influence of dose and fiber type on respiratory malignancy risk in asbestos cement manufacturing, *Am. Rev. Respir. Dis.*, **120**:345–354 (1979).
7. Jones, R. N., J. E. Diem, J. C. Gilson, H. Glindmeyer, and H. Weill, Progression of asbestos radiographic abnormalities: Relationships to measure of dust exposure and annual decline in lung function. Symposium on the Biological Effects of Mineral Fibers, Lyon, 1979. Int. Agency for Research on Cancer (IARC), 1980, pp. 537–543.
8. Comar, C. L., Risk: A pragmatic de minimis approach, *Science,* **203**:4379 (1979).

AUTHOR INDEX

Numbers in brackets are reference numbers and indicate that an author's work is referred to although his name is not cited in the text. Italic numbers give the page on which the complete reference is listed.

B

C

D

E

I

M

N

O

P

Q

R

S

Y

Z

SUBJECT INDEX

O

P

X